Skills Performance Checklists

for

Clinical Nursing Skills & Techniques

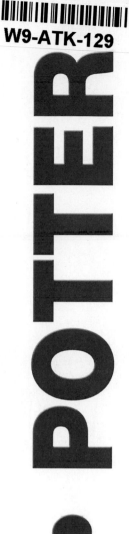
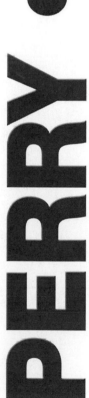

PERRY • POTTER

Skills Performance Checklists

for

Clinical Nursing Skills & Techniques

Prepared by:

Carmen Toca, RN, C, CEN

Assistant Coordinator of Clinical Skills Laboratory
Practical Nursing Program
Union County College
Plainfield, New Jersey

PERRY · POTTER

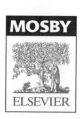

MOSBY

ELSEVIER

7th *edition*

MOSBY
ELSEVIER

11830 Westline Industrial Drive
St. Louis, Missouri 63146

Executive Editor: Susan Epstein
Managing Editor: Jean Sims Fornango
Publishing Services Manager: Anne Altepeter
Senior Project Manager: Beth Hayes

Printed in the United States of America

Last digit is the print number: 9   8   7   6   5   4   3   2

Introduction to Students

The checklists in this book were developed to provide a tool to evaluate your competence at performing the skills presented in *Clinical Nursing Skills & Techniques*. Instructors may check "Satisfactory (S)," "Unsatisfactory (U)," or "Needs Practice (NP)" for each step. Specific instructions or feedback may be provided in the "Comments" column or at the end of the checklist. These checklists may also be used for independent self-evaluation of competency.

Although we understand that each instructor may require slightly different steps in the evaluation of the performance of the specific skill, these checklists have been streamlined to include only the critical steps needed to master each skill. They are not intended to replace the text, which describes and illustrates in detail each step of the nursing skill, as well as the rationale behind it.

The checklists will be a valuable time-saver for instructors or a handy tool for student self-evaluation. Each checklist begins on a separate page and is perforated for easy removal.

Contents

CHAPTER 44: DIAGNOSTIC PROCEDURES

Student _____ Date _____

Instructor _____ Date _____

PERFORMANCE CHECKLIST SKILL 2-1 **ADMITTING PATIENTS**

	S	U	NP	Comments

ROOM PREPARATION

1. Performed hand hygiene before preparing room equipment, furniture, and bed. ___ ___ ___ _____

2. Assembled special equipment. Checked that all equipment operated correctly. ___ ___ ___ _____

ASSESSMENT

1. Greeted patient and family cordially and introduced self by name and job title. ___ ___ ___ _____

2. Arranged for translation service, if necessary. ___ ___ ___ _____

3. Assessed patient's general appearance and condition before beginning admitting procedures. ___ ___ ___ _____

4. Escorted patient and family members to room and introduced roommate. ___ ___ ___ _____

5. Assessed patient's and family members' psychological responses to admitting procedures. ___ ___ ___ _____

6. Assessed patient's vital signs. ___ ___ ___ _____

7. Assessed patient for risk of falling. ___ ___ ___ _____

8. Provided for privacy and prepared patient for examination. ___ ___ ___ _____

9. Obtained a complete nursing history. Identified food, drug, and other substance allergies. ___ ___ ___ _____

10. Conducted physical assessment of appropriate body systems. ___ ___ ___ _____

11. Checked physician's admitting orders. ___ ___ ___ _____

12. Oriented patient and family to nursing division. ___ ___ ___ _____

NURSING DIAGNOSIS

1. Developed appropriate nursing diagnoses based on assessment data. ___ ___ ___ _____

PLANNING

1. Identified expected outcomes. ___ ___ ___ _____

	S	U	NP	Comments

IMPLEMENTATION

1. Informed patient of planned procedures or treatments. _____ _____ _____ _____

2. Allowed patient and family opportunity to ask questions about admission procedures or therapies. _____ _____ _____ _____

3. Collected patient's valuables and explained policy for ensuring safekeeping. _____ _____ _____ _____

4. Allowed patient and family time alone. _____ _____ _____ _____

5. Placed call light within patient's reach; placed bed in low position; raised side rails as needed. _____ _____ _____ _____

6. Performed hand hygiene. _____ _____ _____ _____

EVALUATION

1. Confirmed that patient understands tests and procedures. _____ _____ _____ _____

2. Monitored patient's ability to ambulate independently. _____ _____ _____ _____

3. Checked patient's room setup regularly. _____ _____ _____ _____

4. Assessed for unexpected outcomes. _____ _____ _____ _____

RECORDING AND REPORTING

1. Recorded history and assessment findings. Included information about advance directive. _____ _____ _____ _____

2. Notified physician of patient's admission; reported unusual assessment findings; obtained admission orders, if necessary. _____ _____ _____ _____

3. Began to develop nursing plan of care. _____ _____ _____ _____

Student _____   Date _____

Instructor _____   Date _____

PERFORMANCE CHECKLIST SKILL 2-2 **TRANSFERRING PATIENTS**

	S	U	NP	Comments
ASSESSMENT				
1. Obtained transfer order.	___	___	___	_____
2. Assessed reason for patient's transfer.	___	___	___	_____
3. Explained purpose of transfer. Obtained patient's and family's consent for transfer.	___	___	___	_____
4. Assessed patient's physical condition and determined method and vehicle for transport.	___	___	___	_____
5. Assessed patient's need for analgesic or antiemetic prior to transfer.	___	___	___	_____
6. Assessed if patient's family or significant others had been notified of transfer.	___	___	___	_____
NURSING DIAGNOSIS				
1. Developed appropriate nursing diagnoses based on assessment data.	___	___	___	_____
PLANNING				
1. Identified expected outcomes for transfer.	___	___	___	_____
2. Arranged for transport vehicle.	___	___	___	_____
3. Arranged for placement in new agency.	___	___	___	_____
IMPLEMENTATION				
1. Checked accuracy and completeness of patient's record.	___	___	___	_____
2. Completed nursing care transfer form.	___	___	___	_____
3. Completed medication reconciliation and provided updated medication list to next care provider.	___	___	___	_____
4. Gathered and secured patient's personal items.	___	___	___	_____
5. Attended to any last-minute physical needs of client.	___	___	___	_____
6. Transferred patient to stretcher or wheelchair.	___	___	___	_____
7. Performed final assessment of patient's physical stability.	___	___	___	_____
8. Accompanied patient to transport vehicle.	___	___	___	_____
9. Notified receiving agency of impending transfer and patient's status.	___	___	___	_____

	S	U	NP	Comments

EVALUATION

1. Compared final assessment data with previous finding. — — — _____

2. Inspected patient's alignment and positioning in wheelchair or stretcher. — — — _____

3. Confirmed that patient understands transfer and procedures. — — — _____

4. Determined if receiving agency had questions regarding patient's care. — — — _____

5. Identified unexpected outcomes. — — — _____

RECORDING AND REPORTING

1. Documented patient's status and time, reason, and method of transfer. — — — _____

Student _____ Date _____

Instructor _____ Date _____

PERFORMANCE CHECKLIST SKILL 2-3 **DISCHARGING PATIENTS**

	S	U	NP	Comments

ASSESSMENT

1. Began assessing patient's discharge needs upon admission.

2. Assessed patient's and family members' need for health teaching.

3. Assessed patient and family members for existence of barriers to learning.

4. Assessed existence of environmental factors in patient's home setting.

5. Collaborated with physician and staff in other disciplines about patient's need for referral for home health care services or an extended care facility.

6. Assessed patient's and family's perceptions of continued health care needs outside the hospital.

7. Assessed patient's acceptance of health problems.

8. Consulted with other health team members to determine patient's discharge needs; made appropriate referrals.

NURSING DIAGNOSIS

1. Developed appropriate nursing diagnoses based on assessment data.

PLANNING

1. Identified expected outcomes for patient's discharge.

IMPLEMENTATION
Before Day of Discharge

1. Suggested ways to change physical arrangement of home environment to meet patient's needs.

2. Provided patient and family with information about community health care resources.

3. Conducted teaching sessions related to health care needs.

4. Communicated patient's/family's responses to teaching and proposed discharge plan to other health care team members.

	S	U	NP	Comments

Day of Discharge

1. Allowed patient and family opportunity to ask questions and discuss issues related to home health care.

2. Checked physician's discharge orders.

3. Determined if transportation had been arranged for patient.

4. Assisted patient with dressing and packing personal items.

5. Checked all closets and drawers for belongings; obtained copy of valuables list and had valuables delivered to client; accounted for all valuables.

6. Gave patient prescriptions or medications and reviewed drug information.

7. Provided and discussed discharge instructions and information about follow-up with physician.

8. Assisted patient in making arrangements with business office for bill payment.

9. Assisted patient to wheelchair or stretcher; escorted patient to agency entrance; safely assisted patient into transport vehicle with personal belongings.

10. Notified admitting or appropriate department of discharge time.

EVALUATION

1. Asked patient to describe nature of illness, treatment regimens, and signs and symptoms to be reported to physician.

2. Had patient or family member return demonstrate treatments to be continued at home.

3. Inspected home environment for risks.

4. Identified unexpected outcomes.

RECORDING AND REPORTING

1. Documented patient's discharge.

2. Documented status of patient's health problems at time of discharge.

Student _____ Date _____

Instructor _____ Date _____

PERFORMANCE CHECKLIST SKILL 3-1 **ESTABLISHING THE NURSE-PATIENT RELATIONSHIP**

	S	U	NP	Comments
ASSESSMENT				
1. Assessed patient's behaviors and needs.	___	___	___	_____
2. Determined patient's specific need to communicate.	___	___	___	_____
3. Assessed reason patient needs health care.	___	___	___	_____
4. Assessed factors about self and patient that influence communication.	___	___	___	_____
5. Assessed personal barriers to communication with patient.	___	___	___	_____
6. Assessed patient's language and ability to speak.	___	___	___	_____
7. Assessed patient's literacy level.	___	___	___	_____
8. Assessed patient's ability to hear.	___	___	___	_____
9. Observed patient's pattern of communication and verbal and nonverbal behaviors.	___	___	___	_____
10. Determined available resources for selection of communication methods.	___	___	___	_____
11. Assessed patient's readiness to work toward goals.	___	___	___	_____
12. Considered times of patient's admission, transfer/discharge.	___	___	___	_____
NURSING DIAGNOSIS				
1. Developed appropriate nursing diagnoses based on assessment data.	___	___	___	_____
PLANNING				
1. Identified expected outcomes for communication goals.	___	___	___	_____
2. Prepared for communication throughout all phases of communication.	___	___	___	_____
3. Prepared patient and physical environment.	___	___	___	_____
4. Identified strategies to achieve realistic goals.	___	___	___	_____
5. Summarized pertinent information for aftercare.	___	___	___	_____
IMPLEMENTATION				
Orientation Phase				
1. Created a climate of warmth and acceptance, with consideration of environment and patient's status and needs.	___	___	___	_____

	S	U	NP	Comments
2. Addressed patient by name and introduced self by name and role.	——	——	——	_____
3. Used appropriate nonverbal behaviors.	——	——	——	_____
4. Observed patient's nonverbal behaviors and actively listened to patient.	——	——	——	_____
5. Explained the purpose of the interaction and if the information is to be shared.	——	——	——	_____
6. Identified patient's expectations.	——	——	——	_____
7. Encouraged patient to seek clarification during the interaction.	——	——	——	_____
8. Used therapeutic communication techniques during the interaction.	——	——	——	_____

Working Phase

1. Used effective communication skills.	——	——	——	_____
2. Discussed and prioritized problem areas.	——	——	——	_____
3. Provided information to patient and assisted patient with expressing feelings.	——	——	——	_____
4. Asked questions carefully and allowed sufficient time for patient to answer.	——	——	——	_____
5. Avoided barriers to communication with patient.	——	——	——	_____

Termination Phase

1. Used effective communication skills to discuss discharge/termination issues.	——	——	——	_____
2. Summarized what was discussed with patient.	——	——	——	_____

EVALUATION

1. Observed patient's verbal and nonverbal responses.	——	——	——	_____
2. Noted own responses and effectiveness of therapeutic techniques.	——	——	——	_____
3. Requested feedback from patient on information that was communicated.	——	——	——	_____
4. Summarized and restated information and reinforced patient's strengths.	——	——	——	_____
5. Reinforced patient's strengths; developed action plan.	——	——	——	_____
6. Assessed for unexpected outcomes.	——	——	——	_____

RECORDING AND REPORTING

1. Reported pertinent information to health care team members.	——	——	——	_____
2. Recorded communication pertinent to patient's status and level of understanding.	——	——	——	_____

Student _____ Date _____

Instructor _____ Date _____

PERFORMANCE CHECKLIST SKILL 3-2 **COMMUNICATING WITH AN ANXIOUS PATIENT**

	S	U	NP	Comments

ASSESSMENT

1. Assessed patient for physical, behavioral, and verbal cues indicating anxiety. ___ ___ ___ _____

2. Assessed for possible factors causing patient anxiety. ___ ___ ___ _____

3. Assessed factors influencing communication with patient. ___ ___ ___ _____

4. Assessed own level of anxiety; made conscious effort to remain calm. ___ ___ ___ _____

5. Discussed with family possible causes of patient anxiety. ___ ___ ___ _____

NURSING DIAGNOSIS

1. Developed appropriate nursing diagnoses based on assessment data. ___ ___ ___ _____

PLANNING

1. Identified expected outcomes. ___ ___ ___ _____

2. Prepared for communication. ___ ___ ___ _____

3. Recognized and controlled own anxiety. ___ ___ ___ _____

4. Prepared physical environment to provide quiet, calm area with ample personal space. ___ ___ ___ _____

IMPLEMENTATION

1. Provided brief, simple introduction of self and role. ___ ___ ___ _____

2. Used appropriate nonverbal behaviors and active listening skills. ___ ___ ___ _____

3. Used clear and concise verbal techniques. ___ ___ ___ _____

4. Helped patient acquire alternative coping strategies. ___ ___ ___ _____

5. Provided necessary comfort measures. ___ ___ ___ _____

EVALUATION

1. Observed patient for continuing presence of signs and symptoms and behaviors reflecting anxiety. ___ ___ ___ _____

2. Had patient discuss ways to cope with anxiety in the future. ___ ___ ___ _____

	S	U	NP	Comments
3. Evaluated patient's ability to discuss factors causing anxiety.	——	——	——	———————————
4. Identified unexpected outcomes.	——	——	——	———————————

RECORDING AND REPORTING

	S	U	NP	Comments
1. Recorded cause of patient's anxiety and described signs and symptoms and behaviors exhibited by patient.	——	——	——	———————————
2. Recorded and reported methods used to relieve anxiety and patient's response to them.	——	——	——	———————————

10

Student _____ Date _____

Instructor _____ Date _____

PERFORMANCE CHECKLIST SKILL 3-3 **COMMUNICATING WITH AN ANGRY PATIENT THROUGH DE-ESCALATION**

	S	U	NP	Comments
ASSESSMENT				
1. Observed patient for behaviors or expressions that indicate anger.	___	___	___	_____
2. Assessed factors that influence communication with the angry patient.	___	___	___	_____
3. Considered resources available to assist in communication with the angry patient.	___	___	___	_____
NURSING DIAGNOSIS				
1. Developed appropriate nursing diagnoses based on assessment data.	___	___	___	_____
PLANNING				
1. Identified expected outcomes.	___	___	___	_____
2. Prepared self for interaction with angry patient.	___	___	___	_____
3. Prepared environment to de-escalate the potentially violent patient.	___	___	___	_____
a. Encouraged others to leave the area.	___	___	___	_____
b. Maintained adequate distance from patient.	___	___	___	_____
c. Maintained open exit. Positioned self closest to the door.	___	___	___	_____
d. Made sure gestures were slow and deliberate. Maintained calm, assertive, reassuring voice.	___	___	___	_____
e. Closed door, if necessary.	___	___	___	_____
f. Reduced disturbing factors in room.	___	___	___	_____
g. Took care of patient's physical and emotional needs.	___	___	___	_____
IMPLEMENTATION				
1. Maintained nonthreatening verbal and nonverbal communication with the patient.	___	___	___	_____
2. Responded appropriately to the potentially violent patient.	___	___	___	_____
a. Used therapeutic silence.	___	___	___	_____
b. Answered questions.	___	___	___	_____
c. Remained calm and set limits for patient behavior.	___	___	___	_____

	S	U	NP	Comments

d. Maintained personal space and safety. — — — _____

e. Explored alternatives to anger once patient had been calmed. — — — _____

EVALUATION

1. Observed for continuing behaviors or expressions of anger. — — — _____

2. Noted patient's ability to answer questions and problem-solve. — — — _____

3. Identified unexpected outcomes. — — — _____

RECORDING AND REPORTING

1. Recorded observations related to anger; reported verbal threats to appropriate agency personnel. — — — _____

2. Recorded and reported nursing interventions used and patient's responses. — — — _____

Student _____ Date _____

Instructor _____ Date _____

PERFORMANCE CHECKLIST SKILL 3-4 **COMMUNICATING WITH A DEPRESSED PATIENT**

	S	U	NP	Comments
ASSESSMENT				
1. Assessed patient for physical, behavioral, and verbal cues that indicate depression.	___	___	___	_____
2. Assessed for factors contributing to patient's depression.	___	___	___	_____
3. Assessed factors influencing communication with patient.	___	___	___	_____
4. Conferred with family members about possible reasons for patient's depression.	___	___	___	_____
NURSING DIAGNOSIS				
1. Developed appropriate nursing diagnoses based on assessment data.	___	___	___	_____
PLANNING				
1. Identified expected outcomes.	___	___	___	_____
2. Prepared for communication with patient.	___	___	___	_____
3. Demonstrated awareness of nonverbal cues that influence communication.	___	___	___	_____
4. Prepared environment to decrease stimuli, providing a calming effect.	___	___	___	_____
IMPLEMENTATION				
1. Provided brief, simple introduction of self and purpose of interaction.	___	___	___	_____
2. Created climate of acceptance for patient.	___	___	___	_____
3. Demonstrated honesty and empathy.	___	___	___	_____
4. Used appropriate nonverbal behaviors and active listening skills.	___	___	___	_____
5. Used clear, concise observational statements.	___	___	___	_____
6. Used open-ended questions.	___	___	___	_____
7. Rewarded small decisions and independent actions taken by the patient.	___	___	___	_____
8. Responded therapeutically to anger and encouraged verbal expression of anger.	___	___	___	_____
9. Provided necessary comfort measures.	___	___	___	_____
10. Spent time with withdrawn patient.	___	___	___	_____
11. Asked patient about suicidal ideation and presence of a plan.	___	___	___	_____

	S	U	NP	Comments

EVALUATION

1. Observed for continuing presence of physical signs and symptoms or behaviors reflecting depression.   ___ ___ ___ _____

2. Noted patient's plan for coping with depression and ability to problem-solve.   ___ ___ ___ _____

3. Evaluated patient's ability to discuss factors causing depression.   ___ ___ ___ _____

4. Identified unexpected outcomes.   ___ ___ ___ _____

RECORDING AND REPORTING

1. Recorded observations related to depression; reported suicidal ideations immediately to appropriate agency personnel.   ___ ___ ___ _____

2. Recorded and reported nursing interventions used and patient's responses.   ___ ___ ___ _____

Student _____ Date _____

Instructor _____ Date _____

PERFORMANCE CHECKLIST PROCEDURAL GUIDELINE 4-1 **GIVING A CHANGE-OF-SHIFT REPORT**

	S	U	NP	Comments
IMPLEMENTATION				
1. Gathered pertinent patient information from available sources.	____	____	____	_____
2. Prioritized information.	____	____	____	_____
3. Prepared a detailed description of the patient's current status and progress, including background information, assessment data, nursing diagnoses, interventions, and evaluation.	____	____	____	_____
4. Discussed education progress with patient/caregiver, communication with other disciplines, and family preparation for discharge.	____	____	____	_____
5. Reported significant needs and changes.	____	____	____	_____
6. Reported patient's status post diagnostic or postoperative procedure.	____	____	____	_____
7. Clarified report with oncoming shift.	____	____	____	_____

Student _____ Date _____

Instructor _____ Date _____

PERFORMANCE CHECKLIST PROCEDURAL GUIDELINE 4-2 **DOCUMENTING NURSES' PROGRESS NOTES**

	S	U	NP	Comments

IMPLEMENTATION

1. Completed assessments and interventions and noted responses. ____ ____ ____ _____

2. Identified forms to be maintained and their location. ____ ____ ____ _____

3. Determined information to be documented. ____ ____ ____ _____

4. Documented information in a timely manner using appropriate agency format. ____ ____ ____ _____

5. Determined most effective way to include significant change in status, abnormal finding, new problems, and progress toward goals. ____ ____ ____ _____

6. Signed progress note using full name and status according to agency policy. ____ ____ ____ _____

Student _____ Date _____

Instructor _____ Date _____

PERFORMANCE CHECKLIST PROCEDURAL GUIDELINE 4-3 **INCIDENT REPORTING**

	S	U	NP	Comments
IMPLEMENTATION				
1. Reported accurate, objective, chronological information.	____	____	____	_____
2. Assessed the extent of injury to patient or others.	____	____	____	_____
3. Restored individual's safety, if injured.	____	____	____	_____
4. Notified physician, if injury occurred.	____	____	____	_____
5. Referred nonpatient injury to appropriate setting.	____	____	____	_____
6. Completed incident report correctly and promptly.	____	____	____	_____
7. Documented events of incident in patient's chart correctly.	____	____	____	_____
8. Assessed and implemented ordered therapies in case of injured patient.	____	____	____	_____
9. Sent completed report to designated department.	____	____	____	_____

Student _____ Date _____

Instructor _____ Date _____

PERFORMANCE CHECKLIST SKILL 5-1 **MEASURING BODY TEMPERATURE**

	S	U	NP	Comments

ASSESSMENT
1. Determined need to measure patient temperature. _____ _____ _____ _____

2. Assessed for symptoms that may accompany temperature alteration. _____ _____ _____ _____

3. Assessed for factors that normally influence temperature. _____ _____ _____ _____

4. Determined site and device for most appropriate temperature measurement. _____ _____ _____ _____

5. Determined patient's baseline temperature from patient's record. _____ _____ _____ _____

NURSING DIAGNOSIS
1. Developed appropriate nursing diagnoses based on assessment. _____ _____ _____ _____

PLANNING
1. Identified expected outcomes. _____ _____ _____ _____

2. Explained procedure to patient. _____ _____ _____ _____

IMPLEMENTATION
1. Performed hand hygiene. _____ _____ _____ _____

2. Positioned patient comfortably. _____ _____ _____ _____

3. Obtained temperature reading. _____ _____ _____ _____

Oral Temperature Measurement With Electronic Thermometer

(1) Applied clean gloves (optional). _____ _____ _____ _____

(2) Removed thermometer pack from charging unit. Attached oral thermometer probe stem (blue tip) to thermometer unit. Grasped top of probe stem, being careful not to apply pressure on the ejection button. _____ _____ _____ _____

(3) Slid disposable plastic probe cover over thermometer probe stem until cover locked into place. _____ _____ _____ _____

(4) Asked patient to open mouth; gently placed thermometer probe under tongue in posterior sublingual pocket lateral to center of lower jaw. _____ _____ _____ _____

(5) Asked patient to hold thermometer probe with lips closed. _____ _____ _____ _____

	S	U	NP	Comments

(6) Left thermometer probe in place until audible signal indicated completion and patient's temperature appeared on digital display; removed thermometer probe from under patient's tongue. ____ ____ ____ _____

(7) Pushed ejection button on thermometer probe stem to discard plastic probe cover. ____ ____ ____ _____

(8) Returned thermometer probe stem to storage position of thermometer unit. ____ ____ ____ _____

(9) If gloves worn, removed and disposed of in appropriate receptacle. Performed hand hygiene. ____ ____ ____ _____

(10) Returned thermometer to charger. ____ ____ ____ _____

Rectal Temperature Measurement With Electronic Thermometer

(1) Provided for patient privacy. Assisted patient to side-lying Sims' position. Moved aside bed linen to expose only anal area. Kept patient's upper body and lower extremities covered with sheet or blanket. ____ ____ ____ _____

(2) Applied clean gloves. ____ ____ ____ _____

(3) Removed thermometer pack from charging unit. Attached rectal thermometer probe stem (red tip) to thermometer unit. Grasped top of probe stem, being careful not to apply pressure on the ejection button. ____ ____ ____ _____

(4) Slid disposable plastic probe cover over thermometer probe stem until cover locked into place. ____ ____ ____ _____

(5) Squeezed liberal portion of lubricant onto tissue. Dipped thermometer's blunt end into lubricant, covering 2.5 to 3.5 cm (1 to 1½ inches) for adult. ____ ____ ____ _____

(6) With nondominant hand, separated patient's buttocks to expose anus. Asked patient to breathe slowly and relax. ____ ____ ____ _____

(7) Gently inserted thermometer into anus in direction of umbilicus 3.5 cm (1½ inches) for adult. Did not force thermometer. ____ ____ ____ _____

(8) Withdrew probe immediately if resistance felt during insertion. Never forced thermometer. ____ ____ ____ _____

(9) Held thermometer probe in place until audible signal and patient's temperature appeared on digital display; removed thermometer probe from anus. ____ ____ ____ _____

	S	U	NP	Comments

(10) Pushed ejection button on thermometer stem to discard plastic probe cover. Wiped probe stem with alcohol swab. ____ ____ ____ _____

(11) Returned thermometer stem to storage position of recording unit. ____ ____ ____ _____

(12) Wiped patient's anal area with soft tissue to remove lubricant or feces and discarded tissue. Assisted patient to a comfortable position. ____ ____ ____ _____

(13) Removed and disposed of gloves in appropriate receptacle. Performed hand hygiene. ____ ____ ____ _____

(14) Returned thermometer to charger. ____ ____ ____ _____

Axillary Temperature Measurement With Electronic Thermometer

(1) Provided for patient privacy. Assisted patient to supine or sitting position. Moved clothing or gown away from shoulder and arm. ____ ____ ____ _____

(2) Removed thermometer pack from charging unit. Attached oral thermometer probe stem (blue tip) to thermometer unit. Grasped top of thermometer probe stem, being careful not to apply pressure on the ejection button. ____ ____ ____ _____

(3) Slid disposable plastic probe cover over thermometer stem until cover locked into place. ____ ____ ____ _____

(4) Raised patient's arm away from torso. Inspected for skin lesions and excessive perspiration; if needed, dried axilla. ____ ____ ____ _____

(5) Inserted thermometer probe into center of axilla, lowered arm over probe, and placed arm across patient's chest. ____ ____ ____ _____

(6) Held thermometer probe in place until audible signal and patient's temperature appeared on digital display, removed thermometer probe from axilla. ____ ____ ____ _____

(7) Pushed ejection button on thermometer to discard plastic probe cover. ____ ____ ____ _____

(8) Returned thermometer stem to storage position of recording unit. ____ ____ ____ _____

(9) Assisted patient in assuming a comfortable position, replacing linen or gown. ____ ____ ____ _____

(10) Performed hand hygiene. ____ ____ ____ _____

(11) Returned thermometer to charger. ____ ____ ____ _____

	S	U	NP	Comments

Tympanic Membrane Temperature With
Electronic Thermometer

(1) Assisted patient in assuming comfortable position with head turned toward side, away from nurse. If patient lay on one side, used upper ear. ____ ____ ____ _____

(2) Planned to obtain temperature from patient's right ear; held unit in right hand. ____ ____ ____ _____

(3) Noted if there was an obvious presence of cerumen (ear wax) in the ear canal. ____ ____ ____ _____

(4) Removed thermometer handheld unit from charging base, being careful not to apply pressure to the ejection button. ____ ____ ____ _____

(5) Slid disposable speculum cover over otoscope-like lens tip until it locked into place. Did not touch lens cover. ____ ____ ____ _____

(6) Inserted speculum into ear canal following manufacturer's instructions for tympanic probe positioning:

    (a) Pulled ear pinna backward, up, and out for an adult. ____ ____ ____ _____

    (b) Moved thermometer in a figure-eight pattern. ____ ____ ____ _____

    (c) Fitted speculum tip snugly in canal and pointed toward nose. ____ ____ ____ _____

(7) Depressed scan button on handheld unit. Left thermometer probe in place until audible signal and patient's temperature appeared on digital display. ____ ____ ____ _____

(8) Carefully removed speculum from auditory meatus. Pushed ejection button on handheld unit to discard speculum cover. ____ ____ ____ _____

(9) Waited 2 to 3 minutes before repeating into same ear or repeated measurement into other ear, if temperature was abnormal or second reading was necessary. Considered an alternative site or instrument. ____ ____ ____ _____

(10) Returned handheld unit to thermometer base. ____ ____ ____ _____

(11) Assisted patient in assuming a comfortable position. ____ ____ ____ _____

(12) Informed patient of temperature reading and record measurement. ____ ____ ____ _____

(13) Performed hand hygiene. ____ ____ ____ _____

	S	U	NP	Comments

EVALUATION

1. Established patient's temperature as a baseline if within normal range and no other temperature readings were available. _____ _____ _____ _____

2. Compared patient's temperature with patient's baseline and normal temperature range. _____ _____ _____ _____

3. Took temperature 30 minutes after antipyretics and every 4 hours for patient with fever. _____ _____ _____ _____

4. Identified unexpected outcomes. _____ _____ _____ _____

REPORTING AND RECORDING

1. Recorded and reported temperature correctly. _____ _____ _____ _____

2. Documented alterations and treatments provided and patient's response. _____ _____ _____ _____

3. Reported abnormal findings to nurse in charge or physician. _____ _____ _____ _____

Student _Darcy Brenneman_   Date _9/27/12_

Instructor _____   Date _____

PERFORMANCE CHECKLIST SKILL 5-2   **ASSESSING RADIAL PULSE**

	S	U	NP	Comments
ASSESSMENT				
1. Determined need to assess patient's radial pulse: noted conditions or alterations increasing patient's risk for pulse alterations and assessed for signs and symptoms of cardiovascular alterations.				
2. Identified factors that normally may influence patient's pulse.				
3. Identified patient's baseline heart rate from patient's records.				
NURSING DIAGNOSIS				
1. Developed appropriate nursing diagnoses based on assessment data.				
PLANNING				
1. Identified expected outcomes.				
2. Explained assessment procedure to patient and the need to wait 5 to 10 minutes to assess pulse after patient has been active.				
IMPLEMENTATION				
Radial Pulse				
1. Performed hand hygiene.				
2. Provided privacy.				
3. Assisted patient to a supine or sitting position.				
4. If patient was supine, placed patient's forearm across lower chest with wrist extended and palm down. If patient was sitting, bent patient's elbow 90 degrees and supported lower arm on chair or on nurse's arm. Slightly extended patient's wrist with palm down.				
5. Placed fingertips of first two or middle three fingers over radial pulse.				
6. Lightly compressed against radius, obliterated pulse, then relaxed pressure.				
7. Palpated patient's radial pulse and determined strength of pulse.				
8. Began to count rate when pulse was felt regularly.				
9. With regular rate, counted pulse rate for 30 seconds and converted to minute rate.				

	S	U	NP	Comments

10. With irregular rate, counted pulse rate for 60 seconds. Assessed frequency and pattern of irregularity.

11. Assessed regularity and frequency of any dysrhythmia. Compared bilateral radial pulses.

12. Assisted patient in returning to comfortable position.

13. Discussed findings with patient.

14. Performed hand hygiene.

EVALUATION

1. Established patient's baseline pulse.

2. Compared patient's pulse rate and character with baseline and/or normal range for age-group.

3. Identified unexpected outcomes.

RECORDING AND REPORTING

1. Recorded findings, including site assessed and signs and symptoms of pulse alterations.

2. Recorded and reported abnormal findings to nurse in charge or physician.

Student _____ Date _____

Instructor _____ Date _____

PERFORMANCE CHECKLIST SKILL 5-3 **ASSESSING APICAL PULSE**

	S	U	NP	Comments

ASSESSMENT

1. Determined need to assess apical pulse: Noted conditions or alterations that increase risk for pulse alterations and assessed for signs and symptoms of cardiovascular alterations. ___ ___ ___ _____

2. Identified factors that normally may influence patient's pulse. ___ ___ ___ _____

3. Identified previous baseline apical rate from patient's records. ___ ___ ___ _____

4. Determined any report of latex allergy. ___ ___ ___ _____

NURSING DIAGNOSIS

1. Developed appropriate nursing diagnoses based on assessment data. ___ ___ ___ _____

PLANNING

1. Identified expected outcomes. ___ ___ ___ _____

2. Explained assessment procedure to patient and the need to wait 5 to 10 minutes to assess pulse after patient has been active. ___ ___ ___ _____

IMPLEMENTATION

1. Performed hand hygiene. ___ ___ ___ _____

2. Provided privacy. ___ ___ ___ _____

3. Assisted patient to supine or sitting position. Exposed patient's sternum and left side of chest for auscultation. ___ ___ ___ _____

4. Located anatomical landmarks to identify the point of maximum impulse. ___ ___ ___ _____

5. Warmed diaphragm of stethoscope between hands. ___ ___ ___ _____

6. Placed diaphragm over point of maximum impulse (PMI) and auscultated for normal S_1 and S_2 heart sounds. ___ ___ ___ _____

7. Determined rate of S_1 and S_2 sounds accurately. ___ ___ ___ _____

8. Counted for 30 seconds and multiplied by 2, for regular heart rate. ___ ___ ___ _____

9. With irregular heart rate, or if the patient was receiving cardiovascular medication, counted for 1 minute. ___ ___ ___ _____

10. Assessed regularity for any existing dysrhythmia. ___ ___ ___ _____

	S	U	NP	Comments

11. Replaced patient's gown. Assisted patient in returning to comfortable position.

12. Discussed findings with patient.

13. Performed hand hygiene.

14. Cleaned stethoscope earpieces and diaphragm with alcohol swab.

EVALUATION

1. Established patient's baseline apical rate.

2. Compared patient's apical rate and character with baseline and/or normal range for age-group.

3. Identified unexpected outcomes.

RECORDING AND REPORTING

1. Recorded vital signs appropriately.

2. Documented apical pulse rate before and after administration of specific treatments.

3. Recorded and reported abnormal findings to nurse in charge or physician.

Student _____ Date _____

Instructor _____ Date _____

PERFORMANCE CHECKLIST PROCEDURAL GUIDELINE 5-1 **ASSESSING APICAL-RADIAL PULSE**

	S	U	NP	Comments
STEPS				
1. Determined need to assess for pulse deficit.	___	___	___	_____
2. Performed hand hygiene.	___	___	___	_____
3. Provided for patient privacy.	___	___	___	_____
4. Assisted patient to supine or sitting position. Moved aside bed linen and gown to expose sternum and left side of chest.	___	___	___	_____
5. Located apical and radial pulse sites. If two nurses available, one nurse auscultated the apical pulse and one nurse palpated the radial pulse.	___	___	___	_____
6. The nurse measuring the radial pulse and holding the watch stated "start."	___	___	___	_____
7. Both nurses counted the pulse rate for 60 seconds simultaneously. The nurse taking the radial pulse stated "stop."	___	___	___	_____
8. Subtracted the radial rate from the apical rate to obtain the pulse deficit.	___	___	___	_____
9. Assessed for other signs and symptoms of decreased cardiac output, if a pulse deficit was noted.	___	___	___	_____
10. Discussed findings with patient as needed.	___	___	___	_____
11. Performed hand hygiene, cleaned earpieces and diaphragm of stethoscope with alcohol swab.	___	___	___	_____
12. Recorded apical pulse, radial pulse, and site, and noted the pulse deficit in the nurses' notes. Informed nurse in charge or physician of the presence of a pulse deficit.	___	___	___	_____

Student _____ Date _____

Instructor _____ Date _____

PERFORMANCE CHECKLIST SKILL 5-4 **ASSESSING RESPIRATIONS**

	S	U	NP	Comments

ASSESSMENT

1. Determined need to assess patient's respirations: described conditions that increase patient's risk for respiratory alterations and identified common signs and symptoms of respiratory alteration.

2. Assessed factors that normally influence respirations.

3. Assessed results of pertinent laboratory values.

4. Determined previous baseline respiratory rate (if available) from patient's record.

NURSING DIAGNOSIS

1. Developed appropriate nursing diagnoses based on assessment data.

PLANNING

1. Identified expected outcomes.

2. Waited 5 to 10 minutes before assessing respirations, if patient had been active.

3. Assessed respirations after pulse measurement in adult.

4. Assisted patient to a comfortable position.

IMPLEMENTATION

1. Performed hand hygiene. Provided privacy.

2. Positioned patient and self properly to ensure view of chest wall movement.

3. Placed patient's arm or own hand in relaxed position across abdomen or lower chest.

4. Observed complete respiratory cycle.

5. Correctly began count of respiration rate.

6. Correctly counted respirations for 30 seconds and multiplied by 2 if respirations were regular. If irregular, counted rate for full minute.

7. Assessed respiratory depth.

8. Assessed respiratory rhythm.

9. Replaced patient's gown and covered patient with bed linen.

	S	U	NP	Comments

10. Performed hand hygiene.

11. Discussed findings with patient.

EVALUATION

1. If assessing respirations for the first time, established rate, rhythm, and depth as baseline, if within acceptable range.

2. Compared characteristics of respirations with previous baseline data.

3. Correlated respirations with data from pulse oximetry and ABG (arterial blood gas) measurements, if available.

4. Identified unexpected outcomes.

RECORDING AND REPORTING

1. Recorded respiratory rate, rhythm, and depth.

2. Documented respiratory rate before and after administration of treatments. Indicated type and amount of oxygen therapy.

3. Reported abnormal findings to nurse in charge or physician.

Student _____ Dovey Robinson _____ Date _____ 9/24/12 ____

Instructor _____ T. Brededa _____ Date _____ 9/24/12 ____

PERFORMANCE CHECKLIST SKILL 5-5 **ASSESSING ARTERIAL BLOOD PRESSURE**

	S	U	NP	Comments

ASSESSMENT

1. Determined need to assess patient's blood pressure: identified conditions or alterations that increase patient's risk for blood pressure alterations, identified common signs and symptoms of blood pressure alterations, and determined patient's age.

2. Assessed for factors that normally influence blood pressure.

3. Determined best site for blood pressure assessment.

4. Determined patient's previous baseline blood pressure and site from patient's record. Determine any report of latex allergy.

NURSING DIAGNOSIS

1. Developed appropriate nursing diagnoses based on assessment data.

PLANNING

1. Identified expected outcomes.

2. Explained procedure to patient and had patient rest at least 5 minutes before procedure.

3. Postponed assessment for 30 minutes if patient had recently exercised, smoked, or ingested caffeine.

4. Assisted patient in assuming proper sitting or lying position. Assessed in a comfortable area.

5. Selected appropriate cuff size.

6. Performed hand hygiene.

IMPLEMENTATION

Assessing Blood Pressure by Auscultation—Upper Extremities

1. Positioned patient's forearm at heart level with palm of hand turned up. Feet or legs were not crossed.

2. Removed constricting clothing from around upper arm.

	S	U	NP	Comments

3. Palpated brachial artery, positioned cuff properly above brachial artery, and wrapped deflated cuff evenly and snugly around upper arm. ___ ___ ___ _____

4. Positioned manometer vertically at eye level. ___ ___ ___ _____

5. Measured blood pressure.

   A. Two-step method

      (1) Relocated radial pulse. Palpated the artery distal to the cuff while inflating cuff rapidly to 30 mm Hg above point at which pulse disappeared. Noted point when pulse appeared while deflating cuff slowly. Waited 30 seconds after deflating cuff before auscultation. ___ ___ ___ _____

      (2) Checked stethoscope amplification of sound. ___ ___ ___ _____

      (3) Relocated and applied stethoscope correctly over brachial artery. ___ ___ ___ _____

      (4) Tightened valve of pressure bulb. Quickly inflated cuff to 30 mm Hg above palpated systolic pressure. ___ ___ ___ _____

      (5) Allowed mercury to fall evenly at rate of 2 to 3 mm Hg/sec during auscultation. ___ ___ ___ _____

      (6) Noted point on manometer when first clear sound was heard. ___ ___ ___ _____

      (7) Continued to deflate cuff gradually, noting point at which sound disappeared in adults. Deflated cuff quickly. ___ ___ ___ _____

   B. One-step method

      (1) Placed stethoscope pieces in ears and determined that sounds were clear. ___ ___ ___ _____

      (2) Relocated brachial artery and placed diaphragm of stethoscope over it. ___ ___ ___ _____

      (3) Closed valve of pressure bulb. Quickly inflated cuff to 30 mm Hg above patient's usual systolic blood pressure. ___ ___ ___ _____

      (4) Slowly released pressure bulb valve and allowed mercury or needle of aneroid manometer to fall at a rate of 2 to 3 mm Hg/sec. Noted point on manometer when first clear sound heard. ___ ___ ___ _____

      (5) Continued to deflate cuff gradually, noting point at which sound disappeared in adults. Deflated cuff quickly. ___ ___ ___ _____

6. Used two sets of BP measurements for baseline. ___ ___ ___ _____

7. Removed cuff. ___ ___ ___ _____

	S	U	NP	Comments

8. Repeated procedure on other arm, if first assessment. ____ ____ ____ _____

9. Assisted patient in returning to comfortable position. ____ ____ ____ _____

10. Informed patient of blood pressure reading. ____ ____ ____ _____

11. Performed hand hygiene. ____ ____ ____ _____

12. Cleaned earpieces and diaphragm of stethoscope with alcohol swab. ____ ____ ____ _____

Assessing Blood Pressure—Lower Extremities

1. Assisted patient into prone position (supine optional). ____ ____ ____ _____

2. Removed constricting clothing from around patient's leg. ____ ____ ____ _____

3. Palpated popliteal artery. ____ ____ ____ _____

4. Applied leg cuff to posterior aspect of middle thigh. ____ ____ ____ _____

5. Positioned manometer at eye level. ____ ____ ____ _____

6. Followed Step 5b of one-step method checklist for auscultation of upper extremity. ____ ____ ____ _____

7. Repeated procedure on other leg, if first assessment. ____ ____ ____ _____

8. Assisted patient in returning to comfortable position. ____ ____ ____ _____

9. Informed patient of blood pressure reading. ____ ____ ____ _____

10. Performed hand hygiene. Cleaned earpieces and diaphragm of stethoscope with alcohol swab. ____ ____ ____ _____

Assessing Systolic Blood Pressure by Palpation

1. Followed Steps 1 through 5 of auscultation method for upper or lower extremity. ____ ____ ____ _____

2. Identified approximate systolic pressure by palpating brachial, radial, or popliteal pulse. Inflated cuff to 30 mm Hg above point where pulse disappeared. ____ ____ ____ _____

3. Allowed mercury to fall evenly at rate of 2 to 3 mm Hg/sec. Noted manometer reading when pulse was again palpable. ____ ____ ____ _____

4. Rapidly deflated cuff completely and removed from patient's arm. ____ ____ ____ _____

5. Assisted patient in returning to comfortable position. ____ ____ ____ _____

6. Informed patient of reading. ____ ____ ____ _____

7. Performed hand hygiene. ____ ____ ____ _____

	S	U	NP	Comments

EVALUATION

1. Established blood pressure as baseline, if assessed for first time and found within normal range.

2. Compared patient's blood pressure reading with previous baseline and usual blood pressure for patient's age.

3. Identified unexpected outcomes.

RECORDING AND REPORTING

1. Recorded blood pressure and site appropriately.

2. Documented blood pressure before and after administration of treatments.

3. Documented any signs or symptoms of blood pressure alteration.

4. Reported abnormal findings to nurse in charge or physician.

Student _____ Date _____

Instructor _____ Date _____

PERFORMANCE CHECKLIST PROCEDURAL GUIDELINE 5-2 **NONINVASIVE ELECTRONIC BLOOD PRESSURE MEASUREMENT**

	S	U	NP	Comments
STEPS				
1. Determined the appropriateness of using electronic blood pressure measurement.	___	___	___	_____
2. Determined best site for cuff placement.	___	___	___	_____
3. Assisted patient to comfortable position, either lying or sitting. Plugged in device and placed device near patient, ensuring that connector hose between cuff and machine will reach.	___	___	___	_____
4. Located on/off switch and turned on machine to enable device to self-test computer systems.	___	___	___	_____
5. Selected appropriate cuff size for patient extremity and appropriate cuff for machine.	___	___	___	_____
6. Exposed upper arm fully. Did not place blood pressure cuff over clothing.	___	___	___	_____
7. Prepared blood pressure cuff by manually squeezing all the air out of the cuff and connecting cuff to connector hose.	___	___	___	_____
8. Wrapped flattened cuff snugly around extremity. Made sure the "artery" arrow marked on the outside of the cuff was placed correctly.	___	___	___	_____
9. Verified that connector hose between cuff and machine not kinked.	___	___	___	_____
10. Set the frequency control for automatic or manual, then pressed start button.	___	___	___	_____
11. Observed digital display when deflation completed.	___	___	___	_____
12. Set frequency of blood pressure measurements and upper and lower alarm limits for systolic, diastolic, and mean blood pressure readings.	___	___	___	_____
13. Obtained additional readings, as necessary, by pressing the start button.	___	___	___	_____
14. Left cuff in place if frequent blood pressure measurements required. Removed cuff every 2 hours to assess underlying skin integrity and, if possible, alternated blood pressure sites.	___	___	___	_____
15. Discussed findings with patient. Performed hand hygiene.	___	___	___	_____

	S	U	NP	Comments
16. Compared electronic blood pressure readings with auscultatory blood pressure measurements.	___	___	___	_____
17. Recorded blood pressure and site assessed on vital sign flow sheet or nurses' notes; recorded any signs or symptoms of blood pressure alterations in narrative form in nurses' notes; and reported abnormal findings to nurse in charge or physician.	___	___	___	_____

Student _____ Date _____

Instructor _____ Date _____

PERFORMANCE CHECKLIST SKILL 5-6 **MEASURING OXYGEN SATURATION (PULSE OXIMETRY)**

	S	U	NP	Comments

ASSESSMENT

1. Determined need to measure patient's oxygen saturation. ___ ___ ___ _____

2. Assessed for signs of alteration of oxygen saturation. ___ ___ ___ _____

3. Assessed for factors that influence oxygen saturation measurement. ___ ___ ___ _____

4. Reviewed patient's medical record for order, or agency's policy for standard of care. ___ ___ ___ _____

5. Determined previous baseline SpO_2, if available. ___ ___ ___ _____

6. Determined most appropriate site for sensor. ___ ___ ___ _____

NURSING DIAGNOSIS

1. Developed appropriate nursing diagnoses based on assessment data. ___ ___ ___ _____

PLANNING

1. Identified expected outcomes. ___ ___ ___ _____

2. Obtained equipment and placed at bedside. ___ ___ ___ _____

3. Explained purpose of procedure to patient and family. ___ ___ ___ _____

IMPLEMENTATION

1. Performed hand hygiene. ___ ___ ___ _____

2. Positioned patient comfortably. Instructed patient to breathe normally. ___ ___ ___ _____

3. Removed fingernail polish, if finger site was used. ___ ___ ___ _____

4. Attached sensor probe to selected site. ___ ___ ___ _____

5. Turned on oximeter and observed pulse waveform/intensity display. Watched pulse bar for pulse sensing. Correlated oximeter with radial pulse rate. ___ ___ ___ _____

6. Informed patient that alarm will sound if probe falls off, or if patient removes it. ___ ___ ___ _____

7. Left probe in place until readout reached constant value and full strength. Read oxygen saturation. Assessed skin integrity and relocated probe regularly. ___ ___ ___ _____

	S	U	NP	Comments

8. Turned off power and removed probe when used intermittently.

9. Discussed findings with patient.

10. Assisted patient to comfortable position.

11. Performed hand hygiene.

EVALUATION

1. Established SpO_2 as baseline, if assessed for first time and within normal limits.

2. Compared SpO_2 with previous baseline and normal. Noted use of oxygen therapy.

3. Assessed skin integrity underneath probe regularly.

4. Identified unexpected outcomes.

RECORDING AND REPORTING

1. Recorded SpO_2; identified use of continuous or intermittent pulse oximetry and oxygen therapy, if used.

2. Documented measurements before and after administration of treatments.

3. Reported abnormal findings to nurse in charge or physician.

4. Correlated findings with arterial blood gas measurements, if available.

42

Student _____ Date _____

Instructor _____ Date _____

PERFORMANCE CHECKLIST SKILL 6-1 **GENERAL SURVEY**

	S	U	NP	Comments

ASSESSMENT

1. Noted if patient is experiencing any acute distress.

2. Checked baseline vital signs and assessed factors that alter readings.

3. Determined patient's primary language.

4. Reconfirmed patient's primary reason for seeking health care.

5. Identified patient's normal height and weight. Used growth chart for children age 18 and younger.

6. Reviewed patient's past intake and output records.

7. Determined patient's perceptions about personal health.

8. Assessed patient for latex allergy.

NURSING DIAGNOSIS

1. Developed appropriate nursing diagnosis based on the assessment data.

PLANNING

1. Identified expected outcomes or normal findings.

2. Prepared patient for examination.

IMPLEMENTATION

1. Noted patient's verbal and nonverbal behaviors, level of consciousness, and orientation.

2. Obtained vital sign measurements.

3. Observed patient's overall appearance.

4. Rephrased questions as necessary.

5. Asked patient short, focused questions, if responses inappropriate.

6. Offered simple commands or directions, if patient unable to respond to orientation questions.

7. Assessed affect and mood.

8. Observed interaction with spouse or significant other.

	S	U	NP	Comments

9. Observed for signs of abuse. Made immediate referral as appropriate. ___ ___ ___ _____

10. Assessed posture, positioning, and mobility. ___ ___ ___ _____

11. Assessed speech pace and clarity. ___ ___ ___ _____

12. Observed hygiene and grooming. ___ ___ ___ _____

13. Inspected exposed areas of skin and asked about any changes. ___ ___ ___ _____

14. Inspected skin surface by comparing symmetrical body areas. ___ ___ ___ _____

15. Inspected color of face, oral mucosa, lips, conjunctiva, sclera, and nail beds. ___ ___ ___ _____

16. Palpated skin surfaces for moisture and texture. ___ ___ ___ _____

17. Applied gloves and inspected character of secretions, if present. Removed gloves. ___ ___ ___ _____

18. Palpated skin surfaces for temperature using dorsum of hand. Compared symmetrical body parts. ___ ___ ___ _____

19. Assessed skin turgor. ___ ___ ___ _____

20. Assessed skin for pressure areas. ___ ___ ___ _____

21. Inspected, palpated, and measured any lesions. ___ ___ ___ _____

EVALUATION

1. Observed for evidence of physical or emotional distress. ___ ___ ___ _____

2. Compared assessment findings with previous observations. ___ ___ ___ _____

3. Asked patient if there was information that had not been discussed. ___ ___ ___ _____

4. Identified unexpected outcomes. ___ ___ ___ _____

RECORDING AND REPORTING

1. Recorded vital signs. ___ ___ ___ _____

2. Recorded alterations in patient's general appearance. ___ ___ ___ _____

3. Described patient's behaviors objectively, including subjective reports of signs and symptoms. ___ ___ ___ _____

4. Reported abnormalities and acute symptoms to nurse in charge or physician. ___ ___ ___ _____

Student _____ Date _____

Instructor _____ Date _____

PERFORMANCE CHECKLIST SKILL 6-2 **ASSESSING THE HEAD AND NECK**

	S	U	NP	Comments
ASSESSMENT				
1. Assessed history of headache, dizziness, pain, or stiffness.	___	___	___	_____
2. Determined history of eye disease, diabetes, or hypertension.	___	___	___	_____
3. Questioned experience of blurred vision, flashing lights, or reduced visual field.	___	___	___	_____
4. Determined history of ear pain, itching, discharge, vertigo, tinnitus, or alteration in hearing.	___	___	___	_____
5. Reviewed occupational history.	___	___	___	_____
6. Reviewed history of allergies, nasal discharge, nosebleeds, or postnasal drip.	___	___	___	_____
7. Determined history of tobacco use.	___	___	___	_____
NURSING DIAGNOSIS				
1. Developed appropriate nursing diagnosis based on the assessment data.	___	___	___	_____
PLANNING				
1. Identified expected outcomes.	___	___	___	_____
2. Explained examination to patient.	___	___	___	_____
IMPLEMENTATION				
1. Performed hand hygiene. Positioned and prepared patient for examination.	___	___	___	_____
2. Inspected head; noted head position and facial features.	___	___	___	_____
3. Assessed eyes for position, color, movement, and condition of conjunctiva.				
a. Assessed near and far vision.	___	___	___	_____
b. Tested pupillary reflexes.	___	___	___	_____
4. Assessed hearing.	___	___	___	_____
5. Inspected nose, including mucosa and drainage, if present.	___	___	___	_____
6. Palpated sinuses for tenderness.	___	___	___	_____
7. Assessed mouth and tongue.	___	___	___	_____
8. Inspected and palpated neck. Asked about history of pain or difficulty with movement.	___	___	___	_____

	S	U	NP	Comments

EVALUATION

1. Compared findings with previous observations. ___ ___ ___ _____

2. Had patient identify common symptoms of eye, ear, sinus, and mouth disease as appropriate. ___ ___ ___ _____

3. Had patient list occupational safety precautions as appropriate. ___ ___ ___ _____

4. Identified unexpected outcomes. ___ ___ ___ _____

RECORDING AND REPORTING

1. Recorded observations and findings. ___ ___ ___ _____

2. Reported increased headache, dizziness, or visual changes to nurse in charge or physician. ___ ___ ___ _____

Student _____ Date _____

Instructor _____ Date _____

PERFORMANCE CHECKLIST SKILL 6-3 **ASSESSING THE THORAX AND LUNGS**

	S	U	NP	Comments
ASSESSMENT				
1. Assessed history of tobacco or marijuana use.	___	___	___	_____
2. Assessed for symptoms of respiratory alterations.	___	___	___	_____
3. Determined exposure to environmental pollutants or second-hand cigarette smoke.	___	___	___	_____
4. Reviewed patient history for known risk factors to exposure of tuberculosis and infection with human immunodeficiency virus (HIV) and assessed for signs and symptoms.	___	___	___	_____
5. Assessed for history of allergies and chronic hoarseness.	___	___	___	_____
6. Reviewed family history for risk factors.	___	___	___	_____
NURSING DIAGNOSIS				
1. Developed appropriate nursing diagnosis based on assessment data.	___	___	___	_____
PLANNING				
1. Identified expected outcomes.	___	___	___	_____
IMPLEMENTATION				
1. Performed hand hygiene. Positioned and prepared patient for examination; exposed chest wall for assessment; explained steps of procedure.	___	___	___	_____
2. Posterior thorax:				
a. Stood behind patient and inspected appearance of thorax.	___	___	___	_____
b. Determined rate and rhythm of breathing.	___	___	___	_____
c. Systematically palpated chest wall, costal and intercostal spaces.	___	___	___	_____
d. Palpated chest excursion and identified factors restricting chest expansion.	___	___	___	_____
e. Auscultated breath sounds.	___	___	___	_____
3. Lateral thorax:				
a. Inspected lateral chest wall with patient's arms raised.	___	___	___	_____
b. Extended assessment to lateral sides of chest.	___	___	___	_____
c. Observed patient's respiratory character.	___	___	___	_____

	S	U	NP	Comments

d. Palpated for swelling or tenderness. ___ ___ ___ _____

e. Palpated anterior chest excursion. ___ ___ ___ _____

(f.) Auscultated breath sounds in anterior thorax. ___ ___ ___ _____

4. Anterior thorax:

   a. Inspected accessory muscles of breathing. ___ ___ ___ _____

   b. Inspected spread of angle made by costal margins. ___ ___ ___ _____

EVALUATION

1. Compared findings with normal assessment characteristics of thorax and lungs. ___ ___ ___ _____

2. Had patient identify factors leading to lung disease. ___ ___ ___ _____

3. Identified unexpected outcomes. ___ ___ ___ _____

RECORDING AND REPORTING

1. Recorded observations and findings. ___ ___ ___ _____

2. Recorded respiratory rate and character. ___ ___ ___ _____

3. Recorded characteristics of mucus. ___ ___ ___ _____

4. Reported abnormalities to nurse in charge or physician. ___ ___ ___ _____

Student _____ Date _____

Instructor _____ Date _____

PERFORMANCE CHECKLIST SKILL 6-4 **CARDIOVASCULAR ASSESSMENT**

	S	U	NP	Comments

ASSESSMENT

1. Assessed for risk factors for cardiovascular disease.   ____ ____ ____ _____

2. Determined patient's medication history.   ____ ____ ____ _____

3. Assessed for symptoms of heart disease.   ____ ____ ____ _____

4. Determined presence and character of chest pain.   ____ ____ ____ _____

5. Assessed family history for heart disease.   ____ ____ ____ _____

6. Assessed patient for history of heart problems and vascular problems.   ____ ____ ____ _____

7. Determined if patient experiences symptoms of vascular problems.   ____ ____ ____ _____

8. Determined relationship of symptoms to exertion.   ____ ____ ____ _____

9. Determined if female wears constrictive clothing or crosses legs and feet while sitting or supine.   ____ ____ ____ _____

PLANNING

1. Identified expected outcomes.   ____ ____ ____ _____

IMPLEMENTATION

1. Performed hand hygiene.   ____ ____ ____ _____

2. Assisted patient to comfortable and relaxed position (semi-Fowler's or supine).   ____ ____ ____ _____

3. Explained procedure.   ____ ____ ____ _____

4. Made sure room was quiet.   ____ ____ ____ _____

5. Assessed the heart:

   a. Located anatomical sites to assess the heart.   ____ ____ ____ _____

   b. Stood to patient's right to inspect and palpate.   ____ ____ ____ _____

   c. Inspected epigastric area and palpated abdominal aorta.   ____ ____ ____ _____

   d. Auscultated heart sounds and murmurs.   ____ ____ ____ _____

6. Assessed neck vessels:

   a. Positioned patient comfortably.   ____ ____ ____ _____

   b. Assessed carotid arteries using inspection, palpation, and auscultation.   ____ ____ ____ _____

	S	U	NP	Comments

c. Gently palpated each artery separately. ___ ___ ___ _____

d. Assessed jugular veins separately, measuring from appropriate landmarks. ___ ___ ___ _____

e. Assessed venous pressure and observed for visible jugular pulsation. ___ ___ ___ _____

7. Peripheral vascular assessment:

a. Inspected lower extremities for changes in color and condition. Repositioned patient as needed. ___ ___ ___ _____

b. Palpated and compared symmetrically. ___ ___ ___ _____

c. Assessed mobility of upper and lower extremities. ___ ___ ___ _____

d. Assessed pulses and capillary refill of upper and lower extremities. ___ ___ ___ _____

e. Assessed immobilized patient for pain in lower extremities. ___ ___ ___ _____

f. Donned gloves and palpated femoral pulse. ___ ___ ___ _____

EVALUATION

1. Compared findings with normal assessment characteristics for heart and vascular system. ___ ___ ___ _____

2. If heart sounds were not audible or pulses were not palpable, had another nurse confirm assessment. ___ ___ ___ _____

3 Asked patient to describe behaviors that increase the risk of cardiovascular disease. ___ ___ ___ _____

4. Compared information with previous assessment. ___ ___ ___ _____

5. Identified unexpected outcomes. ___ ___ ___ _____

RECORDING AND REPORTING

1. Recorded all findings for heart and vascular assessment. ___ ___ ___ _____

2. Recorded instructions given to patient and patient's response. ___ ___ ___ _____

3. Reported cardiac or vascular abnormalities to nurse in charge or physician. ___ ___ ___ _____

Student _____ Date _____

Instructor _____ Date _____

PERFORMANCE CHECKLIST SKILL 6-5 **ASSESSING THE ABDOMEN, GENITALIA, AND RECTUM**

	S	U	NP	Comments

ASSESSMENT

1. General patient survey:

   a. Assessed for character of existing abdominal or low back pain. ___ ___ ___ _____

   b. Observed patient for signs of pain associated with positioning. ___ ___ ___ _____

   c. Assessed patient's normal bowel habits. ___ ___ ___ _____

   d. Assessed for history of abdominal surgery or trauma. ___ ___ ___ _____

   e. Assessed for weight change or diet intolerance. ___ ___ ___ _____

   f. Assessed for signs and symptoms of gastrointestinal alterations. ___ ___ ___ _____

   g. Asked whether patient taking any anti-inflammatory medications or antibiotics. ___ ___ ___ _____

   h. Inquired about family history of cancer, kidney disease, alcoholism, hypertension, or heart disease. ___ ___ ___ _____

   i. Reviewed patient's history for risk factors. ___ ___ ___ _____

2. Assessment of female patient:

   a. Determined if patient has signs and symptoms of STI or other pathology. ___ ___ ___ _____

   b. Reviewed history for gynecological or urinary problems. ___ ___ ___ _____

   c. Reviewed risk factors and infection of human papillomavirus (HPV) and availability of vaccine. ___ ___ ___ _____

   d. Reviewed risk factors for ovarian and endometrial cancer. ___ ___ ___ _____

3. Assessment of male patient:

   a. Assessed normal urinary elimination problem. ___ ___ ___ _____

   b. Determined if patient had signs and symptoms of STI. ___ ___ ___ _____

   c. Reviewed signs and symptoms of inguinal hernias. ___ ___ ___ _____

   d. Discussed warning signs and symptoms of testicular cancer. ___ ___ ___ _____

	S	U	NP	Comments

e. Discussed early warning signs of prostate enlargement and prostate cancer. ___ ___ ___ _____

4. Assessment of all patients:

   a. Discussed warning signs and risk factors of colorectal cancer. ___ ___ ___ _____

   b. Inquired and assessed nutritional intake. ___ ___ ___ _____

   c. Assessed medication history. ___ ___ ___ _____

NURSING DIAGNOSIS

1. Formulated appropriate nursing diagnosis based on assessment data. ___ ___ ___ _____

PLANNING

1. Identified expected outcomes. ___ ___ ___ _____

IMPLEMENTATION

1. Prepared patient for abdominal assessment:

   a. Allowed patient to empty bladder before assessment. ___ ___ ___ _____

   b. Correctly draped and positioned patient in a warm room. ___ ___ ___ _____

   c. Explained steps calmly and slowly. ___ ___ ___ _____

   d. Asked patient to identify any tender areas. ___ ___ ___ _____

2. Abdominal assessment:

   a. Identified anatomical landmarks. ___ ___ ___ _____

   b. Inspected skin of abdomen. Questioned patient if bruising present. ___ ___ ___ _____

   c. Noted contour and symmetry of abdomen and condition of umbilicus. ___ ___ ___ _____

   d. If abdomen appeared distended, noted characteristics and assessed flanks. ___ ___ ___ _____

   e. Turned off suction momentarily if a nasogastric tube or intestinal tube was connected. ___ ___ ___ _____

   f. Auscultated bowel sounds systematically with diaphragm of stethoscope. Described characteristics of sounds. Listened for 5 minutes over each quadrant to determine absence of bowel sounds ___ ___ ___ _____

   g. Used bell of stethoscope to auscultate vascular sounds and notified physician if aortic bruit auscultated. ___ ___ ___ _____

   h. Percussed four abdominal quadrants. ___ ___ ___ _____

   i. Percussed abdomen for fluid wave. ___ ___ ___ _____

   j. Percussed over posterior costovertebral angles. ___ ___ ___ _____

	S	U	NP	Comments
k. Performed light palpation of abdomen.	___	___	___	_____
l. Palpated bladder area.	___	___	___	_____
m. Noted characteristics of any masses present.	___	___	___	_____
n. Assessed for rebound tenderness if area was tender on palpation.	___	___	___	_____
o. Performed deep palpation.	___	___	___	_____

3. Female genital examination:

a. Implemented Steps 1a-d.	___	___	___	_____
b. Applied gloves. Positioned patient appropriately.	___	___	___	_____
c. Exposed only perineal area.	___	___	___	_____
d. Inspected surface characteristics of perineum.	___	___	___	_____

4. Male genitalia examination:

a. Implemented Steps 1a-d.	___	___	___	_____
b. Observed surface characteristics, lesions, and parasites.	___	___	___	_____
c. Inspected and palpated penis, scrotum, and testes.	___	___	___	_____

5. Rectal assessment:

a. Female patient remained in dorsal recumbent or Sims' position.	___	___	___	_____
b. Male patient stood and bent forward leaning over examination table; if nonambulatory patient, examined in Sims' position.	___	___	___	_____
c. Inspected the perianal and sacrococcygeal areas by gently retracting the buttocks.	___	___	___	_____

EVALUATION

1. Compared findings with normal assessment characteristics of the abdomen.	___	___	___	_____
2. Asked patient to describe signs and symptoms of colorectal and genitourinary cancer.	___	___	___	_____
3. Identified unexpected outcomes.	___	___	___	_____

RECORDING AND REPORTING

1. Recorded results of assessment.	___	___	___	_____
2. Recorded patient instruction and outcome.	___	___	___	_____
3. Reported abnormalities to nurse in charge or physician.	___	___	___	_____

Student _____ Date _____

Instructor _____ Date _____

PERFORMANCE CHECKLIST SKILL 6-6 **MUSCULOSKELETAL AND NEUROLOGICAL ASSESSMENT**

	S	U	NP	Comments
ASSESSMENT				
1. Reviewed patient's history for risk factors.	___	___	___	_____
2. Asked patient if screened for osteoporosis.	___	___	___	_____
3. Asked patient to describe history of musculoskeletal function/problems.	___	___	___	_____
4. Assessed nature and extent of patient's musculoskeletal pain and ability to perform daily activities.	___	___	___	_____
5. Determined how daily activities affected by alteration.	___	___	___	_____
6. Assessed height decrease in woman older than 50.	___	___	___	_____
7. Determined patient's medication history and current use.	___	___	___	_____
8. Assessed patient's use of alcohol or controlled substances.	___	___	___	_____
9. Determined if patient had a history of seizures.	___	___	___	_____
10. Screened patient for nervous system alterations.	___	___	___	_____
11. Discussed with significant others any changes in patient's behavior.	___	___	___	_____
12. Assessed patient for history of sensory changes.	___	___	___	_____
13. Reviewed history for drug toxicity in older patient.	___	___	___	_____
14. Reviewed past history for head or spinal cord injury, hypertension, or psychiatric disorders.	___	___	___	_____
NURSING DIAGNOSIS				
1. Developed appropriate nursing diagnoses based on assessment data.	___	___	___	_____
PLANNING				
1. Identified expected outcomes based on communication goals.	___	___	___	_____

	S	U	NP	Comments

IMPLEMENTATION

1. Prepared patient:

   a. Integrated musculoskeletal and neurological assessment into other aspects of physical assessment.

   b. Planned time for rest periods during assessment.

2. Musculoskeletal assessment:

   a. Observed patient's ability to use arms and hands.

   b. Assessed muscle strength of upper extremities.

   c. Assessed hand grip strength.

   d. Compared strength of symmetrical muscle groups.

   e. Measured muscle size for patients with decreased strength and muscle atrophy.

   f. Observed patient's position sitting, supine, prone, or standing. Observed joint range of motion.

   g. Inspected gait.

   h. Observed postural alignment.

   i. Observed overall status of extremities.

   j. Gently palpated bones, joints, and surrounding areas where patient reports alterations.

   k. Assessed patient's ability to perform active ROM. Assisted with passive ROM in the presence of weakness.

   l. Palpated joints for swelling, stiffness, tenderness, and heat; noted any redness.

   m. Assessed muscle tone in major muscle groups.

3. Neurological assessment:

   a. Assessed level of consciousness and orientation.

   b. Assessed cranial nerves.

   c. Assessed sensory status of extremities: pain, touch, vibration, and position.

   d. Assessed motor and cerebellar function: gait, Romberg test.

   e. Assessed deep tendon reflexes (DTRs).

	S	U	NP	Comments

g. Palpated each peripheral artery symmetrically and assessed pulses: radial, ulnar, brachial, dorsalis pedis, pedal, posterior tibial, popliteal, and femoral. Used ultrasound instrument for pedal pulses, if necessary. ___ ___ ___ _____

h. Monitored deep tendon reflexes: knee and plantar. Checked for ankle clonus, if indicated. ___ ___ ___ _____

EVALUATION

1. Compared muscle strength and ROM with previous assessments. ___ ___ ___ _____

2. Compared neurological status with previous assessment. ___ ___ ___ _____

3. Evaluated patient's level of discomfort after the procedure. ___ ___ ___ _____

4. Identified unexpected outcomes. ___ ___ ___ _____

RECORDING AND REPORTING

1. Recorded all assessment findings. ___ ___ ___ _____

2. Reported acute pain, sudden muscle weakness, or changes in neurological status or peripheral circulation to nurse in charge or physician. ___ ___ ___ _____

Student _____   Date _____

Instructor _____   Date _____

PERFORMANCE CHECKLIST SKILL 6-7 **ASSESSING INTAKE AND OUTPUT**

	S	U	NP	Comments

ASSESSMENT

1. Identified conditions that could influence a patient's fluid balance status. ___ ___ ___ _____

2. Identified risk of insufficient fluid intake. ___ ___ ___ _____

3. Identified medications that could influence a patient's fluid balance status. ___ ___ ___ _____

4. Assessed patient for signs of dehydration or fluid overload. ___ ___ ___ _____

5. Weighed patient daily. ___ ___ ___ _____

6. Monitored laboratory reports. ___ ___ ___ _____

7. Assessed patient's and family's knowledge of purpose of I&O measurements. ___ ___ ___ _____

NURSING DIAGNOSIS

1. Developed appropriate nursing diagnoses based on assessment data. ___ ___ ___ _____

PLANNING

1. Identified expected outcomes. ___ ___ ___ _____

2. Posted sign indicating I&O was instituted. ___ ___ ___ _____

3. Placed I&O record in established location. ___ ___ ___ _____

IMPLEMENTATION

1. Explained to patient and family the reasons I&O measurements are important. ___ ___ ___ _____

2. Measured and recorded all oral and parenteral fluids and all enteral tube feedings and liquid medicines. ___ ___ ___ _____

3. Instructed patient not to empty urinal, Foley or wound drainage bag, bedpan, or commode. ___ ___ ___ _____

4. Observed color and characteristics of urine. ___ ___ ___ _____

5. Measured and recorded all drainage every 8 hours or as indicated. ___ ___ ___ _____

6. Applied gloves before handling equipment or drainage. Discarded gloves and performed hand hygiene. Recorded output measurements. ___ ___ ___ _____

	S	U	NP	Comments

EVALUATION

1. Observed condition of skin and mucous membranes.

2. Observed characteristics of urinary output and wound drainage.

3. Noted I&O balance.

4. Identified unexpected outcomes.

RECORDING AND REPORTING

1. Calculated and recorded I&O totals in accordance with agency policy.

2. Calculated and recorded 24-hour totals.

3. Documented all assessment findings.

4. Reported to physician alterations in fluid balance and patient status.

Student Daray Brenneman   Date 8/31/12
Instructor _____Korll_____   Date 8/31/12

PERFORMANCE CHECKLIST SKILL 7-1   **HAND HYGIENE**

	S	U	NP	Comments

ASSESSMENT

1. Inspected surface of hands and fingers for cuts or breaks. ___ ___ ___ ___

2. Inspected hands for visible soiling. ___ ___ ___ ___

3. Inspected nails for condition and length. ___ ___ ___ ___

NURSING DIAGNOSIS

1. Developed appropriate nursing diagnoses. ___ ___ ___ ___

PLANNING

1. Identified expected outcomes. ___ ___ ___ ___

IMPLEMENTATION

1. Removed jewelry and pushed clothing or wrist-watch above wrist level. ___ ___ ___ ___

2. Performed hand antisepsis using an instant alcohol waterless antiseptic rub:

   a. Dispensed ample amount of product into palm of hand. ___ ___ ___ ___

   b. Rubbed hands together, covering all surfaces of hands and fingers with antiseptic. ___ ___ ___ ___

   c. Rubbed hands together until the alcohol was dry. Allowed hands to dry completely before applying gloves. ___ ___ ___ ___

3. Performed hand hygiene with antimicrobial soap and water:

   a. Stood at sink without touching sink with hands or uniform. ___ ___ ___ ___

   b. Turned on water. ___ ___ ___ ___

   c. Avoided splashing. ___ ___ ___ ___

   d. Regulated water flow. Adjusted water temperature to "warm." ___ ___ ___ ___

   e. Wet hands and wrists, keeping hands and forearms lower than elbows. ___ ___ ___ ___

   f. Applied antimicrobial soap to hands. ___ ___ ___ ___

   g. Lathered hands and applied friction to skin surfaces for 10 to 15 seconds; interlaced fingers and rubbed palms and backs of hands in circular motion. ___ ___ ___ ___

	S	U	NP	Comments
h. Cleaned thoroughly under fingernails.		___	___	_____
i. Rinsed thoroughly, keeping hands below elbows.		___	___	_____
j. Dried hands thoroughly, wiping from fingers up to wrists and forearms.		___	___	_____
k. Discarded paper towel properly.		___	___	_____
l. Turned off water at sink with paper towel or pedal.		___	___	_____
m. Applied lotion to hands.		___	___	_____

EVALUATION

1. Inspected surface of hands.	___	___	___	_____
2. Identified unexpected outcomes.	___	___	___	_____

Student _____ Date _____

Instructor _____ Date _____

PERFORMANCE CHECKLIST SKILL 7-2 **CARING FOR PATIENTS UNDER ISOLATION PRECAUTIONS**

	S	U	NP	Comments
ASSESSMENT				
1. Reviewed precautions for patient's specific isolation category.	___	___	___	_____
2. Reviewed appropriate laboratory test results.	___	___	___	_____
3. Considered types of care to be delivered to patient.	___	___	___	_____
4. Determined patient's understanding of purpose of isolation and procedures.	___	___	___	_____
5. Determined if patient is allergic to latex.	___	___	___	_____
NURSING DIAGNOSIS				
1. Developed appropriate nursing diagnoses based on patient's isolated status.	___	___	___	_____
PLANNING				
1. Identified expected outcomes.	___	___	___	_____
IMPLEMENTATION				
1. Performed hand hygiene.	___	___	___	_____
2. Prepared equipment and supplies.	___	___	___	_____
3. Determined appropriate barriers to apply.	___	___	___	_____
4. Prepared for entrance into isolation room.				
a. Applied isolation gown correctly, and secured ties at neck and waist.	___	___	___	_____
b. Applied surgical mask or respirator securely over nose and mouth.	___	___	___	_____
c. Applied eyewear or goggles, if needed, to fit snugly around face and eyes.	___	___	___	_____
d. Applied disposable gloves with edges overlying gown cuffs.	___	___	___	_____
5. Entered patient's room. Arranged supplies and equipment.	___	___	___	_____
6. Explained purpose of isolation and necessary precautions to patient and family.	___	___	___	_____
7. Assessed for emotional response to isolation precautions.	___	___	___	_____

	S	U	NP	Comments

8. Assessed vital signs:

   a. Disinfected reusable equipment after removing from room.

   b. Returned stethoscope to clean surface, and cleansed diaphragm/bell with alcohol as needed.

   c. Used individual or disposable thermometer.

9. Administered medications:

   a. Gave oral medication in wrapper or cup.

   b. Properly disposed of wrapper or cup.

   c. Administered injection while wearing gloves.

   d. Discarded syringe and needle in proper receptacle.

   e. Placed reusable syringe on clean towel for removal.

10. Administered hygiene:

   a. Prevented isolation gown from becoming wet.

   b. Assisted in removing patient's gown, and disposed of it appropriately.

   c. Removed linen from bed, and disposed of linen appropriately.

   d. Provided clean linen and towels.

   e. Changed gloves, if necessary. Performed hand hygiene.

11. Collected specimens:

   a. Placed specimen containers on clean paper towel in bathroom.

   b. Followed procedure for specimen collection.

   c. Transferred collected specimen to appropriate container without contaminating container's outer surface. Transferred specimens correctly into plastic bag and applied label.

   d. Checked label for accuracy. Sent specimen to laboratory.

12. Disposed of linen and trash bags:

   a. Used appropriate bags for soiled articles.

   b. Tied bags securely.

	S	U	NP	Comments

13. Removed all reusable equipment and disinfected contaminated surfaces. ___ ___ ___ _____

14. Re-supplied room as needed, with another caregiver handling supplies at door. ___ ___ ___ _____

15. Left isolation room:

   a. Removed gloves by turning them inside out, thereby avoiding contact with contaminated surfaces. ___ ___ ___ _____

   b. Removed eyewear or goggles. ___ ___ ___ _____

   c. Untied neck strings of gown. Allowed gown to fall from shoulders. Pulled gown off correctly and discarded in appropriate receptacle. ___ ___ ___ _____

   d. Untied and removed mask. Disposed of mask. ___ ___ ___ _____

   e. Performed hand hygiene. ___ ___ ___ _____

   f. Picked up wristwatch and stethoscope before leaving room and recorded vital signs. ___ ___ ___ _____

   g. Determined patient's needs before leaving room. ___ ___ ___ _____

   h. Left room and closed door. ___ ___ ___ _____

EVALUATION

1. While in room, determined if patient was offered an opportunity to discuss health problems, course of treatment, and related concerns. ___ ___ ___ _____

2. Identified unexpected outcomes. ___ ___ ___ _____

RECORDING AND REPORTING

1. Documented procedures, education performed or reinforced, and patient's responses to social isolation and education. ___ ___ ___ _____

Student _____ Date _____

Instructor _____ Date _____

PERFORMANCE CHECKLIST PROCEDURAL GUIDELINE 7-1 **SPECIAL TUBERCULOSIS PRECAUTIONS**

	S	U	NP	Comments
1. Assessed potential for infection.	___	___	___	_____
2. Performed hand hygiene.	___	___	___	_____
3. Applied mask and checked fit.	___	___	___	_____
4. Explained purpose of TB isolation to patient, family, and relevant others.	___	___	___	_____
5. Instructed patient to cover mouth with a tissue when coughing and to wear a disposable surgical mask when leaving room.	___	___	___	_____
6. Provided scheduled care.	___	___	___	_____
7. Closed the door upon leaving the room.	___	___	___	_____
8. Removed mask:				
a. If disposable, discarded in the proper receptacle.	___	___	___	_____
b. If reusable, placed in labeled bag for storage and avoided crushing mask.	___	___	___	_____
9. Assessed patient's laboratory data for repeated AFB smears that may be negative.	___	___	___	_____
10. Asked patient and family to identify method of transmission of TB.	___	___	___	_____
11. Assessed any suspected respiratory symptoms in neighboring patients.	___	___	___	_____

Student _____ Date _____

Instructor _____ Date _____

PERFORMANCE CHECKLIST SKILL 8-1 **APPLYING AND REMOVING CAP, MASK, AND PROTECTIVE EYEWEAR**

	S	U	NP	Comments

ASSESSMENT

1. Considered procedure and determined need to apply cap, mask, or eyewear. ___ ___ ___ _____

2. Avoided participating in procedure if had signs or symptoms of an infection. ___ ___ ___ _____

3. Assessed risk of transmitting infection to patient. ___ ___ ___ _____

NURSING DIAGNOSIS

1. Developed appropriate nursing diagnoses based on assessment data. ___ ___ ___ _____

PLANNING

1. Identified expected outcomes. ___ ___ ___ _____

2. Prepared and inspected equipment. ___ ___ ___ _____

IMPLEMENTATION

1. *Applying Cap*

   a. Combed long hair back and secured. ___ ___ ___ _____

   b. Secured hair in place with pins. ___ ___ ___ _____

   c. Applied cap covering hair completely. ___ ___ ___ _____

2. *Applying Mask*

   a. Located top edge of mask. ___ ___ ___ _____

   b. Held mask by top two ties with top edge of mask above nose. ___ ___ ___ _____

   c. Tied top strings at top of back of head properly. ___ ___ ___ _____

   d. Tied two lower strings snugly around neck with mask under chin. ___ ___ ___ _____

   e. Pinched upper metal bar around bridge of nose. ___ ___ ___ _____

3. *Applying Sterile Gloves, If Needed*

4. *Applying Protective Eyewear*

   a. Applied protective eyewear or goggles comfortably and checked vision. ___ ___ ___ _____

   b. Checked that eyewear fit snugly around forehead and face. ___ ___ ___ _____

	S	U	NP	Comments

5. *Disposing of Cap and Mask and Removing Eyewear*

   a. Removed gloves first, if worn.   ____   ____   ____   _____

   b. Untied bottom strings of mask.   ____   ____   ____   _____

   c. Untied top strings of mask; removed and discarded mask.   ____   ____   ____   _____

   d. Removed eyewear without placing hands on soiled lens.   ____   ____   ____   _____

   e. Grasped outer surface of cap and lifted from head.   ____   ____   ____   _____

   f. Discarded cap and mask into receptacle, and washed hands.   ____   ____   ____   _____

EVALUATION

1. Assessed the patient for signs of infection.   ____   ____   ____   _____

2. Identified unexpected outcomes.   ____   ____   ____   _____

RECORDING AND REPORTING

1. Recorded procedure performed and patient status.   ____   ____   ____   _____

Student __Darcy Brenneman__   Date _____

Instructor _____   Date __12/7/12__

PERFORMANCE CHECKLIST SKILL 8-2 **PREPARING A STERILE FIELD**

	S	U	NP	Comments
ASSESSMENT				
1. Verified that procedure required sterile technique.	___	___	___	_____
2. Determined patient's comfort, oxygen, and elimination needs before procedure.	___	___	___	_____
3. Checked integrity of sterile packages.	___	___	___	_____
4. Anticipated number and variety of supplies needed.	___	___	___	_____
NURSING DIAGNOSIS				
1. Developed appropriate nursing diagnoses based on assessment data.	___	___	___	_____
PLANNING				
1. Identified expected outcomes.	___	___	___	_____
2. Completed all priority tasks before beginning procedure.	___	___	___	_____
3. Asked visitors to step out. Discouraged movement by staff.	___	___	___	_____
4. Prepared equipment at beside.	___	___	___	_____
5. Positioned patient comfortably.	___	___	___	_____
6. Explained purpose of procedure and sterile technique.	___	___	___	_____
IMPLEMENTATION				
1. Applied cap, mask, protective eyewear, and gown, as needed.	___	___	___	_____
2. Selected clean, flat, dry work surface above waist level.				_____
3. Performed hand hygiene.				_____
4. *Preparing Sterile Work Surface*				
a. Sterile commercial kit or tray				
(1) Placed kit or package on clean work surface above waist level.	___	___	___	_____
(2) Opened outside cover and removed kit; pulled paper wrapper off and away from body.	___	___	___	_____

	S	U	NP	Comments

(3) Grasped outer surface of tip of outermost flap.

(4) Opened outermost flap away from body.

(5) Grasped outside surface of edge of first side flap.

(6) Opened side flap, pulling to side, allowing it to lie flat on table surface. Kept arm to side and not over sterile surface.

(7) Repeated step (6) for second side flap.

(8) Grasped outside border of last and innermost flap.

(9) Stood away from sterile package and pulled flap back, allowing it to fall flat on table.

b. Sterile linen–wrapped package

(1) Placed package on clean, dry, flat work surface above waist level.

(2) Removed tape seal and unwrapped both layers following same steps as with sterile kit.

(3) Used opened package wrapper as sterile field.

c. Sterile drape

(1) Placed sterile drape pack on flat, dry surface, and opened with sterile technique.

(2) Applied sterile gown and sterile gloves, if indicated.

(3) Using fingertips, picked up folded top edge of sterile drape. Lifted drape from outer cover and let it unfold without touching any object; discarded outer cover.

(4) Allowed drape to unfold, keeping it above waist and work surface and away from body.

(5) With nondominant hand, grasped adjacent corner of drape; held drape straight up and away from body.

(6) Held drape and positioned its bottom half over work surface.

(7) Allowed top half of drape to be placed over work surface last.

	S	U	NP	Comments

5. *Adding Sterile Items*

    a. Opened sterile item.

    b. Peeled wrapper onto the nondominant hand.

    c. Placed item onto sterile field without reaching over sterile field.

    d. Disposed of outer wrapper.

6. *Pouring Sterile Solutions*

    a. Verified contents and expiration date of solution.

    b. Ensured receptacle for solution located near edge of work surface.

    c. Removed seal and cap from bottle in an upward motion.

    d. Poured solution slowly, holding edge of bottle well above and away from edge and 1 to 2 inches above the inside of sterile container.

EVALUATION

1. Identified break in sterile technique.

2. Identified unexpected outcomes.

RECORDING AND REPORTING

1. Recorded sterile procedure performed and patient's status.

12/5/12

Renee 12/5

Student _____ Date _____

Instructor _____ Date _____

PERFORMANCE CHECKLIST SKILL 8-3 **STERILE GLOVING**

_____

	S	U	NP	Comments

ASSESSMENT

1. Considered procedure to be performed and consulted institutional policy on use of gloves. ____ ____ ____ _____

2. Considered patient's risk for infection. ____ ____ ____ _____

3. Examined condition of glove package. ____ ____ ____ _____

4. Inspected condition of hands. ____ ____ ____ _____

5. Determined if patient at risk for allergy to latex. ~~KV~~ ____ ____ _____

NURSING DIAGNOSIS

1. Developed appropriate nursing diagnoses based on assessment data. ____ ____ ____ _____

PLANNING

1. Identified expected outcomes. ____ ____ ____ _____

2. Selected correct size and type of gloves. ____ ____ ____ _____

3. Placed glove package near work area. ____ ____ ____ _____

IMPLEMENTATION

1. *Glove Application*

   a. Performed hand hygiene. ____ ____ ____ _____

   b. Removed outer glove wrapper. ____ ____ ____ _____

   c. Opened inner package, keeping gloves on wrapper's inside surface, and laid package on surface at waist level. ____ ____ ____ _____

   d. Identified right and left gloves. ____ ____ ____ _____

   e. With nondominant hand, grasped inside edge of cuff of glove for dominant hand. ____ ____ ____ _____

   f. Carefully pulled glove over dominant hand with thumb and fingers in proper spaces. ____ ____ ____ _____

   g. With gloved dominant hand, slipped fingers under cuff of second glove. ____ ____ ____ _____

   h. Pulled glove over nondominant hand without contaminating gloved dominant hand. ____ ____ ____ _____

   i. Interlocked fingers of gloved hands to ensure proper fit. ____ ____ ____ _____

	S	U	NP	Comments
2. *Glove Disposal*	KN			
a. Grasped outside of one cuff with other gloved hand, without touching wrist.	___	___	___	_____
b. Pulled glove off, turning it inside out, and placed in palm of gloved hand.	___	___	___	_____
c. Slid fingers of ungloved hand underneath cuff of gloved hand and pulled remaining glove off inside out, and over glove in palm of hand; discarded gloves in receptacle.	___	___	___	_____
d. Performed hand hygiene.	___	___	___	_____

EVALUATION

	S	U	NP	Comments
1. Assessed patient for localized signs of infection.	___	___	___	_____
2. Identified unexpected outcomes.	___	___	___	_____

RECORDING AND REPORTING

	S	U	NP	Comments
1. Recorded procedure performed and patient's response and status.	___	___	___	_____
2. Recorded and reported reaction, treatment, and response to emergency treatment in event of latex allergy.	___	___	___	_____

PE: Kyla van Der Weele

Student Darcy Brenneman   Date 9/14/12

Instructor _____ Kendice Co _____   Date 9/14/12

PERFORMANCE CHECKLIST SKILL 9-1   **USING SAFE AND EFFECTIVE TRANSFER TECHNIQUES**

	S	U	NP	Comments
ASSESSMENT				
1. Assessed patient's physiologic capacity for transfer.	✓ Jw	___	___	___
2. Assessed patient for presence of weakness, dizziness, or postural hypotension.	✓	___	___	___
3. Assessed patient's activity tolerance.	✓	___	___	___
4. Assessed patient's proprioceptive function.	✓	___	___	___
balance/equilibrium				
5. Assessed patient's sensory and cognitive status.	✓	___	___	___
6. Assessed patient for comfort.	✓	___	___	___
7. Assessed patient's cognitive status.	✓	___	___	___
8. Assessed patient's level of motivation.	✓	___	___	___
9. Assessed patient's risk of injury.	✓	___	___	___
10. Determined need for special transfer equipment in the home.	___	___	___	___
11. Determined the number of people needed to transfer.	✓ Jw	___	___	___
NURSING DIAGNOSIS				
1. Developed appropriate nursing diagnoses based on assessment data.	___	___	___	___
PLANNING				
1. Identified expected outcomes.	___	___	___	___
2. Explained procedure to patient.	___	___	___	___
IMPLEMENTATION				
1. Performed hand hygiene.	✓ Jw	___	___	___
2. Assisted patient to sitting position:				
a. Placed patient in supine position.	✓	___	___	___
b. Faced head of bed and removed pillows.	✓	___	___	___
c. Properly placed feet apart to improve balance.	✓	___	___	___
d. Placed hand under patient's shoulders.	✓	___	___	___
e. Placed other hand on bed surface.	✓	___	___	___
f. Raised patient to sitting position (weight shifted to rear leg).	✓	___	___	___
g. Pushed against bed with hand on bed surface.	✓	___	___	___

	S	U	NP	Comments

3. Assisted patient to sitting position on the side of the bed, using electrical bed:

a. Raised head of bed to 30 degrees. ✓

b. Placed patient in side-lying position. ✓

c. Stood in correct position for transfer and turned diagonally to face patient and far corner of bed. ✓

d. Properly placed feet in wide base of support. ✓

e. Placed arm near bed under patient's shoulders. ✓

f. Placed other arm over patient's thighs. ✓

g. Moved patient's lower legs and feet over side of bed and correctly pivoted leg. ✓

h. Shifted weight to elevate patient and remained in front of patient until balance regained. ✓

4. Transferred patient from bed to chair:

a. Assisted patient to sitting position on side of bed, with chair placed correctly. ✓

b. Applied transfer belt or other aids, if needed. ✓

c. Ensured that patient was wearing nonskid shoes; kept weight-bearing leg forward. ✓

d. Stood with feet apart. ✓

e. Flexed knees and hips; aligned knees with patient's knees. ✓

f. Grasped transfer belt at sides. ✓

g. Rocked patient to standing position on count of 3. ✓

h. Used knee to maintain stability of weak (or paralyzed) leg. ✓

i. Pivoted on foot that was farthest from chair. ✓

j. Instructed patient to use arm rests on chair for support. ✓

k. Flexed hips and knees while lowering patient into chair. ✓

l. Assessed patient for proper alignment in sitting position. ✓

m. Provided patient with support and encouragement. ✓

78

	S	U	NP	Comments

5. Performed horizontal transfer from bed to stretcher:

   a. Determined number of staff required for transfer. ____ ____ ____ _____

   b. Lowered the head of the bed as much as tolerated by patient; ensured bed brakes were locked. ____ ____ ____ _____

   c. Crossed patient's arms on chest; lowered side rails. ____ ____ ____ _____

   d. Placed slide board under patient and positioned nurses on sides of the bed. ____ ____ ____ _____

   e. Fan-folded drawsheet on both sides. ____ ____ ____ _____

   f. Turned patient onto side as one unit on the count of 3. ____ ____ ____ _____

   g. Placed slide board under drawsheet. ____ ____ ____ _____

   h. Gently rolled patient back onto the slide board. ____ ____ ____ _____

   i. Lined up the stretcher with the bed. Locked brakes on bed and stretcher. ____ ____ ____ _____

   j. Positioned self and other nurses on side of the stretcher and bed. ____ ____ ____ _____

   k. Fan-folded drawsheet, using count of 3, with two nurses pulling drawsheet with patient onto stretcher and third nurse holding slide board in place. ____ ____ ____ _____

   l. Positioned patient in center of stretcher. Raised head of stretcher. Raised side rails and covered patient. ____ ____ ____ _____

6. Used mechanical/hydraulic lift to transfer patient from bed to chair:

   a. Moved lift to bedside. ____ ____ ____ _____

   b. Placed chair to allow adequate space to maneuver lift. ____ ____ ____ _____

   c. Raised bed to high position. ____ ____ ____ _____

   d. Kept side rail up on side opposite nurse. ____ ____ ____ _____

   e. Rolled patient away from nurse. ____ ____ ____ _____

   f. Placed hammock or a canvas strip under patient to form sling. ____ ____ ____ _____

   g. Raised bed rail. ____ ____ ____ _____

   h. Went to opposite side of bed, lowered side rail. ____ ____ ____ _____

	S	U	NP	Comments

i. Rolled patient to opposite side and pulled hammock through. ___ ___ ___ _____

j. Rolled patient supine onto canvas seat. ___ ___ ___ _____

k. Removed patient's glasses, if applicable. ___ ___ ___ _____

l. Placed lift's horseshoe bar under bed. ___ ___ ___ _____

m. Lowered horizontal bar to sling level; locked valve. ___ ___ ___ _____

n. Attached strap hooks to holes in sling. ___ ___ ___ _____

o. Elevated head of bed. ___ ___ ___ _____

p. Folded patient's arms over chest. ___ ___ ___ _____

q. Pumped handle until patient was lifted from the bed. ___ ___ ___ _____

r. Pulled lift from bed and maneuvered to chair using steering handle. ___ ___ ___ _____

s. Rolled base around chair. ___ ___ ___ _____

t. Released check valve slowly; lowered patient into chair. ___ ___ ___ _____

u. Closed check valve when patient down in chair. ___ ___ ___ _____

v. Removed straps and lift. ___ ___ ___ _____

w. Checked patient for proper alignment. ___ ___ ___ _____

7. Performed hand hygiene. ___ ___ ___ _____

EVALUATION

1. Monitored vital signs. Asked if patient felt dizzy or fatigued. ✓ ___ ___ _____

2. Observed for correct body alignment and presence of pressure points on skin. ✓ ___ ___ _____

3. Observed patient's response to transfer. ✓ ___ ___ _____

4. Asked if patient had pain during transfer. ✓ ___ ___ _____

5. Identified unexpected outcomes. ___ ___ ___ _____

RECORDING AND REPORTING

1. Recorded procedure and observations. ___ ___ ___ _____

2. Reported to appropriate personnel patient's transfer ability, assistance required, and any unusual occurrence. ___ ___ ___ _____

PE: Kyla vanderwell
9/12/12

Student ___Darcy Brenneman___   Date ___9/17/12___

Instructor _____   Date _____

PERFORMANCE CHECKLIST SKILL 9-2 **MOVING AND POSITIONING PATIENTS IN BED**

	S	U	NP	Comments

ASSESSMENT
1. Assessed patient's ROM, body alignment, and comfort level.
2. Assessed for risk factors.
3. Assessed patient's level of consciousness.
4. Assessed skin condition.
5. Assessed for presence of tubes, incisions, and equipment.
6. Assessed patient's ability to assist with positioning.
7. Assessed motivation and ability of patient and family to participate in care.
8. Checked physician's orders before positioning.

NURSING DIAGNOSIS
1. Developed appropriate nursing diagnoses based on assessment data.

PLANNING
1. Identified expected outcomes.
2. Raised level of bed to comfortable working height.
3. Removed pillows and other objects.
4. Obtained extra assistance as needed.
5. Explained procedure to patient.

IMPLEMENTATION
1. Performed hand hygiene.
2. Provided for patient privacy.
3. Put bed in flat position if not contraindicated.
4. Assisted patient to move up in bed (two nurses):
   a. Placed patient on back with head of bed flat. Raised bed to appropriate working height.
   b. Placed pillow at head of bed.
   c. Faced head of bed.
   d. Stood in proper position.

	S	U	NP	Comments

e. Asked patient to flex knees.

f. Instructed patient to flex neck.

g. Instructed patient to push feet into bed surface to assist movement.

h. Maintained own body alignment.

i. Instructed patient to push heels and elevate trunk.

j. Shifted weight while patient elevated trunk.

5. Moved immobile patient up in bed with drawsheet (two nurses):

a. Placed drawsheet under patient.

b. Placed patient on back with bed flat. Raised bed to appropriate working height.

c. Positioned one nurse at each side of patient.

d. Grasped drawsheet firmly near patient.

e. Maintained proper body alignment while shifting weight to move patient and drawsheet to desired position.

6. Realigned patient in proper body alignment:

a. Positioned patient in supported Fowler's position:

(1) Elevated head of bed 45 to 60 degrees.

(2) Rested patient's head against mattress or placed small pillow underneath patient's head.

(3) Placed pillows appropriately to support patient's hands and arms correctly.

(4) Placed pillow at lower back.

(5) Placed small pillow under thighs.

(6) Supported calves with pillows and heels off surface.

b. Positioned hemiplegic patient in supported Fowler's position:

(1) Positioned patient in supine position; elevated head of bed 45 to 60 degrees.

(2) Positioned patient in straight alignment.

(3) Positioned patient's head on pillow with chin slightly forward.

(4) Supported involved arm and hand with arm away from body supporting elbow with pillow and maintaining arch of hand and fingers partially flexed.

82

	S	U	NP	Comments

(5) Maintained leg alignment with tro-chanter rolls. ___ ___ ___ _____

(6) Supported patient's feet in dorsiflexed position. ___ ___ ___ _____

c. Positioned patient in supine position: W

  (1) Placed patient on back with bed flat. ___ ___ ___ _____

  (2) Placed small pillow or rolled towel under small of back. ___ ___ ___ _____

  (3) Placed pillow under upper shoulders, neck, and head. ___ ___ ___ _____

  (4) Placed trochanter rolls along hips and upper thighs. ___ ___ ___ _____

  (5) Placed feet in therapeutic boots or splints. ___ ___ ___ _____

  (6) Placed pillows under pronated arms parallel to body. ___ ___ ___ _____

  (7) Placed handrails to maintain hands in functional position. ___ ___ ___ _____

d. Positioned hemiplegic patient in supine position:

  (1) Placed patient's head on flat bed. ___ ___ ___ _____

  (2) Placed folded towel or pillow under shoulder of affected side. ___ ___ ___ _____

  (3) Placed affected arm away from body with elbow supported and palm up. ___ ___ ___ _____

  (4) Placed folded towel under hip of involved side. ___ ___ ___ _____

  (5) Flexed affected knee 30 degrees supported with pillows. ___ ___ ___ _____

  (6) Maintained feet in dorsiflexion with soft pillows. ___ ___ ___ _____

e. Positioned patient in prone position: W

  (1) Rolled patient to side. ___ ___ ___ _____

  (2) Placed patient on abdomen with bed flat. ___ ___ ___ _____

  (3) Turned patient's head to one side; supported it with a small pillow. ___ ___ ___ _____

  (4) Placed small pillow under patient's abdomen. ___ ___ ___ _____

  (5) Supported patient's arms, flexed them at shoulders on pillows. ___ ___ ___ _____

  (6) Placed pillow under patient's lower legs to elevate toes off bed. ___ ___ ___ _____

	S	U	NP	Comments

f. Positioned hemiplegic patient in prone position:

  (1) Moved patient toward unaffected side. ___ ___ ___ _____

  (2) Rolled patient onto side and placed pillow on patient's abdomen. ___ ___ ___ _____

  (3) Rolled patient onto abdomen. ___ ___ ___ _____

  (4) Turned head toward involved side. ___ ___ ___ _____

  (5) Positioned involved arm properly. ___ ___ ___ _____

  (6) Flexed knees and placed pillows under legs from knees to ankles. ___ ___ ___ _____

  (7) Maintained feet in dorsiflexion. ___ ___ ___ _____

g. Positioned patient in lateral (side-lying) position:

  (1) Lowered head of bed to comfortable level. ___ ___ ___ _____

  (2) Lowered side rail and positioned patient opposite direction to be turned. ___ ___ ___ _____

  (3) Raised side rail, moved to opposite side. ___ ___ ___ _____

  (4) Positioned patient properly and rolled toward nurse. ___ ___ ___ _____

  (5) Placed pillow under patient's head and neck. ___ ___ ___ _____

  (6) Properly aligned patient's shoulders. ___ ___ ___ _____

  (7) Positioned patient's arms in slightly flexed position. ___ ___ ___ _____

  (8) Aligned hips slightly forward. ___ ___ ___ _____

  (9) Supported patient's back with pillows. ___ ___ ___ _____

  (10) Placed pillow under leg from groin to foot. ___ ___ ___ _____

  (11) Maintained foot in dorsiflexion. ___ ___ ___ _____

  (12) Performed hand hygiene. ___ ___ ___ _____

h. Positioned patient in Sims' (semiprone) position:

  (1) Lowered head of bed completely. ___ ___ ___ _____

  (2) Placed patient in supine position. ___ ___ ___ _____

  (3) Rolled patient on side; positioned correctly. ___ ___ ___ _____

  (4) Placed pillow under patient's head. ___ ___ ___ _____

	S	U	NP	Comments
(5) Supported upper arm with pillow.	——	——	——	———————
(6) Supported flexed leg with pillow.	——	——	——	———————
(7) Maintained feet in dorsiflexion.	——	——	——	———————
i. Positioned patient by logrolling (three nurses).				
(1) Placed pillow between patient's knees.	——	——	——	———————
(2) Crossed patient's arms on chest.	——	——	——	———————
(3) Positioned staff correctly on both sides of bed.	——	——	——	———————
(4) Fan-folded drawsheet alongside patient.	——	——	——	———————
(5) Rolled patient on count of 3.	——	——	——	———————
(6) Placed pillows for support.	——	——	——	———————
(7) Leaned patient back on pillows.	——	——	——	———————
(8) Performed hand hygiene.	——	——	——	———————

EVALUATION

	S	U	NP	Comments
1. Assessed patient's body alignment, position, and level of comfort.	——	——	——	———————
2. Measured joint ROM.	——	——	——	———————
3. Assessed for contractures and/or alterations in skin integrity.	——	——	——	———————
4. Identified unexpected outcomes.	——	——	——	———————

RECORDING AND REPORTING

	S	U	NP	Comments
1. Recorded procedure, observations, and patient's ability to assist with repositioning.	——	——	——	———————
2. Reported observations at change of shift.	——	——	——	———————
3. Recorded time and position.	——	——	——	———————

PE: Kyla vanDurwelu

Student _Daray Brenneman_   Date _____

Instructor _____ _Kyndell B_ _____   Date _9/7/12_

PERFORMANCE CHECKLIST FOR PROCEDURAL GUIDELINE 10-1   **PERFORMING RANGE-OF-MOTION EXERCISES**

	S	U	NP	Comments
STEPS				
1. Reviewed patient's medical history and obtained physician's order, if needed.	✓			• Excellent ✓ o pt
2. Performed baseline assessment of joint function.	✓			during exercises on comfort.
3. Determined patient's or caregiver's understanding of exercises.	✓			• Excellent explanation to
4. Assessed for limitations or discomfort during initial ROM.	✓			client as you moved from joint to joint
5. Applied gloves if wound drainage or lesions are present.	✓			
6. Assisted patient to a comfortable position.	✓			
7. Performed exercises slowly and gently, supporting joint with cupped hand.	✓			
8. Completed exercises in a head-to-toe sequence. Repeated each exercise 5 times as tolerated.	✓			
9. Observed patient when performing ROM exercises.	✓			
10. Measured joint motion as needed.	✓			
11. Monitored level of pain during exercises.	✓			

Kyla VanDerWeele

- Body mechanics
- go to midline. neck f/ hyper + flexion
- flexion of shoulder all the way up if tolerated. Shoulder add / abduction.

+ flexion + ext. of thumb

Student _____ Date _____

Instructor _____ Date _____

PERFORMANCE CHECKLIST SKILL 10-1 **PERFORMING ISOMETRIC EXERCISES**

	S	U	NP	Comments

ASSESSMENT

1. Reviewed patient's chart for contraindications. ___ ___ ___ _____

2. Performed baseline assessment of vital signs. ___ ___ ___ _____

3. Assessed patient's baseline muscle strength. ___ ___ ___ _____

4. Assessed patient's nutritional status. ___ ___ ___ _____

5. Assessed patient's comfort level. ___ ___ ___ _____

6. Assessed patient's or caregiver's understanding of exercises. ___ ___ ___ _____

NURSING DIAGNOSIS

1. Developed appropriate nursing diagnoses based on assessment data. ___ ___ ___ _____

PLANNING

1. Identified expected outcomes. ___ ___ ___ _____

2. Explained procedure and demonstrated exercises. ___ ___ ___ _____

3. Assisted patient to comfortable position. ___ ___ ___ _____

IMPLEMENTATION

1. Provided privacy. ___ ___ ___ _____

2. Instructed patient to perform exercises as prescribed:

   a. Gradually increase repetitions. ___ ___ ___ _____

   b. Tighten each muscle group for 5 to 15 seconds, then completely relax for several seconds. ___ ___ ___ _____

   c. Repeat as appropriate for each muscle group. ___ ___ ___ _____

   d. Remind patient to exhale during exertion. ___ ___ ___ _____

3. Had patient perform each isometric exercise correctly:

   a. Quadriceps ___ ___ ___ _____

   b. Gluteal muscles ___ ___ ___ _____

   c. Abdominal muscles ___ ___ ___ _____

   d. Foot muscles ___ ___ ___ _____

   e. Hand grips ___ ___ ___ _____

   f. Biceps ___ ___ ___ _____

   g. Triceps ___ ___ ___ _____

	S	U	NP	Comments

EVALUATION

1. Observed patient's ability to perform exercises. ___ ___ ___ _____

2. Determined patient's level of energy, muscular strength, and comfort. ___ ___ ___ _____

3. Obtained vital signs. ___ ___ ___ _____

4. Identified unexpected outcomes. ___ ___ ___ _____

RECORDING AND REPORTING

1. Recorded performance of isometric exercises and objective and subjective information about muscle strength. ___ ___ ___ _____

2. Reported to nurse in charge or physician patient's tolerance of exercises. ___ ___ ___ _____

90

Student _____ Date _____

Instructor _____ Date _____

PERFORMANCE CHECKLIST SKILL 10-2 **CONTINUOUS PASSIVE MOTION MACHINE**

	S	U	NP	Comments
ASSESSMENT				
1. Assessed the CPM machine for electrical safety.	___	___	___	_____
2. Assessed the setup of the machine before placing on bed.	___	___	___	_____
3. Assessed the patient's pain on a scale of 0 to 10.	___	___	___	_____
4. Assessed patient's baseline vital signs.	___	___	___	_____
5. Assessed patient's ability and willingness to learn about the CPM machine.	___	___	___	_____
6. Assessed patient's condition and ROM limits prescribed by health care provider.	___	___	___	_____
NURSING DIAGNOSIS				
1. Developed appropriate nursing diagnoses based on assessment data.	___	___	___	_____
PLANNING				
1. Identified expected outcomes.	___	___	___	_____
2. Explained procedure and demonstrated CPM machine.	___	___	___	_____
3. Assisted patient to comfortable position.	___	___	___	_____
IMPLEMENTATION				
1. Performed hand hygiene.	___	___	___	_____
2. Provided analgesia as needed before using CPM machine.	___	___	___	_____
3. Applied gloves if wound drainage present.	___	___	___	_____
4. Placed elastic hose on patient, if ordered.	___	___	___	_____
5. Placed CPM machine on bed.	___	___	___	_____
6. Set limits of flexion and extension as prescribed.	___	___	___	_____
7. Set speed control to slow or moderate range.	___	___	___	_____
8. Put machine through one full cycle.	___	___	___	_____
9. Stopped CPM machine when in extension. Placed sheepskin on CPM machine.	___	___	___	_____
10. Placed patient's extremity in CPM machine.	___	___	___	_____
11. Adjusted CPM machine to patient's extremity. Lengthened and shortened appropriate sections of frame, as needed.	___	___	___	_____

	S	U	NP	Comments
12. Centered patient's extremity on frame.	___	___	___	_____
13. Aligned patient's joint with CPM's mechanical joint.	___	___	___	_____
14. Secured patient's extremity on CPM machine with Velcro straps. Applied loosely.	___	___	___	_____
15. Started machine. Stopped machine when in flexed position and checked degree of flexion.	___	___	___	_____
16. Started CPM machine and observed for two full cycles.	___	___	___	_____
17. Made sure patient was comfortable.	___	___	___	_____
18. Provided patient with on/off switch.	___	___	___	_____
19. Instructed patient to turn CPM machine off, if malfunctioning or experiencing pain. Instructed to notify nurse immediately.	___	___	___	_____
20. Discarded gloves and performed hand hygiene.	___	___	___	_____

EVALUATION

	S	U	NP	Comments
1. Inspected bony prominences and areas of skin in contact with machine at least every 2 hours.	___	___	___	_____
2. Asked patient to rate pain on scale of 0 to 10.	___	___	___	_____
3. Assessed patient's comfort, alignment, and positioning at least every 2 hours.	___	___	___	_____
4. Observed patient and CPM machine with each increase in flexion and extension.	___	___	___	_____
5. Identified unexpected outcomes.	___	___	___	_____

RECORDING AND REPORTING

	S	U	NP	Comments
1. Recorded pertinent information about patient's tolerance for CPM machine, rate of cycles per minute, degree of flexion and extension used, condition of extremity and skin, and condition of operative site (if present), and length of time machine is in use.	___	___	___	_____
2. Reported immediately to nurse in charge or physician any resistance to ROM: increased pain, swelling, heat, or redness in joint.	___	___	___	_____

PERFORMANCE CHECKLIST SKILL 10-3 **APPLYING ELASTIC STOCKINGS AND SEQUENTIAL COMPRESSION DEVICE**

	S	U	NP	Comments
ASSESSMENT				
1. Assessed patient's risk factors in Virchow's triad.	✓			
2. Observed for contraindications to use of elastic stockings.	✓			
3. Obtained physician's order.				
4. Assessed patient's or caregiver's understanding of application of elastic stockings and SCD sleeves.	✓			
5. Assessed and documented condition of patient's skin and circulation to the legs.	✓			
6. Assessed patient's or caregiver's understanding of proper care of elastic stockings.				
NURSING DIAGNOSIS				
1. Developed appropriate nursing diagnoses based on assessment data.				
PLANNING				
1. Identified expected outcomes.				
2. Explained procedure and reasons for applying stockings and SCD.				
3. Measured patient's legs to determine proper size for stockings and SCD sleeves.	✓			
IMPLEMENTATION				
1. Performed hand hygiene.	✓			
2. Positioned patient in supine position and elevated head of bed to comfortable level.	✓			
3. Cleansed patient's legs and applied talcum powder to patient's legs and feet.	✓			
4. Applied stockings; properly positioned and smoothed them. Instructed patient not to partially roll stockings back.	✓			
5. Applied SCD sleeves.				
a. Removed SCD sleeves from plastic, unfolded, and flattened.				
b. Arranged SCD sleeve under the patient's leg according to the position indicated on the inner lining of sleeve.				

	S	U	NP	Comments

c. Placed patient's leg on SCD sleeve. Lined up back of ankle with marking on inner lining of sleeve.

d. Positioned back of knee with popliteal opening.

e. Wrapped SCD sleeves securely around patient's leg.

f. Checked fit of SCD sleeves by placing two fingers between patient's leg and sleeve.

7. Attached SCD sleeve's connector to plug on mechanical unit.

8. Turned mechanical unit ON.

9. Monitored functioning of SCD through one full cycle of inflation and deflation.

10. Repositioned patient after procedure, and washed hands.

11. Performed hand hygiene.

12. Removed stockings or SCD sleeves at least once per shift.

13. Removed SCD sleeve when transferring patient.

EVALUATION

1. Inspected stockings for proper fit and wrinkles. ✓

2. Observed circulatory status of lower extremities. ✓

3. Determined patient's response to procedure.

4. Observed patient or caregiver when applying stockings.

5. Inspected SCD for kinks or twisting in tubing.

6. Identified unexpected outcomes.

RECORDING AND REPORTING

1. Recorded pertinent information about stocking/SCD sleeve application and removal, condition of skin, and circulatory status.

2. Reported to physician signs of skin irritation, impaired circulation, or thrombophlebitis.

PE: Kyla Vanderween 9/10/12

Student _Darcy Brenneman_   Date _9/14/12_

Instructor _____   Date _9/14/12_

PERFORMANCE CHECKLIST SKILL 10-4   **ASSISTING WITH AMBULATION AND USE OF CANES, CRUTCHES, AND WALKER**

	S	U	NP	Comments
ASSESSMENT				
1. Reviewed patient's chart.	___	___	___	_____
2. Assessed patient's physical readiness.	✓	___	___	_____
3. Assessed patient's or caregiver's understanding of ambulatory technique.	___	___	___	_____
4. Determined optimal time for ambulation.	___	___	___	_____
5. Assessed degree of assistance needed.	✓	___	___	_____
NURSING DIAGNOSIS				
1. Developed appropriate nursing diagnoses based on assessment data.	___	___	___	_____
PLANNING				
1. Identified expected outcomes.	___	___	___	_____
2. Prepared patient appropriately.	✓	___	___	_____
3. Determined appropriate height of ambulation device.	___	___	___	_____
4. Checked for rubber tips on ambulation device.	___	___	___	_____
5. Made sure that walking surface was clean, dry, well lighted, and unobstructed.	✓	___	___	_____
IMPLEMENTATION				
1. Assisted ambulation with one nurse:				
a. Confirmed patient not feeling light-headed.	✓	___	___	_____
b. Applied gait belt if necessary, assisted patient to standing position, and observed balance.	✓	___	___	_____
c. Positioned self on patient's stronger side and had patient take a few steps. Positioned self on patient's weaker side if assistance device used.	✓	___	___	_____
d. Supported patient at waist. Grasped gait belt, if used.	✓	___	___	_____
e. Took a few steps forward with patient and assessed for strength and balance.	✓	___	___	_____
f. Allowed patient to return to bed or chair if weak or dizzy.	✓	___	___	_____
g. Used appropriate procedure if patient began to fall.	✓	___	___	_____

	S	U	NP	Comments

2. Assisted ambulation with two nurses:

  a. Followed Steps 1a and b.   ✓ ___ ___ _____

  b. Nurses stood on each side of patient.   ✓ ___ ___ _____

  c. Both nurses grasped gait belt in middle of patient's back.   ✓ ___ ___ _____

  d. Stepped in unison with patient.   ✓ ___ ___ _____

  e. Gradually increased distance walked.   ✓ ___ ___ _____

  f. Followed Steps 1f and 1g.   ✓ ___ ___ _____

3. Ambulation with assistive devices:

  a. Assisted patient with crutch walking, using appropriate gait: two-point, three-point, four-point, swing-to, or swing-through gait. ___ ___ ___ _____

  b. Assisted patient in climbing stairs with crutches. ___ ___ ___ _____

  c. Assisted patient in descending stairs with crutches. ___ ___ ___ _____

  d. Assisted patient in ambulating with walker. ___ ___ ___ _____

  e. Assisted patient in ambulating with cane. ___ ___ ___ _____

EVALUATION

1. Assessed patient's response to ambulation, including vital signs and energy level.   ✓ ___ ___ _____

2. Assessed subjective response from patient about experience.   ✓ ✓ ___ _____

3. Assessed gait and body alignment. ___ ___ ___ _____

4. Observed patient's ability to perform self-care activities. ___ ___ ___ _____

5. Identified unexpected outcomes. ___ ___ ___ _____

RECORDING AND REPORTING

1. Recorded type of gait patient used, amount of assistance required, distance walked, and patient's tolerance of activity. ___ ___ ___ _____

2. Immediately reported any injury sustained during procedure, any alteration in vital signs, or an inability to ambulate. ___ ___ ___ _____

PÖ: Kyra vanderwerw
9/12/12

Student _____ Date _____

Instructor _____ Date _____

PERFORMANCE CHECKLIST SKILL 11-1 **ASSISTING WITH CAST APPLICATION**

	S	U	NP	Comments

ASSESSMENT

1. Assessed patient's health status. ___ ___ ___ _____

2. Assessed patient's understanding of cast application. ___ ___ ___ _____

3. Assessed condition of tissues to be casted. ___ ___ ___ _____

4. Determined patient's pain status. ___ ___ ___ _____

5. Determined extent to which patient may use casted extremity. ___ ___ ___ _____

NURSING DIAGNOSIS

1. Developed appropriate nursing diagnoses based on assessment data. ___ ___ ___ _____

PLANNING

1. Identified expected outcomes. ___ ___ ___ _____

2. Instructed patient, parent, or other assistants as needed. ___ ___ ___ _____

IMPLEMENTATION

1. Administered analgesic or muscle relaxant before cast application, if indicated. ___ ___ ___ _____

2. Performed hand hygiene and applied gloves. ___ ___ ___ _____

3. Positioned patient appropriately. ___ ___ ___ _____

4. Prepared skin before casting. ___ ___ ___ _____

5. Explained that warmth may be felt during application. ___ ___ ___ _____

6. Supplied dampened rolls of plaster or synthetic cast roll. ___ ___ ___ _____

7. Supported body part(s) during application of cast. ___ ___ ___ _____

8. Supported body part(s) while casting tape was applied. ___ ___ ___ _____

9. Continued to supply dampened rolls of plaster and tape. ___ ___ ___ _____

10. Supplied stabilization material. ___ ___ ___ _____

11. Assisted with "finishing" of the cast. ___ ___ ___ _____

12. Supplied scissors to trim plaster around edges. ___ ___ ___ _____

	S	U	NP	Comments
13. Facilitated drying of cast. Positioned casted extremity appropriately; handled cast only with palms until dry.	___	___	___	_____
14. Removed gloves. Performed hand hygiene.	___	___	___	_____
15. Covered patient, left casted area uncovered, assisted with transfer; accompanied patient to room.	___	___	___	_____
16. Cleaned equipment. Performed hand hygiene.	___	___	___	_____
17. Explained procedures of exposure for fast drying.	___	___	___	_____
18. Repositioned patient. Maintained heel off surface.	___	___	___	_____
19. Informed patient to notify personnel of alteration in sensation or mobility.	___	___	___	_____
20. Covered synthetic cast with watertight plastic for bathing. Dried with blow dryer on cool setting.	___	___	___	_____

EVALUATION

	S	U	NP	Comments
1. Observed patient for signs of "cast syndrome."	___	___	___	_____
2. Assessed neurovascular status.	___	___	___	_____
3. Observed for edema distal to cast.	___	___	___	_____
4. Assessed temperature of tissues.	___	___	___	_____
5. Compared tissue versus unaffected areas.	___	___	___	_____
6. Inspected skin condition around cast edges.	___	___	___	_____
7. Determined patient's mobility and assisted as necessary with ROM.	___	___	___	_____
8. Assessed patient's subjective response.	___	___	___	_____
9. Smelled the cast edges.	___	___	___	_____
10. Observed patient when verbalizing and performing cast care.	___	___	___	_____
11. Identified unexpected outcomes.	___	___	___	_____

RECORDING AND REPORTING

	S	U	NP	Comments
1. Recorded application of cast, condition of skin, and circulation.	___	___	___	_____
2. Reported abnormal or untoward progression of findings obtained from assessments.	___	___	___	_____

Student _____   Date _____

Instructor _____   Date _____

PERFORMANCE CHECKLIST SKILL 11-2 **ASSISTING WITH CAST REMOVAL**

	S	U	NP	Comments
ASSESSMENT				
1. Assessed patient's understanding of upcoming cast removal.	___	___	___	_____
2. Assessed patient's readiness for cast removal.	___	___	___	_____
3. Asked patient if itching or irritation under cast was felt.	___	___	___	_____
NURSING DIAGNOSIS				
1. Developed appropriate nursing diagnoses based on assessment data.	___	___	___	_____
PLANNING				
1. Identified expected outcomes.	___	___	___	_____
2. Explained procedure to patient and detailed physical sensations to be expected.	___	___	___	_____
IMPLEMENTATION				
1. Applied eye protection for patient and nurse.	___	___	___	_____
2. Applied gloves if indicated and assisted with cast removal.	___	___	___	_____
3. Inspected underlying tissues.	___	___	___	_____
4. Applied enzyme wash to intact skin.	___	___	___	_____
5. Cleansed tissues with warm water and patted dry.	___	___	___	_____
6. Applied lotion to skin.	___	___	___	_____
7. Obtained order and performed ROM exercises within allowed guidelines.	___	___	___	_____
8. Assisted in transfer of patient for return to room or for discharge.	___	___	___	_____
9. Instructed patient to observe for swelling and to elevate the extremity.	___	___	___	_____
10. Cleaned or disposed of equipment appropriately. Removed gloves.	___	___	___	_____
EVALUATION				
1. Inspected underlying skin.	___	___	___	_____
2. Observed patient's behavior and responses.	___	___	___	_____
3. Asked patient to explain and demonstrate exercises.	___	___	___	_____

	S	U	NP	Comments
4. Had patient explain and perform skin care.	——	——	——	_____
5. Identified unexpected outcomes.	——	——	——	_____

RECORDING AND REPORTING

	S	U	NP	Comments
1. Recorded cast removal, condition of tissues under cast, and person removing cast.	——	——	——	_____
2. Reported unexpected outcomes to nurse in charge or physician.	——	——	——	_____

100

Student _____ Date _____

Instructor _____ Date _____

PERFORMANCE CHECKLIST SKILL 11-3 **CARE OF THE PATIENT IN SKIN TRACTION**

	S	U	NP	Comments

ASSESSMENT
1. Assessed patient's health status.
2. Assessed specific tissues to be placed in traction.
3. Assessed patient's understanding of reason for traction.
4. Assessed patient's level of pain.
5. Assessed patient's neurovascular status.

NURSING DIAGNOSIS
1. Developed appropriate nursing diagnoses based on assessment data.

PLANNING
1. Identified expected outcomes.
2. Explained procedure to patient.

IMPLEMENTATION
1. Administered analgesic or muscle relaxant in advance.
2. Prepared patient and area of body to be placed in traction.
3. Positioned patient as requested by physician.
4. Assisted with application of specific traction equipment.
5. Assisted with attachment of bars, ropes, and pulleys.
6. Attached and gently lowered traction weights.
7. Assessed patient's body alignment in traction.
8. Elevated side rails.
9. Returned unused materials to storage area and performed hand hygiene.

EVALUATION
1. Observed patient's participation in self-care.
2. Assessed condition of skin around traction.
3. Inspected entire traction setup and body alignment.
4. Asked if patient understands mobility restrictions.

	S	U	NP	Comments
5. Assessed for level of pain, spasms, or burning sensation.	___	___	___	_____
6. Assessed neurovascular status within 15 minutes after application, then every 1 to 2 hours for 24 hours and as needed.	___	___	___	_____
7. Released skin traction every 4 to 8 hours, and assessed and cleansed skin.	___	___	___	_____
8. Identified unexpected outcomes.	___	___	___	_____

RECORDING AND REPORTING

	S	U	NP	Comments
1. Recorded type of traction, site, skin condition, weight applied, patient's response, and skin assessments.	___	___	___	_____
2. Recorded neurovascular assessment of bilateral body parts.	___	___	___	_____
3. Recorded length of time patient was in or out of traction.	___	___	___	_____
4. Documented instructions given to patient and family.	___	___	___	_____

Student _____ Date _____

Instructor _____ Date _____

PERFORMANCE CHECKLIST SKILL 11-4   **CARE OF THE PATIENT IN SKELETAL TRACTION AND PIN SITE CARE**

	S	U	NP	Comments

ASSESSMENT

1. Assessed patient's health and mobility status. ___ ___ ___ _____

2. Assessed specific tissues to be placed in skeletal traction. ___ ___ ___ _____

3. Assessed patient's understanding of traction. ___ ___ ___ _____

4. Assessed patient's level of pain. ___ ___ ___ _____

5. Observed patient's nonverbal behavior. Encouraged questions. ___ ___ ___ _____

NURSING DIAGNOSIS

1. Developed appropriate nursing diagnoses based on assessment data. ___ ___ ___ _____

PLANNING

1. Identified expected outcomes. ___ ___ ___ _____

IMPLEMENTATION

Traction Setup

1. Positioned patient according to physician's order. ___ ___ ___ _____

2. Prepared specific traction setups. ___ ___ ___ _____

3. Ascertained patient's initial reaction or response to traction. ___ ___ ___ _____

4. Elevated side rails. ___ ___ ___ _____

5. Returned equipment and supplies and performed hand hygiene. ___ ___ ___ _____

6. Ensured skeletal traction maintained continuously. ___ ___ ___ _____

7. *Pin Site Care*

  a. Discussed with physician type and frequency. ___ ___ ___ _____

  b. Performed hand hygiene and applied gloves. ___ ___ ___ _____

  c. Removed and discarded old dressing around pins. Noted condition of tissues around pins. ___ ___ ___ _____

  d. Prepared supplies and applied sterile or clean gloves. ___ ___ ___ _____

	S	U	NP	Comments

e. Used different supplies to clean each pin site. ____ ____ ____ _____

f. Cleaned pin site with chlorhexidine solution on a cotton-tipped applicator. Cleaned in a circular motion outward. ____ ____ ____ _____

g. Rinsed pin site area with normal saline on a cotton-tipped applicator. ____ ____ ____ _____

h. Applied a small amount of topical antibiotic and covered pin site with sterile 2 × 2 split gauze dressing (may be left uncovered). ____ ____ ____ _____

i. Repeated procedure for other pin sites. ____ ____ ____ _____

8. Discarded supplies. Removed and disposed of gloves. Performed hand hygiene. ____ ____ ____ _____

EVALUATION

1. Assessed traction setup and effectiveness, and body alignment. ____ ____ ____ _____

2. Determined patient's response to traction apparatus. ____ ____ ____ _____

3. Determined patient's need for analgesics or muscle relaxants. ____ ____ ____ _____

4. Inspected pin sites. Assessed for indications of infection. ____ ____ ____ _____

5. Assessed for other indications of infection. ____ ____ ____ _____

6. Performed neurovascular checks. ____ ____ ____ _____

7. Assessed for indicators of hypoxemia. ____ ____ ____ _____

8. Checked for fracture blisters. ____ ____ ____ _____

9. Identified unexpected outcomes. ____ ____ ____ _____

RECORDING AND REPORTING

1. Recorded type of traction applied, person applying traction, site, time, weights, and patient's initial response. ____ ____ ____ _____

2. Recorded all findings of skin and neurovascular checks. ____ ____ ____ _____

3. Reported to nurse in charge or physician untoward reactions or unexpected outcomes. ____ ____ ____ _____

4. Documented patient teaching. ____ ____ ____ _____

Student _____ Date _____

Instructor _____ Date _____

PERFORMANCE CHECKLIST SKILL 11-5 **CARE OF THE PATIENT WITH IMMOBILIZATION DEVICES**

	S	U	NP	Comments

ASSESSMENT

1. Reviewed patient's chart for medical history and current status.

2. Assessed patient's previous experience with braces/splints/slings.

3. Assessed patient's baseline level of pain.

4. Assessed patient's understanding of reason for and care of device.

5. Assessed patient's risk for skin breakdown.

6. Referred to occupational or physical therapy consult to determine type and use of device.

7. Assessed patient's additional need for an assistive device.

NURSING DIAGNOSIS

1. Developed appropriate nursing diagnoses based on assessment data.

PLANNING

1. Identified expected outcomes.

IMPLEMENTATION

1. *Preparing to Apply a Splint/Brace/Sling*

   a. Performed hand hygiene.

   b. Explained reasons for the brace/splint/sling, and demonstrated how the device works.

   c. Assisted the patient to a comfortable position, sitting or lying down.

   d. Cleaned the skin with soap and water; rinsed, patted dry, and changed any dressings (if present). Put a thin cotton shirt or gown on the patient, if applying a back brace, and ensured that there were no wrinkles.

   e. Inspected the device for wear, damage, or rough edges.

	S	U	NP	Comments

2. Applied the brace/splint/sling as ordered.

   a. Securing splint with elastic bandage:

      (1) Applied even tension as bandage for splint was wrapped from distal to proximal. ___ ___ ___ _____

      (2) Prevented padding from gathering or bunching. ___ ___ ___ _____

   b. Applying sling using triangular bandage:

      (1) Positioned one end of the bandage over the shoulder of the unaffected arm. ___ ___ ___ _____

      (2) Took the remaining bandage and placed the material against the chest, then under and over the affected arm, cradling the arm. ___ ___ ___ _____

      (3) Positioned the pointed end of the triangle toward the elbow. ___ ___ ___ _____

      (4) Tied the two ends of the triangle at the side of the neck. ___ ___ ___ _____

      (5) Folded the pointed end of the sling at the elbow in the front and secured with a safety pin, closing the end of the sling. ___ ___ ___ _____

      (6) Adjusted the length of the sling by adjusting the amount of material in the knot. ___ ___ ___ _____

      (7) Ensured the sling supported the limb comfortably without interfering with circulation. ___ ___ ___ _____

3. Discussed with patient the prescribed schedule of wear and allowed activities. ___ ___ ___ _____

4. Reiterated the signs of skin breakdown, pressure, or rubbing to report. ___ ___ ___ _____

5. Assisted the patient with finding attractive clothes to fit over immobilizing device. ___ ___ ___ _____

6. Instructed the patient on how to care for the brace/splint/sling. ___ ___ ___ _____

7. Assisted patient to ambulate with brace/splint/sling in place. ___ ___ ___ _____

8. Observed the patient applying and removing the brace/splint and ensuring proper alignment. ___ ___ ___ _____

EVALUATION

1. Inspected areas of the skin underneath the brace/splint/sling for signs of pressure. ___ ___ ___ _____

2. Observed the patient when using the brace/splint/sling. ___ ___ ___ _____

3. Asked the patient to rate level of comfort. ___ ___ ___ _____

106

	S	U	NP	Comments

4. Assessed circulation and sensation of extremity distal to position of brace/splint/sling. ____ ____ ____ _____

5. Asked the patient/family about the ease with which ADLs are performed while wearing the brace/splint/sling. ____ ____ ____ _____

6. Identified unexpected outcomes. ____ ____ ____ _____

RECORDING AND REPORTING

1. Recorded in progress notes type of brace/splint/sling applied, schedule of wear, activity level and movement permitted, and patient's tolerance of procedure. ____ ____ ____ _____

2. Recorded instructions given to patient and family. ____ ____ ____ _____

3. Reported and recorded observations regarding patient's ability to apply, ambulate with, and remove the brace/splint/sling. ____ ____ ____ _____

4. Reported immediately to nurse in charge or physician any injury sustained while ussing the brace/splint/sling. ____ ____ ____ _____

Student _____   Date _____

Instructor _____   Date _____

PERFORMANCE CHECKLIST FOR PROCEDURAL GUIDELINE 12-1   **SELECTION OF PRESSURE-REDUCING SURFACES**

	S	U	NP	Comments
STEPS				
1. Assessed patient's risk for skin breakdown.	___	___	___	_____
2. Assessed patient's existing pressure ulcers, blisters, abnormal reactive hyperemia, and abrasions.	___	___	___	_____
3. Determined need for pressure reduction surface from assessment data.	___	___	___	_____
4. Identified patient factors when selecting appropriate surface.	___	___	___	_____
5. Determined specific device appropriate for patient.	___	___	___	_____
6. Checked agency policy regarding implementation of support surface.	___	___	___	_____
7. Documented pressure ulcer risk assessment and skin assessment.	___	___	___	_____
8. Documented support surface selected and patient response to surface.	___	___	___	_____

Student _____ Date _____

Instructor _____ Date _____

PERFORMANCE CHECKLIST SKILL 12-1 **PLACING A PATIENT ON A SUPPORT SURFACE**

	S	U	NP	Comments
ASSESSMENT				
1. Performed hand hygiene.	___	___	___	_____
2. Determined patient's risk for pressure ulcer formation using assessment tool.	___	___	___	_____
3. Inspected condition of patient's skin.	___	___	___	_____
4. Assessed patient's comfort level.	___	___	___	_____
5. Assessed patient's understanding of purpose of mattress.	___	___	___	_____
6. Checked physician's orders.	___	___	___	_____
NURSING DIAGNOSIS				
1. Developed appropriate nursing diagnoses based on assessment data.	___	___	___	_____
PLANNING				
1. Identified expected outcomes.	___	___	___	_____
2. Explained purpose and procedure to patient.	___	___	___	_____
IMPLEMENTATION				
1. Provided for patient's privacy.	___	___	___	_____
2. Performed hand hygiene and applied gloves, as indicated. Obtained assistance as needed.	___	___	___	_____
3. Correctly applied support surface to bed or prepared alternate bed.				
a. Replacing mattress:				
(1) Applied mattress to bed frame after removing hospital mattress.	___	___	___	_____
(2) Applied sheet over mattress.	___	___	___	_____
b. Preparing an air mattress/overlay:				
(1) Applied deflated mattress over bed.	___	___	___	_____
(2) Secured air mattress over corners of bed mattress.	___	___	___	_____
(3) Attached connector on air mattress to inflation device and inflated mattress to proper air pressure.	___	___	___	_____
(4) Applied sheet over air mattress.	___	___	___	_____

	S	U	NP	Comments

(5) Checked air pump for proper cycling. Kept sharp objects away from mattress. ___ ___ ___ _____

(6) Assisted with patient transfers. ___ ___ ___ _____

  c. Air surface bed:

(1) Obtained and made bed. ___ ___ ___ _____

(2) Placed switch in the "Prevention" mode. ___ ___ ___ _____

  d. Preparing a water mattress: supplemental and self-contained:

(1) Applied unfilled mattress flat over surface of bed mattress (self-contained water mattress would replace bed mattress). ___ ___ ___ _____

(2) Secured water mattress in place. ___ ___ ___ _____

(3) Attached connector on water mattress to water source. Filled mattress to recommended level. ___ ___ ___ _____

(4) Placed sheet over water mattress. ___ ___ ___ _____

(5) Kept sharp objects away from mattress. ___ ___ ___ _____

4. Positioned patient comfortably, and repositioned patient routinely. ___ ___ ___ _____

5. Removed gloves, if worn, and performed hand hygiene. ___ ___ ___ _____

EVALUATION

1. Reassessed patient's risk for pressure sore formation at routine intervals. ___ ___ ___ _____

2. Inspected condition of patient's skin. ___ ___ ___ _____

3. Assessed patient's comfort level. ___ ___ ___ _____

4. Periodically evaluated inflation of mattress. ___ ___ ___ _____

5. Identified unexpected outcomes. ___ ___ ___ _____

RECORDING AND REPORTING

1. Recorded placement of mattress and condition of patient's skin. ___ ___ ___ _____

2. Reported evidence of pressure sores to nurse in charge or physician. ___ ___ ___ _____

Student _____   Date _____

Instructor _____   Date _____

PERFORMANCE CHECKLIST SKILL 12-2 **PLACING A PATIENT ON AN AIR-SUSPENSION BED**

	S	U	NP	Comments
ASSESSMENT				
1. Performed hand hygiene.	___	___	___	_____
2. Determined patient's risk for pressure ulcer development.	___	___	___	_____
3. Identified patients who would benefit from air-suspension therapy.	___	___	___	_____
4. Assessed condition of patient's skin.	___	___	___	_____
5. Assessed patient for pain.	___	___	___	_____
6. Reviewed patient's medical orders.	___	___	___	_____
7. Assessed patient's level of consciousness.	___	___	___	_____
8. Assessed patient's and family members' understanding of purpose of bed.	___	___	___	_____
9. Reviewed patient's serum electrolyte levels, if available.	___	___	___	_____
10. Checked if patient required frequent weight measurement.	___	___	___	_____
NURSING DIAGNOSIS				
1. Developed appropriate nursing diagnoses based on assessment data.	___	___	___	_____
PLANNING				
1. Identified expected outcomes.	___	___	___	_____
2. Explained procedure and purpose of bed to patient and family.	___	___	___	_____
3. Prepared necessary equipment and supplies.	___	___	___	_____
4. Reviewed bed manufacturer's instructions.	___	___	___	_____
5. Premedicated patient as necessary 30 minutes before transfer.	___	___	___	_____
6. Obtained additional personnel needed to transfer patient to bed.	___	___	___	_____
IMPLEMENTATION				
1. Maintained patient's privacy. Performed hand hygiene and applied gloves.	___	___	___	_____
2. Explained steps of transfer.	___	___	___	_____
3. Transferred patient to bed using appropriate transfer techniques.	___	___	___	_____

	S	U	NP	Comments
4. Turned bed on and regulated temperature.	___	___	___	_____
5. Positioned patient and performed ROM exercises as tolerated.	___	___	___	_____
6. Set bed to firm position (Instaflate) when turning or positioning patient in bed.	___	___	___	_____
7. Removed gloves and performed hand hygiene.	___	___	___	_____

EVALUATION

1. Inspected condition of patient's skin.	___	___	___	_____
2. Observed existing pressure ulcers for healing.	___	___	___	_____
3. Asked patient to rate sense of comfort.	___	___	___	_____
4. Assessed patient's orientation.	___	___	___	_____
5. Identified unexpected outcomes.	___	___	___	_____

RECORDING AND REPORTING

1. Recorded type of bed, transfer of patient to bed, tolerance to procedure, condition of skin, and patient/caregiver teaching.	___	___	___	_____
2. Reported to nurse in charge or physician changes in condition of skin and electrolyte levels.	___	___	___	_____
3. Recorded teaching provided and patient/caregiver response.	___	___	___	_____
4. Reported restlessness or change in orientation.	___	___	___	_____

Student _____ Date _____

Instructor _____ Date _____

PERFORMANCE CHECKLIST SKILL 12-3 **PLACING A PATIENT ON AN AIR-FLUIDIZED BED**

	S	U	NP	Comments
ASSESSMENT				
1. Performed hand hygiene.	___	___	___	_____
2. Performed pressure ulcer risk assessment to identify patients who would benefit from air-fluidized therapy.	___	___	___	_____
3. Assessed condition of patient's skin.	___	___	___	_____
4. Assessed patient's comfort level.	___	___	___	_____
5. Assessed patient's level of consciousness.	___	___	___	_____
6. Assessed patient's and family members' understanding of purpose of bed.	___	___	___	_____
7. Reviewed patient's serum electrolyte levels in medical record.	___	___	___	_____
8. Identified patients at risk for complications of air-fluidized therapy.	___	___	___	_____
9. Reviewed patient's medical orders.	___	___	___	_____
NURSING DIAGNOSIS				
1. Developed appropriate nursing diagnoses based on assessment data.	___	___	___	_____
PLANNING				
1. Identified expected outcomes.	___	___	___	_____
2. Explained procedure and purpose of bed to patient and family.	___	___	___	_____
3. Reviewed instructions supplied by bed manufacturer.	___	___	___	_____
4. Premedicated patient as necessary.	___	___	___	_____
5. Obtained any additional personnel needed to transfer patient to bed.	___	___	___	_____
IMPLEMENTATION				
1. Closed patient's room door or bedside curtain.	___	___	___	_____
2. Explained steps of transfer.	___	___	___	_____
3. Performed hand hygiene and applied gloves.	___	___	___	_____
4. Transferred patient to bed.	___	___	___	_____
5. Turned fluidization cycle on and regulated temperature.	___	___	___	_____

	S	U	NP	Comments
6. Positioned patient using foam wedges and performed ROM exercises as appropriate.	___	___	___	_____
7. Correctly set fluidization mode for other therapies.	___	___	___	_____
8. Inspected bony prominences for signs of pressure.	___	___	___	_____
9. Removed gloves, if worn, and performed hand hygiene.	___	___	___	_____

EVALUATION

	S	U	NP	Comments
1. Inspected condition of patient's skin while on bed, and monitored risk assessment.	___	___	___	_____
2. Asked patient to rate level of comfort.	___	___	___	_____
3. Reviewed patient's serum electrolyte levels, monitored body temperature, and noted hydration status of skin and mucous membranes.	___	___	___	_____
4. Measured patient's level of orientation.	___	___	___	_____
5. Identified unexpected outcomes.	___	___	___	_____

RECORDING AND REPORTING

	S	U	NP	Comments
1. Recorded type of bed, transfer of patient to bed, tolerance to procedure, and condition of skin.	___	___	___	_____
2. Reported to nurse in charge or physician changes in condition of skin and electrolyte levels.	___	___	___	_____
3. Recorded teaching provided to patient and family.	___	___	___	_____
4. Reported change in orientation or status.	___	___	___	_____

116

Student _____ Date _____

Instructor _____ Date _____

PERFORMANCE CHECKLIST SKILL 12-4   **PLACING A PATIENT ON A BARIATRIC BED**

	S	U	NP	Comments
ASSESSMENT				
1. Performed hand hygiene.	___	___	___	_____
2. Assessed condition of patient's skin, particularly potential pressure sites.	___	___	___	_____
3. Identified that patient would benefit from the bariatric bed system.	___	___	___	_____
4. Determined patient's and family members' understanding of purpose of bed.	___	___	___	_____
5. Reviewed patient's medical orders.	___	___	___	_____
6. Assessed patient's need to be weighed.	___	___	___	_____
NURSING DIAGNOSIS				
1. Developed appropriate nursing diagnoses based on assessment data.	___	___	___	_____
PLANNING				
1. Identified expected outcomes.	___	___	___	_____
2. Explained procedure and purpose of bed to patient and family.	___	___	___	_____
3. Reviewed instructions supplied by bed manufacturer.	___	___	___	_____
4. Premedicated patient as necessary 30 minutes before transfer.	___	___	___	_____
5. Obtained additional personnel needed to transfer patient to bed.	___	___	___	_____
IMPLEMENTATION				
1. Provided privacy.	___	___	___	_____
2. Performed hand hygiene and applied gloves if indicated.	___	___	___	_____
3. Explained steps of transfer.	___	___	___	_____
4. Placed assistive devices under patient to transfer safely.	___	___	___	_____
5. Covered and positioned patient, and placed hand controls within patient's reach. Attached overhead frame, if needed. Activated out-of-bed alarm when available.	___	___	___	_____

	S	U	NP	Comments

6. Encouraged patient to initiate frequent position changes.   ___ ___ ___ _____

7. Removed gloves, if worn, and performed hand hygiene.   ___ ___ ___ _____

EVALUATION

1. Inspected condition of skin.   ___ ___ ___ _____

2. Asked patient to rate sense of comfort and safety.   ___ ___ ___ _____

3. Evaluated patient's risk for injury.   ___ ___ ___ _____

4. Evaluated patient's ability to move in bed.   ___ ___ ___ _____

5. Identified unexpected outcomes.   ___ ___ ___ _____

RECORDING AND REPORTING

1. Recorded type of bed, transfer of patient to bed, tolerance of procedure, and condition of skin.   ___ ___ ___ _____

2. Reported to nurse in charge or physician changes in condition of skin.   ___ ___ ___ _____

118

Student _____   Date _____

Instructor _____   Date _____

PERFORMANCE CHECKLIST SKILL 12-5 **PLACING A PATIENT ON A ROTOKINETIC BED**

	S	U	NP	Comments
ASSESSMENT				
1. Performed hand hygiene.	___	___	___	_____
2. Determined patient's risk for pressure ulcer formation.	___	___	___	_____
3. Assessed condition of patient's skin.	___	___	___	_____
4. Reviewed medical order.	___	___	___	_____
5. Assessed patient's level of comfort.	___	___	___	_____
6. Assessed patient's level of orientation.	___	___	___	_____
7. Performed pulmonary assessment and obtained vital signs.	___	___	___	_____
8. Assessed patient's and caregiver's understanding of use of Rotokinetic bed.	___	___	___	_____
NURSING DIAGNOSIS				
1. Developed appropriate nursing diagnoses based on assessment data.	___	___	___	_____
PLANNING				
1. Identified expected outcomes.	___	___	___	_____
2. Explained procedure to patient and family.	___	___	___	_____
3. Reviewed manufacturer's instructions.	___	___	___	_____
4. Premedicated patient as needed before transfer.	___	___		_____
5. Obtained additional assistance to transfer patient.	___	___	___	_____
IMPLEMENTATION				
1. Provided privacy. Performed hand hygiene. Applied gloves.	___	___	___	_____
2. Placed Rotokinetic bed in horizontal position; removed all bolsters, straps, and supports. Closed posterior hatches.	___	___	___	_____
3. Unplugged electrical cord and locked hatch.	___	___	___	_____
4. Transferred patient to bed; maintained patient's proper body alignment.	___	___	___	_____

	S	U	NP	Comments
5. Secured thoracic panels, bolsters, head and knee packs, and safety straps.	___	___	___	_____
6. Covered patient with top sheet.	___	___	___	_____
7. Plugged bed in.	___	___	___	_____
8. Had company representative set optional angle as ordered.	___	___	___	_____
9. Gradually increased degree of rotation.	___	___	___	_____
10. Provided adequate space for caregivers and family to move around bed.	___	___	___	_____
11. Stopped bed for patient assessments and procedures.	___	___	___	_____
12. Informed patient of expected sensations and safety measures to prevent falls.	___	___	___	_____

EVALUATION

	S	U	NP	Comments
1. Inspected condition of patient's skin.	___	___	___	_____
2. Inspected pressure ulcers for healing.	___	___	___	_____
3. Observed body alignment and joint range of motion.	___	___	___	_____
4. Auscultated lung sounds and compared with baseline every shift.	___	___	___	_____
5. Determined patient's level of orientation.	___	___	___	_____
6. Asked if patient was experiencing nausea or dizziness.	___	___	___	_____
7. Monitored patient's blood pressure for orthostatic hypotension.	___	___	___	_____
8. Identified unexpected outcomes.	___	___	___	_____

RECORDING AND REPORTING

	S	U	NP	Comments
1. Described skin condition before placement on Rotokinetic bed. Took a photograph, if possible, to use for comparison.	___	___	___	_____
2. Recorded type of bed, time of transfer to bed, degree of rotation, and length of time bed rotation stopped.	___	___	___	_____
3. Documented vital signs and subjective response of patient.	___	___	___	_____
4. Reported unexpected outcomes to the nurse in charge or physician.	___	___	___	_____

Student _____ Date _____

Instructor _____ Date _____

PERFORMANCE CHECKLIST PROCEDURAL GUIDELINE 13-1 **FIRE, ELECTRICAL, RADIATION, AND CHEMICAL SAFETY**

	S	U	NP	Comments

STEPS

1. Reviewed agency guidelines for rapid response to fire, electrical, chemical, and radiation emergencies. ___ ___ ___ _____

2. Familiarized self with location of emergency equipment and responsibilities during an emergency. ___ ___ ___ _____

3. Assessed patient's medical condition, physical and mental status, and activity and mobility levels. ___ ___ ___ _____

4. Assessed patient's and family's knowledge of risks and safety precautions when patients are receiving radioactive implants. ___ ___ ___ _____

5. Assessed if patient receiving radioactive implants is pregnant or will have visitors who are pregnant. ___ ___ ___ _____

6. Fire safety:

   a. Followed the acronym RACE:

     (1) *R*escued or removed patient from immediate danger. ___ ___ ___ _____

     (2) *A*ctivated the alarm following agency policy. ___ ___ ___ _____

     (3) *C*ontained the fire. ___ ___ ___ _____

     (4) *E*vacuated patients. ___ ___ ___ _____

7. Electrical safety:

   a. If patient received a shock, evaluated immediately for presence of pulse; if no pulse, initiated CPR and called for help. ___ ___ ___ _____

   b. Notified emergency personnel and patient's physician. ___ ___ ___ _____

   c. Assessed for thermal injury and any other injury sustained. ___ ___ ___ _____

8. Radiation safety:

   a. Wore radiation exposure dosimeter. ___ ___ ___ _____

   b. Explained treatment plan to patient and family, including radiation safety guidelines for time and distance limits. ___ ___ ___ _____

	S	U	NP	Comments

c. Placed patient in a private room and posted caution sign on outside of door. ___ ___ ___ _____

d. Provided activities and distractions for patient. ___ ___ ___ _____

e. Rotated care providers during patient's length of stay. ___ ___ ___ _____

f. Wore protective lead apron and gloves when entering patient's room. ___ ___ ___ _____

g. Followed agency policy for removal of specimens, trays, dressings, linens, trash, and body fluids. ___ ___ ___ _____

h. Washed gloves after patient care and performed hand hygiene. ___ ___ ___ _____

i. Requested radiation safety officer to conduct survey of radiation sources after patient discharge. ___ ___ ___ _____

9. Chemical safety:

a. Attended to any person exposed to a chemical. ___ ___ ___ _____

b. Notified all personnel in the immediate area and evacuated if necessary. ___ ___ ___ _____

c. Referred to MSDS; turned off electrical and heat sources if material is flammable. ___ ___ ___ _____

d. Used appropriate PPE for cleanup. ___ ___ ___ _____

e. Inspected medical equipment and patient's room for fire, electrical, chemical, or radiation hazards. ___ ___ ___ _____

Student _____ Date _____

Instructor _____ Date _____

PERFORMANCE CHECKLIST SKILL 13-1 **FALL PREVENTION IN A HEALTH CARE FACILITY**

	S	U	NP	Comments
ASSESSMENT				
1. Assessed patient's motor, sensory, and cognitive status to determine fall risk.	___	___	___	_____
2. Reviewed patient's medication history (polypharmacy), including OTCs and herbals.	___	___	___	_____
3. Assessed medical history and factors correlated with fear of falling.	___	___	___	_____
4. Assessed the environment in health care facility and home setting, identifying barriers posing risk for falls.	___	___	___	_____
5. Performed timed "Get Up and Go" test.	___	___	___	_____
6. Determined patient's history of falls by using the acronym SPLATT.	___	___	___	_____
7. Determined patient's knowledge of fall risks and steps for prevention.	___	___	___	_____
8. Applied a color-coded wrist band if high-risk patient.	___	___	___	_____
NURSING DIAGNOSIS				
1. Developed appropriate nursing diagnoses based on assessment data.	___	___	___	_____
PLANNING				
1. Identified expected outcomes.	___	___	___	_____
IMPLEMENTATION				
1. Introduced self to patient by name and role.	___	___	___	_____
2. Identified patient correctly using two identifiers.	___	___	___	_____
3. Explained plan of care.	___	___	___	_____
4. Gathered equipment and performed hand hygiene.	___	___	___	_____
5. Provided privacy. Positioned and draped patient as needed.	___	___	___	_____
6. Adjusted bed and side rails properly.	___	___	___	_____
7. Explained and demonstrated use of call bell/intercom system. Placed call bell within patient's reach.	___	___	___	_____

	S	U	NP	Comments

8. Side rails:

a. Checked agency policy for use. ____ ____ ____ _____

b. Explained to patient and family the main reason for using side rails. ____ ____ ____ _____

c. Kept side rails up and bed in lowest position with wheels locked, as indicated. ____ ____ ____ _____

d. Left one side rail down for oriented, ambulatory patient. ____ ____ ____ _____

9. Provided clear instruction on mobility restrictions and techniques. ____ ____ ____ _____

10. Explained safety measures to patient and family. ____ ____ ____ _____

11. Used gait belt and non-skid, fitted foot wear when ambulating patient. ____ ____ ____ _____

12. Offered hip protector. ____ ____ ____ _____

13. Cleared pathway to bathroom. ____ ____ ____ _____

14. Provided adequate, nonglare lighting. ____ ____ ____ _____

15. Removed unnecessary objects from walkways and stairs. ____ ____ ____ _____

16. Discussed with PT gait training and muscle strengthening exercise. Obtain physician order if needed. ____ ____ ____ _____

17. Discussed with physician medications being taken that influence fall risk. ____ ____ ____ _____

18. Provided safe transport using a wheelchair:

a. Placed wheelchair on patient's strongest side. ____ ____ ____ _____

b. Placed wedge on chair with highest side forward and positioned patient appropriately. ____ ____ ____ _____

c. Secured wheels before transferring patient. ____ ____ ____ _____

d. Properly used footrests and safety devices if available. ____ ____ ____ _____

e. Backed wheelchair into and out of elevator, leading with rear wheels. ____ ____ ____ _____

EVALUATION

1. Monitored patient frequently. Observed modification of patient's environment for safety needs. ____ ____ ____ _____

2. Evaluated patient's ability to use assistive devices. ____ ____ ____ _____

124

	S	U	NP	Comments

3. Asked patient and/or family member to identify safety risks. ____ ____ ____ _____

4. Reassessed motor, sensory, and cognitive status. ____ ____ ____ _____

5. Identified unexpected outcomes. ____ ____ ____ _____

RECORDING AND REPORTING

1. Recorded specific interventions to promote safety. ____ ____ ____ _____

2. Reported specific threats to safety and measures taken to reduce threats to all health care providers. ____ ____ ____ _____

3. Documented instructions given to patient and family. ____ ____ ____ _____

4. Documented patient falls and follow-up. ____ ____ ____ _____

Student _____   Date _____

Instructor _____   Date _____

PERFORMANCE CHECKLIST SKILL 13-2 **DESIGNING A RESTRAINT-FREE ENVIRONMENT**

	S	U	NP	Comments

ASSESSMENT

1. Assessed patient's physical, sensory, and cognitive status, and ability to understand and follow directions; level of combativeness; level of pain; and laboratory test values. ___ ___ ___ _____

2. Reviewed prescribed medications. ___ ___ ___ _____

3. Assessed patient's knowledge of medical condition and treatment. ___ ___ ___ _____

4. Assessed and confirmed risk for wandering. ___ ___ ___ _____

NURSING DIAGNOSIS

1. Developed appropriate nursing diagnoses based on assessment data. ___ ___ ___ _____

PLANNING

1. Identified expected outcomes. ___ ___ ___ _____

IMPLEMENTATION

1. Oriented patient and family to surroundings, introduced to staff, and explained all treatments and procedures. ___ ___ ___ _____

2. Provided same caregiver if possible. Encouraged family and friends to stay with patient. ___ ___ ___ _____

3. Placed patient in room close to staff. ___ ___ ___ _____

4. Provided appropriate visual and auditory stimuli. Assessed availability and use of sensory aid devices. ___ ___ ___ _____

5. Met patient needs as quickly as possible. ___ ___ ___ _____

6. Approached patient in calm, nonthreatening, professional manner. ___ ___ ___ _____

7. Limited number of caregivers interacting with patient. ___ ___ ___ _____

8. Provided scheduled ADL and organized treatments to allow for long, uninterrupted periods. ___ ___ ___ _____

9. Reduced patient's access to tubes and lines, eliminating invasive treatments as soon as possible. ___ ___ ___ _____

10. Employed stress reduction techniques. ___ ___ ___ _____

	S	U	NP	Comments
11. Used a pressure-sensitive bed and chair pads if available.	___	___	___	_____
12. Used various disciplines (e.g., physical therapy) and diversional activities as tolerated.	___	___	___	_____
13. Reviewed medications frequently.	___	___	___	_____

EVALUATION

1. Observed patient for injuries.	___	___	___	_____
2. Observed patient's behavior toward staff and others.	___	___	___	_____
3. Determined the need for continuation of invasive treatments.	___	___	___	_____
4. Identified unexpected outcomes.	___	___	___	_____

RECORDING AND REPORTING

1. Recorded and reported patient behaviors and nursing interventions.	___	___	___	_____

Student **Darcy Brenneman**   Date _____

Instructor _____ _Hrdrll fa_ _____   Date **9/7/12**

PERFORMANCE CHECKLIST SKILL 13-3   **APPLYING PHYSICAL RESTRAINTS**

	S	U	NP	Comments

ASSESSMENT

1. Determined if patient required restraint.   ✓

2. Assessed patient's behavior and ability to understand and follow directions.   ✓

3. Reviewed agency policy and medical orders.   ✓

4. Reviewed manufacturer's instructions for restraint use. Determined appropriate restraint size.   ✓

5. Inspected site for restraint placement.   ✓

NURSING DIAGNOSIS

1. Developed appropriate nursing diagnoses based on assessment data.

PLANNING

1. Identified expected outcome.

IMPLEMENTATION

1. Gathered supplies and performed hand hygiene.   ✓

2. Identified patient using two identifiers.   ✓

3. Approached patient calmly and explained procedure (included family if present).   ✓

4. Provided privacy; positioned patient comfortably.   ✓

5. Adjusted bed to working height.   ✓

6. Assessed skin integrity before placing restraint. Protected skin over bony prominences.   ✓

7. Followed manufacturers' instructions.

8. Correctly applied selected properly fitted restraint:

   a. Belt restraint

   b. Extremity restraint (wrist or ankle)   ✓

   c. Mitten restraint

   d. Elbow restraint

9. Attached restraint appropriately to bed frame or wheelchair.   ✓

10. Secured restraints with quick-release ties.   ✓

Kyla Vanderwum

	S	U	NP	Comments
11. Inserted two fingers under restraint to check for constriction.	✓ 3me	___	___	_____
12. Assessed proper placement of restraint. Removed restraint every 2 hours. Obtained assistance, if necessary, for patient safety.	✓	___	___	_____
13. Secured call bell/intercom within patient's reach.	✓	___	___	_____
14. Left bed in lowest position; locked wheels of bed or chair.	✓	___	___	_____
15. Performed hand hygiene.	✓	___	___	_____

EVALUATION

	S	U	NP	Comments
1. Checked placement of restraint and status of patient and site/extremity every 15 minutes.	✓	___	___	_____
2. Physician assessed patient as per agency protocol.	___	___	___	_____
3. Observed medical equipment for positioning and functioning.	___	___	___	_____
4. Reassessed need for continued use of restraint.	___	___	___	_____
5. Identified unexpected outcomes.	___	___	___	_____

RECORDING AND REPORTING

	S	U	NP	Comments
1. Recorded patient's prior behavior and status; type and specific use of restraint; nursing interventions to promote patient safety; and patient's response to restraint.	___	___	___	_____

Student _____ Date _____

Instructor _____ Date _____

PERFORMANCE CHECKLIST SKILL 13-4 **SEIZURE PRECAUTIONS**

	S	U	NP	Comments

ASSESSMENT

1. Assessed patient's seizure history and precipitating factors. Used family as resource if needed.   ___ ___ ___ _____

2. Assessed patient for medical and surgical conditions that may lead to or exacerbate existing seizure condition.   ___ ___ ___ _____

3. Assessed patient's medication history, adherence, and therapeutic drug levels if applicable.   ___ ___ ___ _____

4. Inspected patient's environment for potential safety hazards. Prepared bed and positioned patient.   ___ ___ ___ _____

5. Prepared emergency equipment.   ___ ___ ___ _____

6. Assessed patient's cultural perspective.   ___ ___ ___ _____

NURSING DIAGNOSIS

1. Developed appropriate nursing diagnoses based on assessment data.   ___ ___ ___ _____

PLANNING

1. Identified expected outcomes.   ___ ___ ___ _____

IMPLEMENTATION

1. Noted time of seizure, remained with patient and called for help. Positioned patient safely. Had staff member bring emergency cart.   ___ ___ ___ _____

2. Provided privacy.   ___ ___ ___ _____

3. Turned patient on side with head flexed slightly forward if possible.   ___ ___ ___ _____

4. Did not restrain patient; loosened clothing.   ___ ___ ___ _____

5. Did not force objects into patient's mouth.   ___ ___ ___ _____

6. Maintained patient's airway and suctioned as needed. Provided oxygen as ordered.   ___ ___ ___ _____

7. Remained with patient, observing sequence and timing of seizure activity. Reassessed patient's status after seizure.   ___ ___ ___ _____

8. Assisted patient to position of comfort and safety in bed after seizure.   ___ ___ ___ _____

9. Explained event and answered patient's and family's questions after seizure.   ___ ___ ___ _____

	S	U	NP	Comments
10. Offered emotional support. Encouraged verbalization.	___	___	___	_____
11. Performed hand hygiene.	___	___	___	_____

EVALUATION

	S	U	NP	Comments
1. Performed a general and focused assessment after seizure. Assessed for injuries during seizure.	___	___	___	_____
2. Determined patient's mental status after seizure.	___	___	___	_____
3. Observed patient's color and respiratory status during and after seizure.	___	___	___	_____
4. Asked patient to verbalize feelings after seizure.	___	___	___	_____
5. Identified unexpected outcomes.	___	___	___	_____

RECORDING AND REPORTING

	S	U	NP	Comments
1. Recorded the timing of seizure activity and sequence of events, including presence of aura, level of consciousness, nursing/medical interventions, and patient status after seizure.	___	___	___	_____
2. Reported seizure episode immediately to nurse in charge or physician.	___	___	___	_____

Student _____   Date _____

Instructor _____   Date _____

PERFORMANCE CHECKLIST SKILL 14-1   **CARE OF THE PATIENT AFTER BIOLOGICAL EXPOSURE**

	S	U	NP	Comments
ASSESSMENT				
1. Conducted a focused health history and physical examination. Reviewed history of patient's presenting symptoms.	___	___	___	_____
2. Measured patient's vital signs.	___	___	___	_____
3. Reviewed results of diagnostic tests and consulted with physician or primary care provider.	___	___	___	_____
4. Assessed patient for other health risks.	___	___	___	_____
5. Assessed patient's immediate psychological response following exposure.	___	___	___	_____
6. Identified resources available.	___	___	___	_____
NURSING DIAGNOSIS				
1. Developed appropriate nursing diagnoses based on assessment data.	___	___	___	_____
PLANNING				
1. Identified expected outcomes.	___	___	___	_____
2. Dispensed timely and accurate information to the patient and family.	___	___	___	_____
IMPLEMENTATION				
1. Performed hand hygiene. Used appropriate PPE.	___	___	___	_____
2. Instituted transmission-based isolation precautions.	___	___	___	_____
3. Decontaminated if indicated. Placed patient's clothing in labeled biohazard bag.	___	___	___	_____
4. Administered oxygen therapy, fluids, medications, antitoxins, nutritional support, and immunizations as ordered.	___	___	___	_____
5. Provided supportive care.	___	___	___	_____
6. Identified all patient contacts for proper follow-up.	___	___	___	_____
7. Counseled patient and family on acute and long-term psychological effects of exposure.	___	___	___	_____
8. Discussed available social support networks.	___	___	___	_____

	S	U	NP	Comments

EVALUATION

1. Observed for improved respiratory status, level of consciousness, and neurological functioning. ____ ____ ____ _____

2. Inspected the condition of the patient's skin, if affected. ____ ____ ____ _____

3. Evaluated the patient for changes that indicate improvement or deterioration of physical and/or psychological status. ____ ____ ____ _____

4. Identified unexpected outcomes. ____ ____ ____ _____

RECORDING AND REPORTING

1. Reported suspected cases of biological incident to appropriate personnel per agency protocol. ____ ____ ____ _____

2. Recorded assessment, interventions, and patient's response. ____ ____ ____ _____

3. Reported unexpected outcomes to physician or nurse in charge. ____ ____ ____ _____

134

Student _____ Date _____

Instructor _____ Date _____

PERFORMANCE CHECKLIST SKILL 14-2 **CARE OF THE PATIENT AFTER CHEMICAL EXPOSURE**

	S	U	NP	Comments

ASSESSMENT

1. Assessed patient's symptoms. Performed focused physical examination. ___ ___ ___ _____

2. Observed for presence of liquid, powder, or odor on patient's skin or clothing. ___ ___ ___ _____

3. Assessed the patient for preexisting medical conditions. ___ ___ ___ _____

4. Assessed patient's immediate psychological response following exposure. ___ ___ ___ _____

5. Identified available resources. ___ ___ ___ _____

NURSING DIAGNOSIS

1. Developed appropriate nursing diagnoses based on assessment data. ___ ___ ___ _____

PLANNING

1. Identified expected outcomes. ___ ___ ___ _____

2. Explained care to patient and family. ___ ___ ___ _____

IMPLEMENTATION

1. Gathered appropriate supplies and PPE. Performed hand hygiene. ___ ___ ___ _____

2. Had only trained personnel participate in decontamination. ___ ___ ___ _____

3. Provided privacy. ___ ___ ___ _____

4. Decontaminated the patient.

   a. Acted quickly, cut off patient's contaminated clothing, and disposed of clothing in properly labeled biohazard bag. ___ ___ ___ _____

   b. Used copious amounts of soap and water to wash patient thoroughly. ___ ___ ___ _____

   c. Rinsed eyes with plain water for 10 to 15 minutes, as necessary. Removed contact lenses (did not re-insert) and placed with clothing. Washed and reapplied eyeglasses. ___ ___ ___ _____

5. Initiated treatment for chemical agent per MSDS and agency protocol. ___ ___ ___ _____

6. Established and maintained airway. ___ ___ ___ _____

7. Controlled bleeding if present. ___ ___ ___ _____

	S	U	NP	Comments
8. Provided supportive care.	___	___	___	_____
9. Counseled patient and family on acute and long-term psychological effects of exposure.	___	___	___	_____

EVALUATION

	S	U	NP	Comments
1. Observed for improved respiratory status, level of consciousness, and neurological functioning.	___	___	___	_____
2. Inspected the condition of the patient's skin.	___	___	___	_____
3. Evaluated patient's level of orientation, ability to problem-solve, and perception of condition.	___	___	___	_____
4. Assessed for unexpected outcomes.	___	___	___	_____

RECORDING AND REPORTING

	S	U	NP	Comments
1. Reported suspected cases of a toxic chemical event to physician or emergency officer.	___	___	___	_____
2. Recorded patient's status and response to treatment and/or comfort measures.	___	___	___	_____
3. Reported any unexpected outcomes to physician or nurse in charge.	___	___	___	_____

136

Student _____ Date _____

Instructor _____ Date _____

PERFORMANCE CHECKLIST SKILL 14-3 CARE OF THE PATIENT AFTER RADIATION EXPOSURE

	S	U	NP	Comments
ASSESSMENT				
1. Assessed patient's symptoms. Performed focused physical examination.	___	___	___	_____
2. Assessed the patient for secondary traumatic wounds.	___	___	___	_____
3. Assessed the patient for preexisting medical conditions.	___	___	___	_____
4. Determined patient's allergies, specifically iodine.	___	___	___	_____
5. Assessed patient's immediate psychological response following exposure.	___	___	___	_____
6. Identified available resources.	___	___	___	_____
NURSING DIAGNOSIS				
1. Developed appropriate nursing diagnoses based on assessment data.	___	___	___	_____
PLANNING				
1. Identified expected outcomes.	___	___	___	_____
2. Explained care to patient and family.	___	___	___	_____
IMPLEMENTATION				
1. Performed hand hygiene.	___	___	___	_____
2. Had only trained personnel participate in decontamination.	___	___	___	_____
3. Provided privacy.	___	___	___	_____
4. Decontaminated patient				
a. Removed patient's clothing.	___	___	___	_____
b. Washed patient's skin thoroughly with soap and water.	___	___	___	_____
c. Had radiation tech resurvey the patient after washing. Rewash as necessary.	___	___	___	_____
d. Isolated and covered any area of skin still positive for radiation by using plastic bag or wrap.	___	___	___	_____
5. Bagged and tagged patient's clothing and placed in biohazard container.	___	___	___	_____

	S	U	NP	Comments

6. Prepared to possibly obtain specimens for laboratory analysis. ____ ____ ____ _____

7. Treated symptoms as indicated. Provided IV fluids, antidiarrheal/antiemetic medication, and potassium iodide unless contraindicated. ____ ____ ____ _____

EVALUATION

1. Observed for improved fluid balance, respiratory and GI status, skin integrity, and neurological functioning. ____ ____ ____ _____

2. Monitored CBC and other laboratory tests. ____ ____ ____ _____

3. Evaluated patient's level of consciousness, orientation, and ability to relate events. ____ ____ ____ _____

4. Identified unexpected outcomes. ____ ____ ____ _____

RECORDING AND REPORTING

1. Recorded patient's status and response to treatment and/or comfort measures. ____ ____ ____ _____

2. Reported presence of open wound and any suspected radioactive fragments to physician or nurse in charge. ____ ____ ____ _____

3. Reported any unexpected outcomes to physician or nurse in charge. ____ ____ ____ _____

Student _____   Date _____

Instructor _____   Date _____

PERFORMANCE CHECKLIST SKILL 15-1 **PROVIDING PAIN RELIEF**

	S	U	NP	Comments
ASSESSMENT				
1. Assessed patient's risk for pain.	___	___	___	_____
2. Asked patient if experiencing pain/discomfort and response to previous therapies or treatments.	___	___	___	_____
3. Assessed need for pharmacological interventions.	___	___	___	_____
4. Assessed physical, behavioral, and emotional signs and symptoms of pain.	___	___	___	_____
5. Assessed characteristics of pain—PQRSTU.	___	___	___	_____
NURSING DIAGNOSIS				
1. Developed appropriate nursing diagnoses based on assessment data.	___	___	___	_____
PLANNING				
1. Identified expected outcomes.	___	___	___	_____
2. Adjusted environmental factors affecting patient's comfort and provided privacy.	___	___	___	_____
3. Explained steps to be taken to minimize pain stimuli.	___	___	___	_____
IMPLEMENTATION				
1. Performed hand hygiene and applied gloves.	___	___	___	_____
2. Administered pain-relieving medications as ordered.	___	___	___	_____
3. Removed any painful stimuli:				
a. Positioned patient so that area of discomfort is accessible.	___	___	___	_____
b. Smoothed wrinkled bed linen.	___	___	___	_____
c. Loosened constrictive bandages or devices.	___	___	___	_____
d. Repositioned underlying tubes, wires, or equipment.	___	___	___	_____
4. Discussed, demonstrated, and assisted patient with technique.	___	___	___	_____
5. Provided psychosocial intervention to assist patient to relax.	___	___	___	_____
6. Removed and disposed of gloves and performed hand hygiene.	___	___	___	_____

	S	U	NP	Comments

EVALUATION

1. Evaluated patient's level of comfort within 1 hour of analgesic intervention. ___ ___ ___ _____

2. Compared current level of pain versus personal goal. ___ ___ ___ _____

3. Compared patient's ability to function and perform ADLs. ___ ___ ___ _____

4. Evaluated presence of analgesic side effects. ___ ___ ___ _____

5. Identified unexpected outcomes. ___ ___ ___ _____

RECORDING AND REPORTING

1. Reported to nurse in charge or physician changes in character of pain or patient status, inadequate pain relief, and adverse effects of medication. ___ ___ ___ _____

2. Recorded assessment, interventions, and patient's response. ___ ___ ___ _____

Student _____ Date _____

Instructor _____ Date _____

PERFORMANCE CHECKLIST SKILL 15-2 **PATIENT-CONTROLLED ANALGESIA**

	S	U	NP	Comments
ASSESSMENT				
1. Assessed patient's cognitive ability.	___	___	___	_____
2. Assessed patient for physical, behavioral, and emotional signs and symptoms of pain or discomfort.	___	___	___	_____
3. Assessed characteristics of pain.	___	___	___	_____
4. Assessed environment for factors that contribute to pain.	___	___	___	_____
5. Inspected incision on postoperative patient.	___	___	___	_____
6. Assessed patency of existing IV infusion line.	___	___	___	_____
7. Assessed venipuncture site and surrounding areas for signs of infiltration or inflammation.	___	___	___	_____
8. Assessed response to previous pain management strategies.	___	___	___	_____
9. Checked physician's orders for dose and frequency of PCA-delivered medication. Had second RN confirm physician's order and PCA setup.	___	___	___	_____
10. Determined patient's history of drug allergies.	___	___	___	_____
NURSING DIAGNOSIS				
1. Developed appropriate nursing diagnoses based on assessment data.	___	___	___	_____
PLANNING				
1. Identified expected outcomes.	___	___	___	_____
2. Explained purpose and demonstrated functioning of PCA.	___	___	___	_____
3. Checked infuser and patient control module for accurate labeling or evidence of leaking.	___	___	___	_____
4. Set the PCA pump to deliver prescribed dosage and lockout interval.	___	___	___	_____
5. Maintained patient's privacy.	___	___	___	_____
6. Positioned patient comfortably.	___	___	___	_____

	S	U	NP	Comments

IMPLEMENTATION

1. Performed hand hygiene.

2. Followed the "six rights" to ensure correct medication; checked patient's ID using two identifiers.

3. Attached drug reservoir to infusion device and primed tubing.

4. Applied gloves.

5. Attached needleless adapter to tubing of patient control module.

6. Cleansed injection port of IV line with alcohol.

7. Inserted needleless adapter into injection port nearest IV site.

8. Secured connection and immobilized PCA tubing.

9. Administered loading dose of analgesia as prescribed.

10. Disposed of gloves and supplies. Performed hand hygiene.

11. Determined patient's understanding of PCA system through return demonstration or repeated instructions.

12. Monitored and recorded PCA use per agency policy.

13. Disposed of empty cassette or syringe per agency policy.

14. If PCA was discontinued before completion, two RNs were required to witness and record wastage per institutional policy.

15. Maintained a secondary infusion.

EVALUATION

1. Used pain rating scale to evaluate comfort level.

2. Observed for signs of adverse reactions.

3. Had patient demonstrate a dose delivery.

4. Periodically checked infusion rate and site.

5. Assessed for unexpected outcomes.

RECORDING AND REPORTING

1. Recorded on medication record drug, dose, and time initiated; included concentration and diluent. Noted basal dose, demand, and lockout time.

2. Recorded periodic assessment of patient status on PCA medication record.

3. Reported to appropriate staff adverse reactions and pain status.

142

Student _____ Date _____

Instructor _____ Date _____

PERFORMANCE CHECKLIST SKILL 15-3 **EPIDURAL ANALGESIA**

	S	U	NP	Comments
ASSESSMENT				
1. Assessed patient's comfort and current medical condition and appropriateness of epidural analgesia.	—	—	—	_____
2. Determined use of anticoagulants.	—	—	—	_____
3. Determined and identified herbals used.	—	—	—	_____
4. Checked patient's history of drug allergies.	—	—	—	_____
5. Assessed patient for physical, behavioral, and emotional signs and symptoms of pain or discomfort.	—	—	—	_____
6. Assessed characteristics of pain and provocative factors.	—	—	—	_____
7. Assessed patient's baseline sedation response to present analgesic dose.	—	—	—	_____
8. Checked rate, pattern, and depth of respirations and blood pressure.	—	—	—	_____
9. Assessed baseline motor and sensory function.	—	—	—	_____
10. Determined if epidural catheter was secured to patient's skin.	—	—	—	_____
11. Checked physician's order for medication, dosage, and infusion method.	—	—	—	_____
12. If continuous infusion, checked infusion pump for proper calibration and operation.	—	—	—	_____
13. If continuous infusion, checked patency of tubing.	—	—	—	_____
14. Kept patient IV intact for 24 hours after analgesia ended.	—	—	—	_____
NURSING DIAGNOSIS				
1. Developed appropriate nursing diagnoses based on assessment data.	—	—	—	_____
PLANNING				
1. Identified expected outcomes.	—	—	—	_____
2. Identified patient ID using two identifiers.	—	—	—	_____
3. Explained purpose and function of epidural analgesia and expectations of patient during procedure.	—	—	—	_____

	S	U	NP	Comments

4. Attached "epidural line" label to tubing and epidural catheter.

5. Used tubing without Y-port for continuous infusions.

6. Provided for patient's privacy.

IMPLEMENTATION

1. Washed hands and applied clean gloves.

2. Administered continuous infusion:

   a. Attached container of preservative-free medication to infusion pump and primed tubing.

   b. Attached proximal end of tubing to pump.

   c. Used sterile gloves to connect to epidural catheter.

   d. Checked pump for calibration and operation per agency protocol.

3. Administered bolus dose:

   a. Checked physician's order and gathered equipment.

   b. Prepared medication as ordered.

   c. Assisted nurse anesthetist or anesthesiologist with procedure.

4. Repositioned patient for comfort. Monitored vital signs and pain level.

5. Removed gloves. Performed hand hygiene.

EVALUATION

1. Evaluated comfort level and compared with baseline assessment data.

2. Checked insertion site.

3. Observed for signs of adverse reactions.

4. Assessed respiratory and neurological status.

5. Monitored vital signs.

6. Monitored intake and output (I&O).

7. Identified unexpected outcomes.

	S	U	NP	Comments

RECORDING AND REPORTING

1. Recorded drug, dose, and time given and person administering (if injection) or time initiated and ended (if infusion). Specified concentration and diluent, pump settings, and demand usage. ___ ___ ___ _____

2. Recorded any supplemental analgesic requirements. ___ ___ ___ _____

3. Recorded regular periodic assessment of patient's status. ___ ___ ___ _____

4. Reported to physician any adverse reactions or complications. ___ ___ ___ _____

Student _____   Date _____

Instructor _____   Date _____

PERFORMANCE CHECKLIST SKILL 15-4 **LOCAL INFUSION PUMP ANALGESIA**

	S	U	NP	Comments
ASSESSMENT				
1. Assessed surgical dressing and catheter insertion site.	___	___	___	_____
2. Assessed catheter connections for patency.	___	___	___	_____
3. Assessed characteristics of patient's pain.	___	___	___	_____
4. Assessed for blood backing up in tubing.	___	___	___	_____
5. Reviewed label information on device and compared medication administration record versus physician's order.	___	___	___	_____
6. Determined patient's extremity activity per physician's orders.	___	___	___	_____
7. Assessed for signs of local anesthetic toxicity.	___	___	___	_____
8. Determined patient's knowledge of infusion pump.	___	___	___	_____
NURSING DIAGNOSIS				
1. Developed appropriate nursing diagnosis based on assessment data.	___	___	___	_____
PLANNING				
1. Identified expected outcomes.	___	___	___	_____
IMPLEMENTATION				
1. Taught patient or family how to safely remove catheter.				
a. Performed hand hygiene and applied clean gloves.	___	___		_____
b. Positioned patient appropriately.	___	___		_____
c. Removed surgical dressing.	___	___	___	_____
d. Grasped catheter firmly and pulled outward from skin in steady motion.				
(1) Stopped pulling when resistance occurred. Repositioned extremity and tried again.	___	___	___	_____
(2) Stopped pulling when resistance continued, covered area with sterile dressing and notified physician.	___	___	___	_____

	S	U	NP	Comments

e. Looked for mark at end of catheter.

f. Placed sterile dressing over area and applied pressure as soon as catheter was removed.

g. Discarded soiled dressing and gloves.

h. Performed hand hygiene.

EVALUATION

1. Asked patient to rate pain during infusion, using appropriate scale.

2. Observed for signs of adverse drug reactions.

3. Observed patient's position, mobility, relaxation, participation in ADLs, and other non-verbal behaviors.

4. Inspected condition of surgical dressing.

5. Identified unexpected outcomes.

Student _____ Date _____

Instructor _____ Date _____

PERFORMANCE CHECKLIST SKILL 15-5 **NONPHARMACOLOGICAL AIDS TO PROMOTE COMFORT**

	S	U	NP	Comments

ASSESSMENT
1. Had patient identify level of pain or comfort. ___ ___ ___ _____

2. Assessed patient for physiological, behavioral, and emotional signs and symptoms of pain or discomfort. ___ ___ ___ _____

3. Assessed characteristics of pain. ___ ___ ___ _____

4. Examined site of patient's pain. ___ ___ ___ _____

5. Assessed patient's understanding and willingness to participate in pain relief program. ___ ___ ___ _____

6. Assessed types of distraction activities in which the patient is interested. ___ ___ ___ _____

7. Assessed patient's language level and identified terms to be used. ___ ___ ___ _____

NURSING DIAGNOSIS
1. Developed appropriate nursing diagnoses based on assessment data. ___ ___ ___ _____

PLANNING
1. Identified expected outcomes. ___ ___ ___ _____

2. Explained purpose of technique and expectations of patient during procedure. ___ ___ ___ _____

3. Planned to perform technique in a comfortable environment after patient's rest period. ___ ___ ___ _____

4. Assisted patient to comfortable position. ___ ___ ___ _____

IMPLEMENTATION
1. *Massage*

   a. Performed hand hygiene. ___ ___ ___ _____

   b. Adjusted bed to high position and lowered side rail. ___ ___ ___ _____

   c. Placed patient in comfortable position. ___ ___ ___ _____

   d. Exposed only area to be massaged. ___ ___ ___ _____

   e. Warmed lotion in hands. Checked for sensitivities or allergies to lotion. ___ ___ ___ _____

   f. Used techniques of effleurage, petrissage, and friction on muscle groups. ___ ___ ___ _____

	S	U	NP	Comments

g. Encouraged patient to breathe deeply and relax during massage.

h. Massaged patient's scalp and temples.

i. Massaged muscles at base of patient's head.

j. Massaged patient's hands and arms.

k. Placed patient in prone position, unless contraindicated.

l. Massaged patient's neck, as appropriate.

m. Massaged patient's back, keeping hands in contact with skin.

n. Massaged patient's feet, as appropriate, with patient in supine position.

o. Told patient when massage completed.

p. Completed procedure by having patient breathe deeply and slowly resume activity.

q. Removed excess lotion from patient's body.

r. Returned bed to low position and adjusted side rails appropriately.

s. Performed hand hygiene.

2. *Progressive Relaxation*

a. Instructed patient to breathe slowly and deeply.

b. Instructed patient to close eyes, if desired.

c. Instructed patient on alternating tightening and relaxation of muscle groups.

d. Asked patient to relax and breathe deeply after each muscle group completed.

e. Explained expected sensations.

f. Instructed patient to breathe deeply and move around slowly after a few minutes of rest after completion of exercise.

3. *Deep Breathing*

a. Assisted patient to a comfortable position.

b. Instructed patient to put one hand on the chest and one on the abdomen.

c. Instructed patient to inhale deeply, allowing the abdomen to rise, and to continue to breathe while allowing chest to expand.

	S	U	NP	Comments

d. Patient told to pause for a few seconds and exhaled slowly through pursed lips. ____ ____ ____ _____

e. Repeated 4 to 6 times or as tolerated. ____ ____ ____ _____

4. *Guided Imagery*

   a. Directed patient through exercise. ____ ____ ____ _____

   b. Directed patient imagery with suggestions for pleasant and relaxing sensory experiences. ____ ____ ____ _____

   c. On completion, instructed patient to breathe deeply, open eyes, and move around slowly. ____ ____ ____ _____

   d. Provided uninterrupted practice time for patient. ____ ____ ____ _____

5. *Distraction*

   a. Directed patient's attention from pain. ____ ____ ____ _____

   b. Asked patient to close eyes or focus on a single object. ____ ____ ____ _____

   c. Instructed/guided patient in slow, rhythmical breathing. ____ ____ ____ _____

   d. Continued skill with method of choice (e.g., music, conversation). ____ ____ ____ _____

EVALUATION

1. Determined patient's physiological and behavioral responses to technique. ____ ____ ____ _____

2. Used pain rating scale to evaluate patient's comfort level. ____ ____ ____ _____

3. Observed patient's performance of techniques. ____ ____ ____ _____

4. Identified unexpected outcomes. ____ ____ ____ _____

REPORTING AND RECORDING

1. Recorded procedure, technique, preparation given to patient, and patient's response. ____ ____ ____ _____

2. Recorded alterations in patient's condition (e.g., vital signs). ____ ____ ____ _____

3. Reported to nurse in charge patient's response to techniques. ____ ____ ____ _____

4. Reported any unusual responses to techniques. ____ ____ ____ _____

PE: Kyla vanderweele

Student _____ Date _____

Instructor _____ Date _____

PERFORMANCE CHECKLIST SKILL 16-1 **SUPPORTING PATIENTS AND FAMILIES IN GRIEF**

	S	U	NP	Comments

ASSESSMENT

1. Found private location or provided privacy in patient's room.   ___ ___ ___ _____

2. Established quiet presence; sat near patient. Established eye contact depending on culture.   ___ ___ ___ _____

3. Considered influence of patient's age, gender, race, culture, and socioeconomic status on communication.   ___ ___ ___ _____

4. Began to interview patient/family using honest, open communication, listening skills, and observation of patient's concerns.   ___ ___ ___ _____

5. Determined quality and meaning of the patient's grief experience.   ___ ___ ___ _____

6. Encouraged patient to describe loss and its effects. Determined how much time passed since loss occurred and described nature of loss.   ___ ___ ___ _____

7. Asked patient to describe coping strategies used in the past.   ___ ___ ___ _____

8. Determined how patient's illness has affected family members.   ___ ___ ___ _____

9. Assessed patient's spiritual needs and resources.   ___ ___ ___ _____

NURSING DIAGNOSIS

1. Developed appropriate nursing diagnoses based on assessment data.   ___ ___ ___ _____

PLANNING

1. Identified expected outcomes.   ___ ___ ___ _____

IMPLEMENTATION

1. Showed empathetic understanding of patient's strengths.   ___ ___ ___ _____

2. Offered information about the patient's illness and corrected any misinformation.   ___ ___ ___ _____

3. Discussed best use of resources by family members for patient to remain as independent as possible.   ___ ___ ___ _____

4. Encouraged patient to engage in supportive relationships with family and friends.   ___ ___ ___ _____

	S	U	NP	Comments

5. Worked with patient in focusing on ways to achieve short-term goals.

6. Offered frequent sessions that allowed patient and family opportunities to further express grief, fears, or concerns.

7. Helped patient and family identify and solve caregiving problems.

8. Offered to instruct patient on relaxation strategies.

9. Encouraged visits with friends and family to reminisce with life stories, events, and photographs.

10. Encouraged spiritual guidance.

EVALUATION

1. Had patient describe activities engaged in with family/friends.

2. Observed patient's behaviors during ongoing interactions.

3. Discussed with patient perceptions of benefits gained from stress-relieving strategies.

4. Discussed with patient progress toward meeting defined short-term goals.

5. Identified unexpected outcomes.

RECORDING AND REPORTING

1. Recorded approaches used in grief support and patient's response.

2. Reported patient's grief expressions and reactions. Identified changes in physical health status.

Student _____ Date _____

Instructor _____ Date _____

PERFORMANCE CHECKLIST SKILL 16-2 **SYMPTOM MANAGEMENT AT THE END OF LIFE**

	S	U	NP	Comments

ASSESSMENT

1. Asked patient to describe symptoms that are being experienced. Gave patient time to describe symptoms. ___ ___ ___ _____

2. Assessed pain level. ___ ___ ___ _____

3. Used the PQRST criteria for assessing the character of pain. ___ ___ ___ _____

4. Assessed patient's respirations and breathing pattern. ___ ___ ___ _____

5. Assessed the condition of the skin. ___ ___ ___ _____

6. Assessed patient's oral cavity. ___ ___ ___ _____

7. Assessed patient's bowel elimination. ___ ___ ___ _____

8. Assessed patient's urinary elimination. ___ ___ ___ _____

9. Asked if patient was experiencing nausea, vomiting, or decreased appetite. ___ ___ ___ _____

10. Assessed daily food and fluid intake. Weighed patient. ___ ___ ___ _____

11. Assessed patient's level of fatigue using analog scale. ___ ___ ___ _____

12. Assessed patient's status and reviewed medical record if exhibiting signs of terminal restlessness. ___ ___ ___ _____

NURSING DIAGNOSIS

1. Developed appropriate nursing diagnoses based on assessment data. ___ ___ ___ _____

PLANNING

1. Identified expected outcomes. ___ ___ ___ _____

2. Explained procedures to be performed and involved patient in schedule of activities. ___ ___ ___ _____

IMPLEMENTATION

1. Implemented pharmacological and nonpharmacological pain relief measures. ___ ___ ___ _____

2. Provided general comfort measures, including bathing, skin care, and repositioning. ___ ___ ___ _____

3. Provided oral hygiene as appropriate for patient's status. ___ ___ ___ _____

	S	U	NP	Comments

4. Treated nausea with antiemetics (as ordered). Avoided coffee, milk, and fruit juices.

5. Provided a bowel management program: high-fiber diet, increased fluids, daily exercise, and suppository (if ordered).

6. Provided low-residue diet, assessed for impaction, and conferred with physician on medication orders for patient with diarrhea.

7. Conferred with physician regarding use of urinary catheter or diapers for total incontinence.

8. Had patient identify tasks that he/she wished to perform and assisted patient to conserve energy.

9. Provided adequate ventilation and oxygenation: positioned patient, suctioned as necessary, administered oxygen (as ordered), and kept room cool with low humidity.

10. Controlled terminal restlessness with environmental manipulation and pharmacological intervention.

EVALUATION

1. Used pain rating scale to evaluate comfort level.

2. Asked patient to describe comfort of oral cavity.

3. Inspected character of bowel elimination.

4. Inspected condition of skin.

5. Asked patient to rate level of fatigue on scale of 0 to 10.

6. Assessed patient's respirations.

7. Observed patient's behavior.

8. Assessed for unexpected outcomes.

RECORDING AND REPORTING

1. Recorded patient symptoms.

2. Recorded types of interventions provided and patient responses.

3. Recorded interventions that were repeatedly successful in controlling patient's symptoms.

Student _____ Date _____

Instructor _____ Date _____

PERFORMANCE CHECKLIST SKILL 16-3 **CARE OF A BODY AFTER DEATH**

	S	U	NP	Comments

ASSESSMENT

1. Confirmed with physician regarding the time of death. Determined need for autopsy. ____ ____ ____ _____

2. Determined presence of family members. Asked if family wished to view the body. ____ ____ ____ _____

3. Approached next of kin for tissue donation and processed forms. ____ ____ ____ _____

4. Allowed time for family/significant others to ask questions. ____ ____ ____ _____

5. Determined if family members had special requests for preparation or viewing of the body. ____ ____ ____ _____

6. Made arrangements for staff, minister, or others to stay with family during preparation of body. ____ ____ ____ _____

7. Checked orders for collection of specimens. ____ ____ ____ _____

8. Determined general condition of body. ____ ____ ____ _____

NURSING DIAGNOSIS

1. Developed appropriate nursing diagnoses based on assessment data. ____ ____ ____ _____

PLANNING

1. Identified expected outcomes. ____ ____ ____ _____

2. Had body placed in private room or moved roommate to another area. ____ ____ ____ _____

3. Gathered needed equipment. ____ ____ ____ _____

IMPLEMENTATION

1. Assisted family/significant other present about notifying others. Called the funeral home. ____ ____ ____ _____

2. Consulted agency policy regarding care of the body if tissue donation was made. ____ ____ ____ _____

3. Performed hand hygiene and applied PPE. ____ ____ ____ _____

4. Identified the body according to agency policy. ____ ____ ____ _____

5. Removed all tubes according to agency policy. Dressed any wounds with small dressing and paper tape. ____ ____ ____ _____

6. Inserted into mouth patient's dentures, if worn. ____ ____ ____ _____

7. Positioned patient appropriately. ____ ____ ____ _____

	S	U	NP	Comments
8. Placed small pillow under patient's head.	___	___	___	_____
9. Closed patient's eyelids.	___	___	___	_____
10. Determined if family wanted patient left unshaven; otherwise, shave male patient.	___	___	___	_____
11. Washed soiled body parts.	___	___	___	_____
12. Removed soiled dressings and replaced with clean gauze dressings and paper tape.	___	___	___	_____
13. Placed absorbent pad under patient's buttocks.	___	___	___	_____
14. Placed clean gown on body.	___	___	___	_____
15. Brushed and combed patient's hair.	___	___	___	_____
16. Accounted for all valuables in patient's room.	___	___	___	_____
17. Prepared patient and room for viewing, if requested by family.	___	___	___	_____
18. Allowed time for family/significant others to view body in private.	___	___	___	_____
19. Removed all linen and patient's gown and placed body in shroud.	___	___	___	_____
20. Attached label to outside of body bag or shroud, noting if patient had transmissible infection.	___	___	___	_____
21. Arranged for transportation of body.	___	___	___	_____

EVALUATION

	S	U	NP	Comments
1. Observed family's response to loss.	___	___	___	_____
2. Noted appearance and condition of patient's skin during body preparation.	___	___	___	_____
3. Identified unexpected outcomes.	___	___	___	_____

RECORDING AND REPORTING

	S	U	NP	Comments
1. Recorded time of death, resuscitative measures taken (if applicable), and person who pronounced death.	___	___	___	
2. Recorded any special preparation of body and type of organ/tissue donation or autopsy.	___	___	___	
3. Recorded names of morgue, funeral home, and chaplain, and relationship to deceased of individual family members who are involved in decisions.	___	___	___	
4. Recorded how valuables and personal belongings were handled and who received them. Secured signatures as required by agency policy.	___	___	___	
5. Recorded personal articles or medical devices left on the body.	___	___	___	
6. Recorded time body was transported and destination of body. Noted location of identifying tags.	___	___	___	

PERFORMANCE CHECKLIST SKILL 17-1 **BATHING AND PERSONAL HYGIENE**

	S	U	NP	Comments
ASSESSMENT				
1. Assessed patient's preference and tolerance for bathing.	___	___	___	_____
2. Assessed patient's visual status, ability to sit without support, hand grasp, and ROM of extremities.	___	___	___	_____
3. Assessed for presence of equipment (e.g., intravenous [IV] line or oxygen tubing).	___	___	___	_____
4. Asked if patient has noticed any problems related to condition of skin and genitalia.	___	___	___	_____
5. Assessed condition of patient's skin.	___	___	___	_____
6. Identified risks for skin impairment.	___	___	___	_____
7. Assess patient's knowledge of skin hygiene.	___	___	___	_____
8. Checked physician's therapeutic bath order for type of solution, length of time for bath, and body part to be attended.	___	___	___	_____
9. Reviewed orders for specific precautions concerning patient's movement or positioning.	___	___	___	_____
NURSING DIAGNOSIS				
1. Developed appropriate nursing diagnoses based on assessment data.	___	___	___	_____
PLANNING				
1. Identified expected outcomes.	___	___	___	_____
2. Explained procedure to patient and asked for patient's suggestions.	___	___	___	_____
3. Adjusted room temperature and ventilation for patient's comfort and provided for patient's privacy during bath.	___	___	___	_____
4. Prepared necessary equipment and supplies.	___	___	___	_____
IMPLEMENTATION				
1. *Complete or Partial Bed Bath*				
a. Offered bedpan or urinal before bath.	___	___	___	_____
b. Gathered all supplies, performed hand hygiene, and applied gloves.	___	___	___	_____
c. Adjusted bed height, lowered side rail, and assisted patient to a comfortable position.	___	___	___	_____

	S	U	NP	Comments

d. Used bath blanket properly while removing top linens of bed. Disposed of soiled linen correctly. ___ ___ ___ _____

e. Removed patient's gown correctly. ___ ___ ___ _____

f. Checked temperature of bath water and patient's tolerance. Warmed bath lotion, if desired. ___ ___ ___ _____

g. Removed pillow if allowed and raised head of bed; placed a towel under patient's head and a towel over patient's chest. ___ ___ ___ _____

h. Washed face:

(1) Inquired if patient was wearing contact lenses. If so, performed eye care. ___ ___ ___ _____

(2) Formed mitt with washcloth. Immersed mitt in water and wrung thoroughly. ___ ___ ___ _____

(3) Washed patient's eyes with plain warm water, using a clean area of cloth for each eye, bathing from inner to outer canthus. Soaked any crusts on eyelid for 2 to 3 minutes with damp cloth before attempting removal. Dried around eyes gently and thoroughly. ___ ___ ___ _____

(4) Asked if patient would prefer to use soap on face. Otherwise, washed, rinsed, and dried forehead, cheeks, nose, neck, and ears without using soap. Asked men if they would like to be shaved. ___ ___ ___ _____

i. Provided eye care for the unconscious patient:

(1) Cleansed the eyelids with a washcloth from the inner to outer canthus using plain warm water. ___ ___ ___ _____

(2) Instilled prescribed eye drops or ointment per physician's order. ___ ___ ___ _____

(3) In absence of blink reflex, kept eyes closed. ___ ___ ___ _____

j. Washed trunk and upper extremities:

(1) Removed bath blanket from patient's arm. Placed bath towel lengthwise under arm. Bathed with minimal soap and water using long, firm strokes from distal to proximal (fingers to axilla). ___ ___ ___ _____

(2) Raised and supported arm above head (if possible) to wash, rinse, and dry axilla thoroughly. Applied deodorant or powder to underarms if desired or needed. ___ ___ ___ _____

160

	S	U	NP	Comments

(3) Moved to other side of bed and repeated steps a and b with other arm.

(4) Covered patient's chest with bath towel and folded bath blanket down to umbilicus. Bathed chest using long, firm strokes. Took special care with skin under female patient's breasts. Rinsed and dried well.

k. Washed hands and nails:

(1) Folded bath towel in half and laid it on bed beside patient. Placed basin on towel. Immersed patient's hand in water. Allowed hand to soak for 3 to 5 minutes (if needed) before cleansing fingernails. Removed basin and dried hand well. Repeated for other hand.

l. Checked temperature of bath water and changed water if necessary; otherwise continued.

m. Washed the abdomen:

(1) Placed bath towel lengthwise over chest and abdomen. (Two towels may be needed.) Folded bath blanket down to just above pubic region. Bathed, rinsed, and dried abdomen with special attention to umbilicus and skinfolds of abdomen and groin. Kept abdomen covered between washing and rinsing. Dried well.

(2) Applied clean gown or pajama top.

n. Washed the lower extremities:

(1) Covered chest and abdomen with top of bath blanket. Exposed near leg by folding blanket toward midline. Kept perineum draped.

(2) Placed bath towel under leg, while supporting leg at knee and ankle. If appropriate, placed patient's foot in a basin to soak while washing and rinsing.

(3) Washed leg using long, firm strokes from ankle to knee, then knee to thigh. Did not rub or massage the back of the calf. Dried well. Washed between toes of foot. Cleansed foot, making sure to bathe between toes. Cleaned and clipped nails, adhering to agency policy as needed. Dried toes and feet completely. Removed and discarded towel.

	S	U	NP	Comments

(4) Raised side rail, moved to opposite side of bed, lowered side rail, and repeated steps for other leg and foot. Applied moisturizing lotion to dry skin. When finished, covered patient with bath blanket. _____ _____ _____ _____

(5) Raised side rail and changed bath water. Removed contaminated gloves. _____ _____ _____ _____

o. Washed back:

(1) Reapplied clean gloves. Assisted patient to a comfortable position Placed towel along side. _____ _____ _____ _____

(2) If fecal material was present, enclosed in toilet tissue and removed with disposable wipe. _____ _____ _____ _____

(3) Washed, rinsed, and dried back from neck to buttocks. Assessed skinfolds. Removed soiled linens. Made bed. Removed gloves. Performed hand hygiene. _____ _____ _____ _____

p. Gave back rub with lotion. Determined patient's sensitivities or allergies to product. _____ _____ _____ _____

q. Repositioned patient and assisted in grooming. _____ _____ _____ _____

r. Cleaned and replaced bathing supplies. Placed bed in safe position with call light and personal belongings next to patient. _____ _____ _____ _____

s. Performed hand hygiene. _____ _____ _____ _____

RECORDING AND REPORTING

1. Recorded procedure and amount of assistance and patient participation. _____ _____ _____ _____

2. Recorded condition of skin, joints, and muscles. _____ _____ _____ _____

3. Reported findings to charge nurse or health care provider. _____ _____ _____ _____

PE: Kyla vanderwell 9/12/12

Student _____ Date _____

Instructor _____ Date _____

PERFORMANCE CHECKLIST PROCEDURAL GUIDELINE 17-1 **PERINEAL CARE**

	S	U	NP	Comments
STEPS				
1. Performed hand hygiene and applied gloves.	_____	_____	_____	_____
2. *Perineal Care for the Female*				
a. Observed patient's ability to maneuver and handle washcloth. Allowed patient to clean perineum on own.	_____	_____	_____	_____
b. Assisted patient to dorsal recumbent position. Placed waterproof pad under buttocks.	_____	_____	_____	_____
c. Draped patient for privacy.	_____	_____	_____	_____
d. Folded lower corner of bath blanket up between patient's legs onto abdomen. Washed and dried patient's upper thighs.	_____	_____	_____	_____
e. Washed labia majora. Wiped in direction from perineum to rectum. Repeated on opposite side using separate section of washcloth. Rinsed and dried area thoroughly.	_____	_____	_____	_____
f. Gently separated labia with nondominant hand to expose urethral meatus and vaginal orifice. Washed downward from pubic area toward rectum in one smooth stroke. Used separate section of cloth for each stroke. Cleansed thoroughly around labia minora, clitoris, and vaginal orifice. Avoided tension on indwelling catheter if present, and cleaned area around it thoroughly.	_____	_____	_____	_____
g. Rinsed area thoroughly. If patient used bedpan, poured warm water over perineal area. Dried thoroughly, using front-to-back method.	_____	_____	_____	_____
h. Assisted to a comfortable position.	_____	_____	_____	_____
3. *Perineal Care for Male*				
a. Observed patient's ability to maneuver and handle washcloth. Allowed patient to cleanse perineum on own.	_____	_____	_____	_____
b. Assisted patient to supine position.	_____	_____	_____	_____
c. Folded lower half of bath blanket up to expose upper thighs. Washed and dried patient's thighs.	_____	_____	_____	_____

	S	U	NP	Comments

d. Covered thighs with bath towels. Raised bath blanket up to expose genitalia. Raised penis and placed bath towel underneath. Grasped shaft of penis. Retracted foreskin if present. Deferred care if patient had an erection.

e. Washed tip of penis at urethral meatus first. Using circular motion, cleansed from meatus outward. Discarded washcloth and repeated with clean cloth until penis was clean. Rinsed and dried.

f. Returned foreskin to its natural position.

g. Cleansed shaft of penis and scrotum by having patient abduct legs. Paid special attention to underlying surface of penis. Lifted scrotum carefully and washed underlying skinfolds. Rinsed and dried thoroughly.

h. Folded bath blanket back over patient's perineum and assisted patient to comfortable position.

4. Observed perineal area for signs of persistent irritation and redness.

5. Disposed of gloves. Performed hand hygiene.

PE: Kayla Vanderwelle 9/12/12

Student _____ Date _____

Instructor _____ Date _____

PERFORMANCE CHECKLIST PROCEDURAL GUIDELINE 17-2 **USE OF DISPOSABLE BED BATH, TUB, OR SHOWER**

	S	U	NP	Comments

STEPS

1. *Bag Bath*

   a. Warmed the package contents in a microwave following package directions. ___ ___ ___ _____

   b. Used a single towel for each general body part cleansed. Followed the same order of cleansing as in the total or partial bed bath. ___ ___ ___ _____

   c. Allowed the skin to air dry for 30 seconds. Lightly covered patient with a bath towel to prevent chilling. ___ ___ ___ _____

   d. Used an extra bag bath if necessary or conventional wash cloths, soap, and water, and towels for excessive soiling. ___ ___ ___ _____

2. *Tub Bath or Shower*

   a. Considered patient's condition and reviewed medical orders. ___ ___ ___ _____

   b. Scheduled use of shower or tub. ___ ___ ___ _____

   c. Cleaned tub or shower according to agency policy; provided rubber bath mat or disposable mat to prevent slipping. ___ ___ ___ _____

   d. Arranged all hygienic aids, toilet items, and linen within reach of patient. ___ ___ ___ _____

   e. Assisted patient into tub or shower. ___ ___ ___ _____

   f. Placed "Occupied" sign on bathroom door. ___ ___ ___ _____

   g. Filled tub halfway, adjusted water temperature, and instructed patient on use of faucets. If patient was taking a shower, turned shower on and adjusted water temperature before patient entered shower stall. ___ ___ ___ _____

   h. Used shower seat or chair, if necessary. ___ ___ ___ _____

   i. Instructed patient on use of safety bars and cautioned patient against use of bath oil in tub water. ___ ___ ___ _____

   j. Cautioned patient against remaining in tub for longer than 20 minutes and checked on patient every 5 minutes. ___ ___ ___ _____

   k. Returned to bathroom when patient signaled, and knocked before entering. ___ ___ ___ _____

		S	U	NP	Comments
l.	Drained water from tub; placed bath towel over patient's shoulders; assisted patient in getting out of tub and with drying.	——	——	——	———————————
m.	Assisted patient in donning clean gown or pajamas.	——	——	——	———————————
n.	Assisted patient to room and comfortable position.	——	——	——	———————————
o.	Cleaned tub or shower according to policy. Removed soiled linen, discarded of disposable equipment properly.	——	——	——	———————————
p.	Performed hand hygiene.	——	——	——	———————————

Student _____   Date _____

Instructor _____   Date _____

PERFORMANCE CHECKLIST SKILL 17-2   **ORAL HYGIENE**

	S	U	NP	Comments

ASSESSMENT

1. Performed hand hygiene. Applied gloves.   ___ ___ ___ _____

2. Assessed the oral cavity.   ___ ___ ___ _____

3. Identified presence of common oral problems.   ___ ___ ___ _____

4. Removed gloves and performed hand hygiene.   ___ ___ ___ _____

5. Assessed patient's risk for oral hygiene problems.   ___ ___ ___ _____

6. Determined patient's oral hygiene practices.   ___ ___ ___ _____

7. Assessed patient's ability to grasp and manipulate toothbrush.   ___ ___ ___ _____

NURSING DIAGNOSIS

1. Developed appropriate nursing diagnoses based on assessment data.   ___ ___ ___ _____

PLANNING

1. Identified expected outcomes.   ___ ___ ___ _____

2. Prepared equipment at bedside.   ___ ___ ___ _____

3. Explained procedure to patient and discussed preferences.   ___ ___ ___ _____

IMPLEMENTATION

1. Arranged equipment on paper towels on bedside table.   ___ ___ ___ _____

2. Raised bed to comfortable working position, lowered side rail, and positioned patient on side near nurse in semi-Fowler's or side-lying position.   ___ ___ ___ _____

3. Placed towel over patient's chest. Applied gloves.   ___ ___ ___ _____

4. Applied toothpaste to brush and moistened paste.   ___ ___ ___ _____

5. Held or had patient hold toothbrush at 45-degree angle to gum line and used short strokes to brush tooth surfaces from gum to crown; held brush parallel to teeth to clean biting surfaces; brushed sides of teeth, moving bristles back and forth.   ___ ___ ___ _____

	S	U	NP	Comments
6. Held or had patient hold brush at 45-degree angle and lightly brushed tongue surface.	___	___	___	_____
7. Provided water for patient to rinse mouth thoroughly. Offered mouthwash for gargling and rinsing.	___	___	___	_____
8. Assisted in wiping patient's mouth.	___	___	___	_____
9. Allowed patient to floss.	___	___	___	_____
10. Allowed patient to rinse mouth thoroughly with tepid water after flossing.	___	___	___	_____
11. Repositioned patient comfortably after procedure.	___	___	___	_____
12. Disposed of equipment and soiled linen properly.	___	___	___	_____
13. Performed hand hygiene.	___	___	___	_____

EVALUATION

	S	U	NP	Comments
1. Assessed patient's comfort level.	___	___	___	_____
2. Applied gloves and inspected condition of oral cavity.	___	___	___	_____
3. Asked patient to describe proper oral hygiene techniques.	___	___	___	_____
4. Observed patient brushing.	___	___	___	_____
5. Identified unexpected outcomes.	___	___	___	_____

RECORDING AND REPORTING

	S	U	NP	Comments
1. Recorded procedure on flowsheet. Included condition of oral cavity.	___	___	___	_____
2. Reported any unusual findings to nurse in charge or physician.	___	___	___	_____

Student _____ Date _____

Instructor _____ Date _____

PERFORMANCE CHECKLIST PROCEDURAL GUIDELINE 17-3 **CARE OF DENTURES**

	S	U	NP	Comments
STEPS				
1. Determined patient's ability to clean dentures.	____	____	____	_____
2. Added tepid water to emesis basin or sink lined with washcloth.	____	____	____	_____
3. Applied clean gloves.	____	____	____	_____
4. Removed dentures.	____	____	____	_____
5. Thoroughly brushed all denture surfaces with denture or regular toothbrush and dentifrice.	____	____	____	_____
6. Rinsed dentures thoroughly with tepid water.	____	____	____	_____
7. Reinserted dentures according to patient's preferences (moistened denture before reinsertion); checked to see if denture adhesive was needed for proper seal.	____	____	____	_____
8. If not in use, stored dentures in labeled denture cup containing tepid water.	____	____	____	_____
9. Disposed of gloves. Cleaned and stored supplies after procedure. Performed hand hygiene.	____	____	____	_____

Student _____ Date _____

Instructor _____ Date _____

PERFORMANCE CHECKLIST SKILL 17-3 **PERFORMING MOUTH CARE FOR THE UNCONSCIOUS OR DEBILITATED PATIENT**

	S	U	NP	Comments
ASSESSMENT				
1. Performed hand hygiene. Applied clean gloves.	___	___	___	_____
2. Assessed for presence of gag reflex.	___	___	___	_____
3. Conducted physical assessment of oral cavity.	___	___	___	_____
4. Removed gloves. Performed hand hygiene.	___	___	___	_____
5. Assessed patient's risk for oral hygiene problems.	___	___	___	_____
NURSING DIAGNOSIS				
1. Developed appropriate nursing diagnoses based on assessment data.	___	___	___	_____
PLANNING				
1. Identified expected outcomes.	___	___	___	_____
2. Positioned patient on side with head turned toward dependent side and head of bed lowered. Unless contraindicated, raised side rail.	___	___	___	_____
3. Explained procedure to patient.	___	___	___	_____
4. Performed hand hygiene and applied clean gloves.	___	___	___	_____
5. Properly arranged equipment and turned on suction device.	___	___	___	_____
6. Closed curtain or room door for privacy.	___	___	___	_____
IMPLEMENTATION				
1. Raised bed and lowered side rail to have easy access to patient; raised side rail when patient was unattended.	___	___	___	_____
2. Positioned patient on side of bed near student; kept patient positioned on side with head turned toward mattress unless contraindicated.	___	___	___	_____
3. Removed dentures, if present.	___	___	___	_____
4. Placed towel under patient's face and positioned emesis basin under patient's chin.	___	___	___	_____
5. Placed oral airway if patient was uncooperative.	___	___	___	_____

	S	U	NP	Comments
6. Cleansed mouth.		___	___	_____
7. Used toothette for patient without teeth.		___	___	_____
8. Suctioned secretions as necessary.		___	___	_____
9. Applied water-soluble jelly to lips.		___	___	_____
10. Informed patient that procedure was completed.		___	___	_____
11. Raised side rail. Removed gloves and disposed of them in proper receptacle.		___	___	_____
12. Repositioned patient safely and comfortably after procedure.		___	___	_____
13. Disposed of equipment and soiled linen properly.		___	___	_____
14. Performed hand hygiene.		___	___	_____

EVALUATION

	S	U	NP	Comments
1. Applied gloves and inspected patient's oral cavity.	___	___	___	_____
2. Assessed patient's level of comfort and cleanliness.	___	___	___	_____
3. Assessed patient's respirations on an ongoing basis.	___	___	___	_____
4. Identified unexpected outcomes.	___	___	___	_____

RECORDING AND REPORTING

	S	U	NP	Comments
1. Recorded procedure, including description of the condition of the oral cavity and patient's ability to assist.	___	___	___	_____
2. Reported any unusual findings to nurse in charge or physician.	___	___	___	_____

PE: Kyla VanderWeele 9/12/12

Student _____ Date _____

Instructor _____ Date _____

PERFORMANCE CHECKLIST SKILL 17-4 **HAIR CARE (COMBING AND SHAVING)**

	S	U	NP	Comments

ASSESSMENT

1. Assessed patient's hair and scalp. ___ ___ ___ _____

2. Assessed patient's hair care/shaving product preferences. ___ ___ ___ _____

3. Reviewed medical history for presence of bleeding tendencies. ___ ___ ___ _____

4. Assessed patient's ability to manipulate razor. ___ ___ ___ _____

NURSING DIAGNOSIS

1. Developed appropriate nursing diagnosis based on assessment data. ___ ___ ___ _____

PLANNING

1. Identified expected outcomes. ___ ___ ___ _____

2. Positioned patient comfortably with head of bed elevated 45 to 90 degrees. ___ ___ ___ _____

3. Arranged supplies at bedside table; adjusted light. ___ ___ ___ _____

4. Performed hand hygiene. ___ ___ ___ _____

IMPLEMENTATION

1. Combing/brushing hair:

   a. Parted hair into sections. ___ ___ ___ _____

   b. Combed from scalp toward hair ends. ___ ___ ___ _____

   c. Moistened hair with water. ___ ___ ___ _____

   d. Loosened tangles with fingers. ___ ___ ___ _____

   e. Used wide-tooth comb to comb hair into shape. ___ ___ ___ _____

2. Shaving with a disposable razor:

   a. Placed towel over patient's chest and shoulders. ___ ___ ___ _____

   b. Ran warm water into basin; checked temperature. ___ ___ ___ _____

   c. Applied dampened cloth to patient's face for several seconds. ___ ___ ___ _____

   d. Applied shaving cream/soap to patient's face. ___ ___ ___ _____

	S	U	NP	Comments

e. Shaved patient's face; rinsed razor in warm water cream/soap accumulated. ___ ___ ___ _____

f. Rinsed face thoroughly with warm water when shaving completed. ___ ___ ___ _____

g. Dried face thoroughly, applied lotion when requested. ___ ___ ___ _____

h. Returned equipment to proper place; discarded soil linens into laundry; performed hand hygiene. ___ ___ ___ _____

3. Shaving with an electric razor:

a. Placed towel over patient's chest and shoulders. ___ ___ ___ _____

b. Applied skin conditioner/preshave. ___ ___ ___ _____

c. Held skin taut while shaving with downward strokes. ___ ___ ___ _____

d. Applied aftershave when requested. ___ ___ ___ _____

e. Performed steps 2g and h above (for disposable razor). ___ ___ ___ _____

4. Moustache and beard care:

a. Placed towel over patient's chest and shoulders. ___ ___ ___ _____

b. Combed beard as needed. ___ ___ ___ _____

c. Held mirror; allowed patient to trim with scissors as needed. ___ ___ ___ _____

EVALUATION

1. Asked patient how hair and scalp felt. ___ ___ ___ _____

2. Inspected condition of shaved area and skin under beard/moustache. ___ ___ ___ _____

3. Asked patient how face felt. ___ ___ ___ _____

4. Asked if patient was happy with degree of participation. ___ ___ ___ _____

5. Identified any unexpected outcomes. ___ ___ ___ _____

RECORDING AND REPORTING

1. Reported unusual findings to nurse in charge. ___ ___ ___ _____

Student _____ Date _____

Instructor _____ Date _____

PERFORMANCE CHECKLIST PROCEDURAL GUIDELINE 17-4 **SHAMPOOING HAIR OF A BED-BOUND PATIENT**

	S	U	NP	Comments
STEPS				
1. Determined no contraindications to procedure.	___	___	___	_____
2. Applied clean gloves; inspected hair and scalp.	___	___	___	_____
3. Protected bed linen with waterproof pad; properly positioned patient supine with shampoo trough under head and washbasin at end of trough.	___	___	___	_____
4. Placed rolled towel under patient's neck; draped patient's shoulders with towel.	___	___	___	_____
5. Brushed and combed patient's hair.	___	___	___	_____
6. Checked water temperature.	___	___	___	_____
7. Provided patient with towel to cover eyes during shampooing.	___	___	___	_____
8. Rinsed hair thoroughly before shampooing.	___	___	___	_____
9. Lathered hair thoroughly; worked from hairline toward back of neck to sides of head; used fingertips to massage scalp.	___	___	___	_____
10. Rinsed hair thoroughly.	___	___	___	_____
11. Applied conditioner or cream rinse as patient desired.	___	___	___	_____
12. Used bath towel to wrap patient's head and dried moisture from around eyes, face, and neck.	___	___	___	_____
13. Dried hair and scalp thoroughly.	___	___	___	_____
14. Combed hair to remove tangles and completed drying.	___	___	___	_____
15. Applied oil or conditioner if desired.	___	___	___	_____
16. Provided specific care for patient with coarse, curly hair.	___	___	___	_____
17. Brushed and styled hair with patient in comfortable position.	___	___	___	_____
18. Returned equipment to its proper place, disposed of soiled linen, and performed hand hygiene.	___	___	___	_____

Student _____   Date _____

Instructor _____   Date _____

PERFORMANCE CHECKLIST PROCEDURAL GUIDELINE 17-5 **SHAMPOOING HAIR USING A DISPOSABLE SHAMPOO PRODUCT**

	S	U	NP	Comments
STEPS				
1. Explained procedure to the patient.	___	___	___	_____
2. Positioned patient comfortably.	___	___	___	_____
3. Performed hand hygiene.	___	___	___	_____
4. Combed hair to remove tangles.	___	___	___	_____
5. Applied product cap to patient head, tucking all hair into cap.	___	___	___	_____
6. Massaged head thoroughly through cap, per product directions.	___	___	___	_____
7. Discarded cap into the trash.	___	___	___	_____
8. Towel-dried hair as requested.	___	___	___	_____
9. Brushed patient's hair to smooth.	___	___	___	_____
10. Performed hand hygiene.	___	___	___	_____

Student _____ Date _____

Instructor _____ Date _____

PERFORMANCE CHECKLIST SKILL 17-5 **PERFORMING NAIL AND FOOT CARE**

	S	U	NP	Comments

ASSESSMENT

1. Inspected all surfaces of hands, feet, and nails. ___ ___ ___ _____

2. Assessed circulatory status of toes, feet, and fingers. ___ ___ ___ _____

3. Observed patient's gait and determined relationship to local foot or nail problems. ___ ___ ___ _____

4. Assessed female patient's use of nail polish or polish removal. ___ ___ ___ _____

5. Assessed type of footwear worn by patient. ___ ___ ___ _____

6. Identified patient's risk for foot or nail problems. ___ ___ ___ _____

7. Assessed patient's use of home remedies for foot problems. ___ ___ ___ _____

8. Assessed patient's ability to perform foot and nail care. ___ ___ ___ _____

9. Assessed patient's knowledge of foot and nail care practices. ___ ___ ___ _____

NURSING DIAGNOSIS

1. Developed appropriate nursing diagnoses based on assessment data. ___ ___ ___ _____

PLANNING

1. Identified expected outcomes. ___ ___ ___ _____

2. Explained procedure to patient. ___ ___ ___ _____

3. Obtained physician's order to cut nails, if required by agency policy. ___ ___ ___ _____

IMPLEMENTATION

1. Performed hand hygiene and arranged supplies on over-bed table. ___ ___ ___ _____

2. Closed room door or curtain for privacy. ___ ___ ___ _____

3. Assisted patient to chair (when possible); placed bath mat under patient's feet. ___ ___ ___ _____

4. Prepared washbasin with water; tested water temperature. ___ ___ ___ _____

5. Placed washbasin on bath mat on floor and helped patient place feet in basin; put call light within reach, unless contraindicated. ___ ___ ___ _____

	S	U	NP	Comments
6. Adjusted over-bed table to low position and placed it over patient's lap.	——	——	——	————————
7. Filled emesis basin with water and tested temperature; placed emesis basin on over-bed table.	——	——	——	————————
8. Instructed patient to position fingertips in basin, with arms in comfortable position, unless contraindicated.	——	——	——	————————
9. Instructed patient to soak hands and feet (unless contraindicated) for 10 minutes.	——	——	——	————————
10. Cleaned debris from under fingernails while fingers were immersed; removed emesis basin and dried fingers thoroughly.	——	——	——	————————
11. Filed fingernails straight across and even with top of fingers. See agency policy.	——	——	——	————————
12. Used soft cuticle brush to clean around cuticles and push back overgrowth.	——	——	——	————————
13. Moved over-bed table away from patient.	——	——	——	————————
14. Applied gloves before giving foot care; scrubbed calluses of feet with washcloth.	——	——	——	————————
15. Cleaned, filed, and trimmed toenails.	——	——	——	————————
16. Applied lotion to feet and hands and assisted patient back to bed and into comfortable position.	——	——	——	————————
17. Properly disposed of gloves and soiled linen, cleaned and returned equipment and supplies to proper place, performed hand hygiene.	——	——	——	————————

EVALUATION

	S	U	NP	Comments
1. Inspected nails and skin surfaces after soaking.	——	——	——	————————
2. Asked patient to explain or demonstrate nail care.	——	——	——	————————
3. Assessed patient's walk after nail care.	——	——	——	————————
4. Identified unexpected outcomes.	——	——	——	————————

RECORDING AND REPORTING

	S	U	NP	Comments
1. Recorded procedure and observations related to condition of nails and feet.	——	——	——	————————
2. Reported to nurse in charge or physician the presence of foot ulcers or other breaks.	——	——	——	————————

Student _____ Date _____

Instructor _____ Date _____

PERFORMANCE CHECKLIST PROCEDURAL GUIDELINE 17-6 **MAKING AN UNOCCUPIED BED**

	S	U	NP	Comments
STEPS				
1. Assessed potential for patient incontinence or excess drainage on linen. Applied gloves if needed.	___	___	___	_____
2. Verified patient's activity orders and assessed patient's ability to get out of bed.	___	___	___	_____
3. Lowered side rails; adjusted bed to a comfortable working height.	___	___	___	_____
4. Removed soiled linens and placed in laundry bag without shaking or fanning.	___	___	___	_____
5. Repositioned mattress toward head of bed; cleaned any moisture off mattress with appropriate disinfectant. Dried thoroughly.	___	___	___	_____
6. Applied all bottom linens on one side before moving to opposite side.	___	___	___	_____
7. Applied drawsheet as needed.	___	___	___	_____
8. Moved to opposite side of bed and smoothed bottom linens on that side.	___	___	___	_____
9. Smoothed drawsheet over bottom linens as needed.	___	___	___	_____
10. Moved to side of bed where linen was placed and applied all top linen to one side of bed at a time.	___	___	___	_____
11. Correctly made horizontal toe pleat in top sheet.	___	___	___	_____
12. Tucked in remaining portion of top sheet under foot of mattress (optional). Placed blanket correctly on bed. Placed bedspread over bed.	___	___	___	_____
13. Made cuff out of top edge of sheet, blanket, and bedspread.	___	___	___	_____
14. Made a modified mitered corner at bottom edge of mattress.	___	___	___	_____
15. Moved to opposite side of bed to complete application of top linen.	___	___	___	_____
16. Correctly applied a clean pillowcase over pillow.	___	___	___	_____

	S	U	NP	Comments

17. Placed pillow at center of head of bed; placed call light within patient's reach. Returned bed to low, comfortable height. Assisted patient into bed. ___ ___ ___ _____

18. Placed patient's personal items within easy reach. Removed and discarded supplies properly. Removed gloves and performed hand hygiene. ___ ___ ___ _____

Student _Darcy Brenneman_   Date _9/17/12_

Instructor _____   Date _____

PERFORMANCE CHECKSLIST PROCEDURAL GUIDELINE 17-7   **MAKING AN OCCUPIED BED**

	S	U	NP	Comments
STEPS				
1.) Determined if patient has been incontinent, or if excess drainage is on linen.	✓	___	___	_____
2.) Assessed restrictions affecting patient's positioning and movement during bed making.		___	___	_____
3.) Performed hand hygiene and donned gloves, if needed.		___	___	_____
4. Assembled equipment and clean linen on bedside table. Closed curtain or room door.		___	___	_____
6. Adjusted bed to comfortable working height; lowered head of bed, and removed call light.		___	___	_____
7. Loosened top linen at foot of bed.		___	___	_____
8. Removed bedspread and blanket first. Folded each into a square for reuse; otherwise, disposed of in linen bag.		___	___	_____
9. Covered patient with bath blanket and removed top sheet without exposing body parts. Discarded sheet into linen bag.		___	___	_____
10. Assisted patient to side-lying position. Elevated side rail. Checked patency of medical devices.		___	___	_____
11. Loosened bottom linen from head to foot of bed. Fan-folded soiled bottom linen and drawsheet and tucked them under patient's shoulders, back, and buttocks.	✓	___	___	_____
12. Cleaned soiled mattress with appropriate disinfectant. Dried thoroughly.		___	___	_____
13. Applied clean linen to exposed half of bed. Applied clean mattress pad (if used).		___	___	_____
14. Pulled bottom sheet down smoothly and tucked tightly under mattress. Mitered corners.		___	___	_____
15. Put drawsheet in place correctly (optional).		___	___	_____
16. Placed waterproof pad on bed, as needed.		___	___	_____
17. Assisted patient to roll slowly over linen. Raised side rail on working side and moved to other side of bed.		___	___	_____

	S	U	NP	Comments

18. Lowered side rail and loosened edges of soiled linen from underneath mattress. Pulled soiled linen from bed. — W — — — —————————

19. Discarded linen correctly into linen bag. Cleaned mattress, if necessary. — — — — —————————

20. Pulled clean linen over mattress from head to foot. — — — — —————————

21. Assisted patient in rolling to supine on bottom linens. — — — — —————————

22. Mitered top corner of bottom sheet. — — — — —————————

23. Tucked all bottom linens under mattress. — — — — —————————

24. Smoothed fan-folded drawsheet and tucked under mattress. — — — — —————————

25. Placed top sheet over patient and unfolded from head to foot. Made horizontal pleat at foot.

26. Removed bath blanket and discarded it into linen bag. — — — — —————————

27. Placed blanket correctly on bed. — W — — — —————————

28. Placed bedspread correctly on bed. — — — — —————————

29. Made cuff out of top edge of sheet, blanket, and bedspread.

30. Tucked top sheet, blanket, and spread under mattress.

31. Made modified mitered corner with top sheet, blanket, and spread at bottom corner. — — — — —————————

32. Raised side rail. Made other side of bed. — — — — —————————

33. Applied clean pillowcase to pillow. Repositioned pillow under patient's head. — — — — —————————

34. Placed call light within patient's reach and returned bed to comfortable position. Opened room curtains, and placed patient's personal items within easy reach. Returned bed to a safe, comfortable height. — — — — —————————

35. Discarded linen bag properly. Removed gloves and performed hand hygiene. — — — — —————————

PT: Kyla VanDerWeele

Student _____ Date _____

Instructor _____ Date _____

PERFORMANCE CHECKLIST FOR SKILL 18-1 **RISK ASSESSMENT, SKIN ASSESSMENT, AND PREVENTION STRATEGIES**

	S	U	NP	Comments

ASSESSMENT

1. Identified patient's risk for pressure ulcer formation.

2. Selected risk assessment tool.

3. Performed and repeated risk assessment.

4. Obtained patient's "Risk Score."

5. Assessed condition of patient's skin, particularly over potential pressure sites.

6. Observed patient for preferred positions when in bed or chair.

7. Assessed patient's ability to initiate and assist with position changes.

8. Assessed patient and caregiver understanding of risk for development of pressure ulcers.

NURSING DIAGNOSIS

1. Developed appropriate nursing diagnoses based on assessment data.

PLANNING

1. Identified expected outcomes.

2. Explained procedure(s) and purpose to patient and family.

3. Performed hand hygiene and prepared needed equipment and supplies.

IMPLEMENTATION

1. Implemented recommendations for prevention and management of pressure ulcers.

2. Provided for patient's privacy.

3. Applied clean gloves.

4. Assisted patient to change position.

5. Assessed for redness in area that was under pressure. Palpated areas of discoloration or mottling.

6. Did not massage areas of redness or discoloration.

	S	U	NP	Comments

7. Kept head of bed at 30 degrees or lower when positioning patient in bed. ____ ____ ____ _____

8. Removed gloves and disposed of them properly. Performed hand hygiene. ____ ____ ____ _____

EVALUATION

1. Assessed condition of skin areas at risk for change in color and texture. ____ ____ ____ _____

2. Assessed patient's tolerance of position changes. ____ ____ ____ _____

3. Compared subsequent risk assessment scores. ____ ____ ____ _____

4. Identified unexpected outcomes. ____ ____ ____ _____

RECORDING AND REPORTING

1. Recorded patient's risk score. ____ ____ ____ _____

2. Recorded appearance of skin area under pressure. ____ ____ ____ _____

3. Recorded positions, turning intervals, and other preventive measures. ____ ____ ____ _____

4. Reported need for additional consultations for the high-risk patient. ____ ____ ____ _____

Student _____ Date _____

Instructor _____ Date _____

PERFORMANCE CHECKLIST SKILL 18-2 **TREATMENT OF PRESSURE ULCERS**

	S	U	NP	Comments

ASSESSMENT

1. Assessed patient's level of comfort and need for pain medication. ___ ___ ___ _____

2. Determined presence of allergies to topical agents. ___ ___ ___ _____

3. Reviewed physician's order for topical agent or dressing. ___ ___ ___ _____

4. Performed hand hygiene and applied clean gloves; provided privacy. ___ ___ ___ _____

5. Positioned patient to allow dressing removal. ___ ___ ___ _____

6. Assessed pressure ulcer and surrounding skin to determine stage and color of pressure ulcer. ___ ___ ___ _____

7. Assessed tissue in wound bed. ___ ___ ___ _____

8. Used tool for wound assessment. ___ ___ ___ _____

9. Removed gloves and disposed of them properly. Performed hand hygiene. ___ ___ ___ _____

8. Performed a general assessment of patient. ___ ___ ___ _____

9. Assessed patient's and support persons' understanding of pressure ulcer characteristics and purpose of treatment. ___ ___ ___ _____

NURSING DIAGNOSIS

1. Developed appropriate nursing diagnoses based on assessment data. ___ ___ ___ _____

PLANNING

1. Identified expected outcomes. ___ ___ ___ _____

2. Promoted nutritional needs. ___ ___ ___ _____

3. Protected patient's overall skin. ___ ___ ___ _____

4. Explained procedure and its purpose to patient and family. ___ ___ ___ _____

5. Prepared necessary equipment and supplies. Selected appropriate dressing. ___ ___ ___ _____

IMPLEMENTATION

1. Assembled needed supplies at bedside. Provided privacy. Performed hand hygiene and applied gloves. Opened sterile packages and topical solution containers. ___ ___ ___ _____

	S	U	NP	Comments
2. Removed patient's bed linen and gown to expose ulcer and surrounding skin; kept remaining body parts draped.	——	——	——	_____
3. Gently cleansed skin surrounding ulcer with warm water and soap.	——	——	——	_____
4. Rinsed and dried area thoroughly.	——	——	——	_____
5. Performed hand hygiene.	——	——	——	_____
6. Changed gloves.	——	——	——	_____
7. Cleansed ulcer thoroughly with normal saline or prescribed cleansing agent.	——	——	——	_____
8. Applied topical agents if prescribed:				
a. Applied enzymes.	——	——	——	_____
b. Applied hydrogel agents.	——	——	——	_____
c. Applied calcium alginates.	——	——	——	_____
9. Repositioned patient comfortably off pressure ulcer.	——	——	——	_____
10. Disposed of soiled supplies. Removed gloves. Performed hand hygiene.	——	——	——	_____

EVALUATION

	S	U	NP	Comments
1. Inspected condition of skin surrounding pressure ulcer.	——	——	——	_____
2. Inspected ulcer and dressing. Monitored for signs and symptoms of infection.	——	——	——	_____
3. Compared subsequent ulcer measurements.	——	——	——	_____
4. Used an appropriate scale to measure healing.	——	——	——	_____
5. Identified unexpected outcomes.	——	——	——	_____

RECORDING AND REPORTING

	S	U	NP	Comments
1. Recorded appearance of ulcer.	——	——	——	_____
2. Described type of topical agent and dressing applied, including patient's response.	——	——	——	_____
3. Reported worsening of ulcer to nurse in charge or physician.	——	——	——	_____

Student _____   Date _____

Instructor _____   Date _____

PERFORMANCE CHECKLIST PROCEDURAL GUIDELINE 19-1 **EYE CARE FOR COMATOSE PATIENTS**

	S	U	NP	Comments

STEPS

1. Assessed patient's eyes for drainage, irritation, redness, and lesions.   ___ ___ ___ _____

2. Assessed for blink reflex.   ___ ___ ___ _____

3. Performed eye examination, noting symmetry of movements.   ___ ___ ___ _____

4. Explained procedure to patient and family.   ___ ___ ___ _____

5. Positioned patient supine, unless contraindicated.   ___ ___ ___ _____

6. Performed hand hygiene and applied gloves.   ___ ___ ___ _____

7. Used washcloth or cotton ball moistened in water or saline; wiped from inner canthus to outer canthus; used clean washcloth/cotton ball for each eye.   ___ ___ ___ _____

8. Instilled eye medication/lubrication as prescribed.   ___ ___ ___ _____

9. Applied and secured eye patches if absent blink reflex.   ___ ___ ___ _____

10. Discarded excess materials; removed and disposed of gloves; performed hand hygiene.   ___ ___ ___ _____

11. Removed eye patches (if used) every 4 hours and reassessed eyes.   ___ ___ ___ _____

12. Notified physician of any alterations.   ___ ___ ___ _____

Student _____   Date _____

Instructor _____   Date _____

PERFORMANCE CHECKLIST PROCEDURAL GUIDELINE 19-2 **TAKING CARE OF CONTACT LENSES**

	S	U	NP	Comments

STEPS

1. Determined if contact lenses were in place.

2. Assessed patient's ability to manipulate and hold lenses; determined length of time patient usually wears lenses and routine for cleaning and storing.

3. Assessed for eye discomfort or unusual visual signs and symptoms.

4. Reviewed patient's medication history, including OTC and herbals.

5. Explained procedure to patient

6. Assembled equipment and verified expiration date for solutions.

7. Made sure nails were short and smooth before beginning.

8. Positioned patient appropriately.

9. *Removing Lenses*

   a. Performed hand hygiene. Applied gloves and placed towel just below patient's face.

   b. Removed lenses using technique appropriate to type of lens in use.

   c. Inspected eyes for redness, pain, swelling of eyelids, discharge, and excess tearing.

10. *Cleaned and Stored Lenses*

   a. Applied 1 to 2 drops of cleaner to lens in palm of hand. Used fingertips to distribute cleansing solution over lens surfaces for 20 to 30 seconds.

   b. Rinsed lens thoroughly in recommended rinsing solution.

   c. Placed lenses in correct storage case compartment for left/right lens.

   d. Filled case with recommended solution.

   e. Secured and labeled storage case.

	S	U	NP	Comments

11. *Inserting Lenses*

   a. Performed hand hygiene and applied gloves. ___ ___ ___ _____

   b. Placed towel over patient's chest. ___ ___ ___ _____

   c. Inserted lens using appropriate technique for type of lens in use. ___ ___ ___ _____

12. Determined if lens was centered correctly. ___ ___ ___ _____

13. Instructed patient to cover other eye to see if vision is clear and comfortable. ___ ___ ___ _____

14. Repeated steps to insert lens in other eye. ___ ___ ___ _____

15. Discarded soiled supplies, rinsed storage case, allowed to air dry, and performed hand hygiene. ___ ___ ___ _____

16. Asked if lenses felt comfortable. ___ ___ ___ _____

17. Identified unexpected outcomes. ___ ___ ___ _____

Student _____ Date _____

Instructor _____ Date _____

PERFORMANCE CHECKLIST PROCEDURAL GUIDELINE 19-3 **TAKING CARE OF AN ARTIFICIAL EYE**

	S	U	NP	Comments
STEPS				
1. Determined which eye is artificial.	___	___	___	_____
2. Assessed patient's routines for prosthesis care.	___	___	___	_____
3. Assessed patient's ability to remove, clean, and replace prosthesis.	___	___	___	_____
4. Inspected condition of eyelids and eye socket before and after removing prosthesis.	___	___	___	_____
5. Discussed procedure with patient.	___	___	___	_____
6. Assembled supplies at bedside.	___	___	___	_____
7. *Removing Prosthesis*				
a. Positioned patient appropriately. Provided privacy.	___	___	___	_____
b. Performed hand hygiene. Applied gloves.	___	___	___	_____
c. Placed towel below patient's face.	___	___	___	_____
d. Retracted lower eyelid against lower orbital ridge.	___	___	___	_____
e. Exerted slight pressure below eyelid to loosen prosthesis.	___	___	___	_____
f. Removed prosthesis and placed in palm of hand.	___	___	___	_____
g. Noted presence and position of colored dot at margin of prosthesis.	___	___	___	_____
h. Cleaned prosthesis with mild soap and water or normal saline.	___	___	___	_____
i. Inspected condition of prosthesis.	___	___	___	_____
j. Stored prosthesis in labeled container when not used.	___	___	___	_____
8. *Cleaned Eyelid Margins and Socket*				
a. Washed and rinsed eyelid margins with mild soap and water. Wiped from inner to outer canthus, using clean section of cloth with each wipe.	___	___	___	_____
b. Retracted upper and lower eyelid margins with thumb and index finger.	___	___	___	_____

	S	U	NP	Comments
c. Gently irrigated socket with sterile saline. Noted presence of discharge or odor.	___	___	___	_____
d. Removed excess moisture with gauze pads.	___	___	___	_____

9. *Inserting Prosthesis*

	S	U	NP	Comments
a. Moistened prosthesis in water or sterile saline.	___	___	___	_____
b. Retracted upper eyelid with index finger or thumb of nondominant hand.	___	___	___	_____
c. Held prosthesis with dominant hand so that iris faced outward and colored dot was properly oriented.	___	___	___	_____
d. Gently slid prosthesis up under upper eyelid and then pushed down lower lid to allow prosthesis to slip into place.	___	___	___	_____
e. Asked patient if prosthesis felt comfortable.	___	___	___	_____

	S	U	NP	Comments
10. Inspected eyelids and sockets for signs of infection, excessive tearing, discharge, itching, or lashes turned toward the prosthesis.	___	___	___	_____
11. Observed patient performing procedure.	___	___	___	_____
12. Instructed patient to inspect eye socket, eye prosthesis for integrity and to report any changes to health care provider.	___	___	___	_____

PERFORMANCE CHECKLIST SKILL 19-1 **EYE IRRIGATION**

	S	U	NP	Comments
ASSESSMENT				
1. Reviewed physician's order.	___	___	___	_____
2. Assessed reason for eye irrigation.	___	___	___	_____
3. Performed a complete eye examination.	___	___	___	_____
4. Established baseline pain level.	___	___	___	_____
5. Assessed patient's ability to cooperate.	___	___	___	_____
NURSING DIAGNOSIS				
1. Developed appropriate nursing diagnoses based on assessment data.	___	___	___	_____
PLANNING				
1. Identified expected outcomes.	___	___	___	_____
2. Discussed procedure with patient.	___	___	___	_____
3. Checked accuracy and completeness of MAR; compared label of eye irrigation solution versus MAR.	___	___	___	_____
4. Checked patient's identification by reading bracelet and asking for name and birth date.	___	___	___	_____
5. Assembled supplies at patient bedside.	___	___	___	_____
6. Assisted patient to side-lying position on side of affected eye or supine position for bilateral irrigation.	___	___	___	_____
IMPLEMENTATION				
1. Performed hand hygiene. Applied gloves.	___	___	___	_____
2. Removed any contact lens if present.	___	___	___	_____
3. Placed towel just below patient's face and emesis basin just below patient's cheek.	___	___	___	_____
4. Cleaned visible secretions or foreign material from eyelids and lashes, wiping from inner to outer canthus.	___	___	___	_____
5. Gently retracted eyelids. Held open by applying pressure to orbit, not to eyeball.	___	___	___	_____
6. Held solution-filled bulb, dropper, or tubing approximately 1 inch (2.5 cm) from inner canthus.	___	___	___	_____

	S	U	NP	Comments

7. Asked patient to look toward brow. Gently irrigated with a steady stream toward the lower conjunctival sac.

8. Reinforced the importance of the procedure and encouraged patient using calm, confident, soft voice.

9. Allowed patient to blink periodically.

10. Continued for prescribed volume and/or time or until secretions cleared.

11. Blotted excess moisture from eyelids and face with gauze or towel.

12. Disposed of soiled supplies, removed gloves, and performed hand hygiene.

EVALUATION

1. Observed for verbal and nonverbal signs of anxiety during irrigation.

2. Assessed patient's comfort level after irrigation.

3. Inspected eye for movement, reaction to light, and accommodation.

4. Asked patient if vision is clear.

5. Identified unexpected outcomes.

RECORDING AND REPORTING

1. Recorded condition of eye, type and amount of irrigation solution, duration of irrigation, and patient's report of pain and visual symptoms.

2. Reported continuing symptoms of pain or blurred vision.

Student _____ Date _____

Instructor _____ Date _____

PERFORMANCE CHECKLIST SKILL 19-2 **EAR IRRIGATIONS**

	S	U	NP	Comments

ASSESSMENT

1. Reviewed physician's order, including solution to be instilled and affected ear(s). ___ ___ ___ _____

2. Reviewed medical record and inspected pinna and external auditory structures for redness, swelling, drainage, abrasions, and presence of cerumen and foreign objects. Cleared ear canal as needed. ___ ___ ___ _____

3. Asked if patient was experiencing discomfort. ___ ___ ___ _____

4. Explained procedure to patient. ___ ___ ___ _____

NURSING DIAGNOSIS

1. Developed appropriate nursing diagnoses based on assessment data. ___ ___ ___ _____

PLANNING

1. Identified expected outcomes. ___ ___ ___ _____

2. Checked accuracy and completeness of MAR; compared label of irrigation solution versus MAT. ___ ___ ___ _____

3. Checked patient's identification; asked for name and birth date. ___ ___ ___ _____

4. Instilled a few drops of mineral oil or softener into ear twice a day for several days before irrigation, if needed. ___ ___ ___ _____

5. Explained procedure to patient. ___ ___ ___ _____

IMPLEMENTATION

1. Performed hand hygiene; arranged supplies at bedside; applied gloves. ___ ___ ___ _____

2. Provided for patient privacy. ___ ___ ___ _____

3. Assisted patient to an appropriate position; placed towel under patient's head and shoulders; placed emesis basin under ear to be irrigated. ___ ___ ___ _____

4. Poured irrigation solution into basin. ___ ___ ___ _____

5. Gently cleaned auricle and outer ear canal with moistened cotton applicator. ___ ___ ___ _____

6. Filled irrigating syringe with appropriate amount of solution. ___ ___ ___ _____

	S	U	NP	Comments

7. Gently pulled pinna in correct direction for age of patient.

8. Instilled irrigation solution slowly into ear canal. Kept tip of syringe from occluding ear canal. Continued until canal was cleansed or solution was used completely.

9. Dried outer ear canal with cotton ball. Left cotton loosely in place for 5 to 10 minutes.

10. Assisted patient into sitting position.

11. Removed gloves, disposed of supplies, and performed hand hygiene.

EVALUATION

1. Asked patient if there was discomfort during procedure.

2. Asked patient about sensations of dizziness or light-headedness.

3. Reinspected condition of exterior structure of ear and canal.

4. Measured patient's hearing acuity.

5. Reviewed with patient purpose of procedure and proper ear care.

6. Noted any unexpected outcomes.

RECORDING AND REPORTING

1. Recorded in nurses' notes and/or MAR procedure, amount of instillation, time of administration, and ear receiving irrigation.

2. Recorded appearance of external ear and level of hearing acuity.

3. Recorded unexpected findings to nurse in charge or physician.

Student _____   Date _____

Instructor _____   Date _____

PERFORMANCE CHECKLIST SKILL 19-3 **CARE OF HEARING AIDS**

	S	U	NP	Comments

ASSESSMENT

1. Determined whether patient can hear clearly with use of aid.   ___ ___ ___ _____

2. Determined if patient is able to manipulate and hold hearing aid.   ___ ___ ___ _____

3. Assessed patient's knowledge of and routines for cleaning and caring for hearing aid.   ___ ___ ___ _____

4. Assessed patient for any unusual physical or auditory signs/symptoms.   ___ ___ ___ _____

5. Assessed patient for perceived ability to deal with social situations and events.   ___ ___ ___ _____

NURSING DIAGNOSIS

1. Developed appropriate nursing diagnoses based on assessment data.   ___ ___ ___ _____

PLANNING

1. Identified expected outcomes.   ___ ___ ___ _____

2. Discussed procedure with patient. Explained all steps before removing aid.   ___ ___ ___ _____

3. Assembled supplies at bedside. Placed towel over work area.   ___ ___ ___ _____

4. Had patient assume supine, side-lying, or sitting position in bed or chair.   ___ ___ ___ _____

IMPLEMENTATION

1. *Removing and Cleaning Hearing Aid*

   a. Performed hand hygiene. Applied clean gloves if needed.   ___ ___ ___ _____

   b. Determined type of hearing aid and proper handling. Turned hearing aid volume off if indicated. Grasped aid securely and gently removed device along natural ear contour.   ___ ___ ___ _____

   c. Held aid over towel and wiped exterior to remove cerumen.   ___ ___ ___ _____

   d. Inspected all openings in aid for accumulated cerumen. Carefully removed cerumen with wax loop or other device supplied with the hearing aid.   ___ ___ ___ _____

   e. Inspected ear mold for rough edges.   ___ ___ ___ _____

	S	U	NP	Comments

f. Opened battery door and placed hearing aid in labeled storage container.

    ——— ——— ——— ————————————

g. Repeated Steps d. through f. for other aid.

    ——— ——— ——— ————————————

h. Assessed ear for redness, tenderness, discharge, and odor.

    ——— ——— ——— ————————————

i. Provided ear hygiene and skin care.

    ——— ——— ——— ————————————

j. Disposed of towel; removed gloves and performed hand hygiene.

    ——— ——— ——— ————————————

2. *Inserting Hearing Aid*

a. Performed hand hygiene and applied clean gloves, if needed.

    ——— ——— ——— ————————————

b. Removed hearing aid from storage case and checked/replaced battery.

    ——— ——— ——— ————————————

c. Turned aid off and volume control down.

    ——— ——— ——— ————————————

d. Identified hearing aid as right or left.

    ——— ——— ——— ————————————

e. Held aid correctly to prepare for insertion into ear. Followed natural ear contour and guided aid into place.

    ——— ——— ——— ————————————

f. Anchored any separate pieces.

    ——— ——— ——— ————————————

g. Adjusted volume to comfortable level.

    ——— ——— ——— ————————————

h. Closed and stored case. Removed gloves, if worn, and performed hand hygiene.

    ——— ——— ——— ————————————

EVALUATION

1. Assessed patient's comfort level after removal or insertion.

    ——— ——— ——— ————————————

2. Determined patient's ability to hear with aid in place.

    ——— ——— ——— ————————————

3. Observed patient performing insertion, removal, and cleaning.

    ——— ——— ——— ————————————

4. Identified unexpected outcomes.

    ——— ——— ——— ————————————

RECORDING AND REPORTING

1. Documented removal and storage of aid.

    ——— ——— ——— ————————————

2. Recorded and reported to staff any indications of infection or injury, decreased hearing acuity, and communication problems.

    ——— ——— ——— ————————————

Student __Darcy Brenneman__   Date __10/12/12__

Instructor __PBecker RN__   Date

PERFORMANCE CHECKLIST SKILL 21-1   **ADMINISTERING ORAL MEDICATIONS**

	S	U	NP	Comments

ASSESSMENT

1. Assessed whether oral medications should be contraindicated for patient.

2. Assessed risk for aspiration.

3. Assessed historical data for medication, allergies, diet, and current use.

4. Reviewed assessment and laboratory data.

5. Assessed extent of patient's knowledge regarding health status and medications.

6. Assessed patient's fluid preference and any interaction with prescribed medications.

7. Determined if medication can be given with preferred fluid.

8. Checked accuracy and completeness of MAR versus prescriber's order. Clarified incomplete or unclear orders.

9. Recopied or reprinted parts of MAR that were illegible.

NURSING DIAGNOSIS

1. Developed appropriate nursing diagnoses based on assessment data.

PLANNING

1. Identified expected outcomes.

2. Identified patient.

3. Explained procedure.

IMPLEMENTATION

1. *Prepared Medications*

    a. Performed hand hygiene.

    b. Arranged supplies.

    c. Unlocked medicine drawer/cart or accessed automated system.

    d. Prepared medications for one patient at a time.

	S	U	NP	Comments

e. Compared drug label versus MAR or form when selecting medication from supply or unit dose drawer. _____ _____ _____ _____

f. Calculated dosage correctly and double-checked. _____ _____ _____ _____

g. Prepared solid tablets or capsules in medicine cup correctly. Left unit doses in wrappers. _____ _____ _____ _____

h. Properly identified tablets to be cut. _____ _____ _____ _____

i. Applied gloves. _____ _____ _____ _____

j. Correctly prepared tablets with pill-crushing device if patient had difficulty swallowing. _____ _____ _____ _____

k. Correctly poured liquid medication without contaminating bottle cap or soiling bottle label.

(1) Gently shook container. If medication was in a multidose bottle, removed bottle cap from multidose bottle and placed cap upside down on work surface. _____ _____ _____ _____

(2) Held bottle with label against palm of hand while pouring. _____ _____ _____ _____

(3) Placed medication cup at eye level and filled to desired level on scale. _____ _____ _____ _____

(4) Poured the desired volume of liquid so that base of meniscus was level with line on scale. _____ _____ _____ _____

(5) Discarded any excess liquid into sink. Wiped lip and neck of bottle with paper towel and recapped the bottle. _____ _____ _____ _____

(6) Drew small amounts of liquid into a calibrated oral syringe, if available. Did not use a hypodermic syringe or a syringe with a needle or syringe cap. _____ _____ _____ _____

l. Checked expiration date on all medications. _____ _____ _____ _____

m. Checked previous controlled substance count and compared with previous count before preparing medication. _____ _____ _____ _____

n. Compared MAR with prepared drugs. _____ _____ _____ _____

o. Labeled medication with patient's name. Did not leave drugs unattended. _____ _____ _____ _____

2. *Administered Medications*

a. Properly identified patient. Administered at correct time. _____ _____ _____ _____

b. Explained purpose and action of each medicine. Discussed potential side effects and action to be taken. _____ _____ _____ _____

c. Assisted patient to a sitting position, unless contraindicated. Assessed gag reflex.

   (1) For *tablets:* Allowed patient, if able, to hold solid medications in hand or cup before placing in mouth. Offered water or juice to help patient swallow medications.

   (2) For *sublingually* administered medications: Had patient place medication under tongue and allow it to dissolve completely. Cautioned patient against swallowing tablet.

   (3) For *buccally* administered medications: Had patient place medication in mouth against mucous membranes until it dissolved.

d. Cautioned patient against chewing or swallowing lozenges.

e. For *powdered* medications: Mixed with liquids at bedside and gave to patient to drink.

f. Gave effervescent powders and tablets immediately after dissolving.

g. Assisted patient as needed with placing medication in mouth.

h. If tablet fell, discarded it and repeated procedure.

i. Remained with patient and confirmed that medication had been taken.

j. Offered snack after administration of highly acidic medications.

k. Assisted patient in returning to comfortable position.

l. Disposed of soiled supplies and performed hand hygiene.

3. *Recorded Medication Administration*

a. Returned MAR or forms to appropriate place.

EVALUATION

1. Evaluated patient's response to medications in a timely manner after administration.

2. Determined patient's or family member's level of knowledge gained about the medication.

3. Identified unexpected outcomes.

	S	U	NP	Comments

RECORDING AND REPORTING

1. Accurately recorded medications in medication record.
2. Recorded and reported if drug was withheld.
3. Reported unexpected findings to nurse in charge or physician.

PE: Kyla VanderWeele

PERFORMANCE CHECKLIST SKILL 21-2 **ADMINISTERING MEDICATIONS BY NASOGASTRIC TUBE**

	S	U	NP	Comments
ASSESSMENT				
1. Checked accuracy and completeness of MAR versus medication order.	___	___	___	_____
2. Assessed for contraindications to patient receiving oral medication.	___	___	___	_____
3. Assessed patient's medical history, history of allergies, medications, and diet.	___	___	___	_____
4. Reviewed assessment and laboratory data that may influence drug administration.	___	___	___	_____
5. Verified placement of nasogastric tube before administration of medications.	___	___	___	_____
NURSING DIAGNOSIS				
1. Developed appropriate nursing diagnoses based on assessment data.	___	___	___	_____
PLANNING				
1. Identified expected outcomes.	___	___	___	_____
2. Explained procedure to patient.	___	___	___	_____
IMPLEMENTATION				
1. Performed hand hygiene.	___	___	___	_____
2. Prepared medications for administration through tube. Prepared 50 to 100 mL of tepid water in graduated container. Assessed for fluid restriction.				
a. *Tablets/pills:* If applicable, used a crushing device. If not crushable, alerted the physician for a substitution.	___	___	___	_____
b. *Capsules/gelcaps:* Verified that contents can be expressed from the covering.	___	___	___	_____
3. Identified patient using two identifiers.	___	___	___	_____
4. Assisted patient to high-Fowler's position.	___	___	___	_____
5. Applied clean gloves.	___	___	___	_____
6. Verified placement of nasogastric tube.	___	___	___	_____
7. Checked for residual, noted aspirate, and returned aspirate to patient.	___	___	___	_____

	S	U	NP	Comments

8. Pinched NG tube. Drew up 30 mL of water in syringe. Reinserted syringe and flushed tube. Pinched NG tube again.

9. Removed bulb or plunger of syringe.

10. Administered first dose through syringe.

   a. Administered single dose of medication and flushed with 30 mL of water.

   b. Administered multiple medications with a 10-mL rinse with water between doses.

   c. Followed last dose of medication with 30 to 60 mL of water.

11. Clamped off and capped end of tube until next feeding.

12. Stopped continuous tube feeding for 1 hour following medication administration.

13. Assisted patient to comfortable position, with head of bed elevated for 1 hour after medication administration.

14. Removed gloves, disposed of supplies, and rinsed graduated container. Performed hand hygiene.

EVALUATION

1. Returned within 30 minutes to determine patient's response to medications or to reinstitute continuous tube feedings.

2. Identified unexpected outcomes.

RECORDING AND REPORTING

1. Recorded method used to check tube placement, volume of aspirate, and pH of aspirate (if indicated).

2. Recorded actual time of drug administration on MAR or computer printout.

3. Recorded total amount of fluid on I & O sheet.

4. Recorded and reported if drug was withheld.

5. Reported unexpected findings.

206

PERFORMANCE CHECKLIST SKILL 21-3   **ADMINISTERING SKIN APPLICATIONS**

	S	U	NP	Comments

ASSESSMENT

1. Assessed condition of patient's skin. Applied clean gloves if needed.

2. Inspected area where medication is to be applied. Cleaned skin as needed.

3. Assessed for presence of drug allergy/latex allergy.

4. Checked accuracy and completeness of MAR versus medication order.

5. Determined amount of topical agent required and directions for use.

6. Assessed patient's knowledge regarding medication therapy.

7. Assessed patient's ability to self-administer medication.

NURSING DIAGNOSIS

1. Developed appropriate nursing diagnoses based on assessment data.

PLANNING

1. Identified expected outcomes.

2. Prepared medication for application. Compared label versus MAR.

3. Identified patient correctly.

4. Explained procedure to patient.

IMPLEMENTATION

1. Performed hand hygiene. Arranged supplies at bedside and applied gloves.

2. Closed door or curtain for privacy, positioned patient comfortably, and exposed site.

3. *Topical Agent*

    a. Creams, ointments, or oil-based lotions

      (1) Softened medications by placing in gloved hand.

      (2) Spread gently over affected area.

      (3) Explained that skin may feel greasy, not to remove.

	S	U	NP	Comments

b. Antianginal ointment

(1) Measured proper dose on paper measuring guide. ___ ___ ___ _____

(2) Removed previous dose paper. Cleansed and assessed skin. ___ ___ ___ _____

(3) Applied over smooth (hairless) skin surface. Rotated sites of application. ___ ___ ___ _____

(4) Dated and initialed dose paper; noted time. ___ ___ ___ _____

(5) Secured dose paper with hypoallergenic tape. ___ ___ ___ _____

c. Transdermal patches

(1) Located and removed old patch. Cleansed area ___ ___ ___ _____

(2) Dated and initialed outer side of patch and noted time ___ ___ ___ _____

(3) Verified specific instructions for placement. ___ ___ ___ _____

(4) Removed protective covering and applied ensuring proper adherence. ___ ___ ___ _____

d. Aerosol spray

(1) Shook container vigorously. ___ ___ ___ _____

(2) Followed manufacturer's instructions for preparation and application. ___ ___ ___ _____

(3) Protected patient's airway, preventing inhalation. ___ ___ ___ _____

(4) Sprayed evenly over affected area. ___ ___ ___ _____

e. Suspension-based lotion

(1) Shook vigorously. ___ ___ ___ _____

(2) Applied evenly using a gauze dressing. ___ ___ ___ _____

(3) Explained to patient that area will feel cool and dry. ___ ___ ___ _____

f. Powder

(1) Thoroughly dried skin surface. ___ ___ ___ _____

(2) Fully exposed area and skin folds. ___ ___ ___ _____

(3) Protected patient from in haling powder. ___ ___ ___ _____

(4) Dusted area with a thin coating of medication. ___ ___ ___ _____

(5) Covered skin area with dressing when ordered. ___ ___ ___ _____

(6) Assisted patient in returning to a comfortable position after application. ___ ___ ___ _____

(7) Removed gloves and properly disposed of soiled supplies. Performed hand hygiene. ___ ___ ___ _____

	S	U	NP	Comments

EVALUATION

1. Evaluated patient's or caregiver's knowledge of prescribed medication.   ___ ___ ___ _____

2. Had patient keep a diary of dosages taken.   ___ ___ ___ _____

3. Observed patient administering medication.   ___ ___ ___ _____

4. Evaluated condition of patient's skin between applications.   ___ ___ ___ _____

5. Identified unexpected outcomes.   ___ ___ ___ _____

RECORDING AND REPORTING

1. Recorded condition of patient's skin before applying topical agent.   ___ ___ ___ _____

2. Recorded application of topical agent.   ___ ___ ___ _____

3. Recorded and reported if drug was withheld.   ___ ___ ___ _____

4. Reported any adverse effects, abnormalities of skin condition, and patient response to nurse in charge or physician.   ___ ___ ___ _____

PE: Kyra vanderwell

Student __Darcy Brenneman__   Date __10/26/12__

Instructor _____ _Kendee Rw_   Date __10/26/12__

PERFORMANCE CHECKLIST SKILL 21-4   **ADMINISTERING EYE MEDICATIONS**

	S	U	NP	Comments

ASSESSMENT

1. Reviewed accuracy and completeness of MAR with medication order.

2. Assessed condition of patient's eye.

3. Determined patient's history of allergies.

4. Assessed patient for symptoms of visual alteration.

5. Assessed patient's level of consciousness.

6. Assessed patient's knowledge regarding drug therapy.

7. Assessed patient's ability to self-administer medication.

NURSING DIAGNOSIS

1. Developed appropriate nursing diagnoses based on assessment data.

PLANNING

1. Identified expected outcomes.

2. Prepared medication for instillation.

3. Identified patient correctly.

4. Explained procedure to patient.

IMPLEMENTATION

1. Performed hand hygiene, arranged supplies at bedside, and applied clean gloves.

2. Positioned patient supine or in chair with head slightly hyperextended, unless contraindicated.

3. Washed existing crusts and drainage from eyelids before drug administration.

4. Instructed patient to look up.

5. Placed cotton ball or tissue below lower lid margin.

6. Retracted lower lid downward to expose conjunctival sac.

a. Instilled eye drops.

  (1) Placed cotton ball or tissue below lower lid margin and pressed down to expose conjunctival sac.

  (2) With dominant hand resting on patient's forehead, held filled medication eye dropper approximately 1 to 2 cm (½ to ¾ inch) above conjunctival sac.

  (3) Dropped prescribed number of medication drops into conjunctival sac.

  (4) If patient blinked or closed eye or if drops fell on outer lid margins, repeated procedure.

  (5) After instilling drops, asked patient to close eye gently.

  (6) Applied gentle pressure with a clean tissue to patient's nasolacrimal duct for 30 to 60 seconds, for drugs with a systemic effect.

b. Instilled eye ointment.

  (1) Held ointment applicator above lower lid margin, applied thin ribbon of ointment evenly along inner edge of lower eyelid on conjunctiva from the inner to outer canthus.

  (2) Had patient close eye and rub lid lightly in circular motion with cotton ball, if rubbing is not contraindicated.

c. Intraocular disk

  (1) Application

    (a) Opened package containing the disk. Gently pressed fingertip against the disk so that it adhered to the finger. Positioned the convex side of the disk on fingertip.

    (b) With other hand, gently pulled the patient's lower eyelid away from the eye. Asked patient to look up.

    (c) Placed the disk in the conjunctival sac, so that it floated on the sclera between the iris and lower eyelid.

    (d) Pulled the patient's lower eyelid out and over the disk.

212

	S	U	NP	Comments
(2) Removal				
(a) Gently pulled on the patient's lower eyelid to expose the disk.	___	___	___	_____
(b) Used forefinger and thumb of opposite hand, pinched the disk, and lifted it out of the patient's eye.	___	___	___	_____
7. Wiped away excess medication on eyelids.	KV *Jnd*	___	_____
8. Applied eye patch, when appropriate.	___	___	_____
9. Assisted patient to comfortable position.	___	___	_____
10. Disposed of soiled supplies properly. Removed gloves and performed hand hygiene.	___	✓	___	_____

EVALUATION

	S	U	NP	Comments
1. Evaluated patient's response to medication.	___	___	___	_____
2. Evaluated effects of medication by assessing for visual changes or side effects.	___	___	___	_____
3. Determined patient's level of understanding of medication.	___	___	___	_____
4. Had patient demonstrate self-administration.	___	___	___	_____
5. Identified unexpected outcomes.	___	___	___	_____

RECORDING AND REPORTING

	S	U	NP	Comments
1. Recorded medication on medication record.	___	___	___	_____
2. Recorded appearance of eye.	___	___	___	_____
3. Recorded and reported if drug was withheld.	___	___	___	_____
4. Reported any undesired effects to nurse in charge or physician.	___	___	___	_____

PE: Kyla VanDerWeele

Student Darcy Brenneman   Date 10/26/12

Instructor _Kimber D_   Date 10/26/12

PERFORMANCE CHECKLIST SKILL 21-5   **ADMINISTERING EAR DROPS**

	S	U	NP	Comments
ASSESSMENT				
1. Checked accuracy and completeness of MAR versus medication order.				
2. Assessed condition of external ear.	W			
3. Assessed patient for symptoms of ear discomfort or hearing impairment.				
4. Assessed patient's level of cooperation.				
5. Assessed patient's knowledge of drug therapy.				
6. Assessed patient's ability to self-administer medication.				
NURSING DIAGNOSIS				
1. Developed appropriate diagnoses based on assessment data.				
PLANNING				
1. Identified expected outcomes.	W			
2. Compared MAR versus order and medication label.				
3. Identified patient correctly.				
4. Explained procedure to patient.				
IMPLEMENTATION				
1. Performed hand hygiene and arranged supplies at bedside. Applied gloves if necessary.				
2. Warmed medication.				
3. Assisted patient to bedside chair or to side-lying position with ear to be treated facing up.				
4. Straightened ear canal according to patient's age.				
5. Wiped out cerumen and drainage with cotton-tipped applicator, as needed.				
6. Instilled ordered number of drops, holding dropper 1 cm (½ inch) above ear canal.				
7. With patient in side-lying position for a few minutes, applied gentle pressure to tragus.				
8. Placed cotton ball in outer ear canal, if prescribed.				

	S	U	NP	Comments

9. Removed cotton ball after 15 minutes, if pre-scribed.

10. Disposed of soiled supplies properly, removed gloves (if worn), and performed hand hygiene.

11. Assisted patient to comfortable position.

EVALUATION

1. Asked patient whether there was discomfort during instillation.

2. Evaluated condition of external ear between drug instillations.

3. Evaluated patient's hearing acuity.

4. Asked patient to explain technique for instilling ear drops.

5. Had patient demonstrate self-administration.

6. Identified unexpected outcomes.

RECORDING AND REPORTING

1. Recorded drug administration correctly on medication form.

2. Recorded condition of ear canal.

3. Reported change in patient's hearing acuity.

4. Recorded and reported if drug was withheld.

5. Reported unexpected findings to nurse in charge or physician.

PE: Kyla vanDerWeele

Student _____ Date _____

Instructor _____ Date _____

PERFORMANCE CHECKLIST SKILL 21-6 **ADMINISTERING NASAL INSTILLATIONS**

	S	U	NP	Comments
ASSESSMENT				
1. Checked accuracy and completeness of MAR versus medication record.	____	____	____	_____
2. Determined affected nasal sinus.	____	____	____	_____
3. Assessed patient's history to determine contraindication of drug.	____	____	____	_____
4. Assessed condition of nares and sinuses.	____	____	____	_____
5. Assessed patient's knowledge regarding use of nasal instillations.	____	____	____	_____
NURSING DIAGNOSIS				
1. Developed appropriate nursing diagnoses based on assessment data.	____	____	____	_____
PLANNING				
1. Identified expected outcomes.	____	____	____	_____
2. Compared MAR versus order and medication label.	____	____	____	_____
3. Identified patient correctly.	____	____	____	_____
4. Explained procedure to patient.	____	____	____	_____
IMPLEMENTATION				
1. Performed hand hygiene and arranged supplies and medications at bedside. Applied clean gloves if drainage present.	____	____	____	_____
2. Instructed patient to blow nose gently, unless contraindicated.	____	____	____	_____
3. Administered nasal medication.				
a. Nose drops				
(1) Assisted patient to supine position.	____	____	____	_____
(2) Positioned head properly to access specific nasal passages.	____	____	____	_____
(3) Supported patient's head with nondominant hand	____	____	____	_____
(4) Instructed patient to breathe through mouth.	____	____	____	_____
(5) Held dropper 1 cm (½ inch) above nares and instilled prescribed drops.	____	____	____	_____
(6) Had patient remain supine for 5 minutes.	____	____	____	_____

	S	U	NP	Comments

b. Nasal sprays

(1) Determined number of sprays to administer.

(2) Positioned patient with head tilted slightly forward.

(3) Inserted tip of spray into nostril and occluded the other. Pointed tip toward the turbinate.

(4) Instructed patient to inhale with mouth closed and sprayed into nostril.

(5) Repeated above steps for other nostril, if ordered.

(6) Offered tissue to blot runny nose, and warned against blowing nose for several minutes.

(7) Assisted patient to a comfortable position.

EVALUATION

1. Observed patient for side effects of medication.

2. Evaluated patient's ability to breathe through nose.

3. Inspected condition of nasal passages.

4. Asked patient to review knowledge regarding use of decongestant and methods of administration.

5. Had patient demonstrate self-administration.

6. Identified unexpected outcomes.

RECORDING AND REPORTING

1. Recorded medication administration correctly on medication administration record.

2. Recorded patient's response to medication.

3. Recorded and reported if drug was withheld.

4. Reported any unusual side effects to nurse in charge or physician.

Student _____ Date _____

Instructor _____ *Hynda* _____ Date *10/26/12*

PERFORMANCE CHECKLIST SKILL 21-7   **USING METERED-DOSE INHALERS**

	S	U	NP	Comments

ASSESSMENT

1. Assessed patient's respiratory status.

2. Assessed patient's readiness and ability to learn.

3. Assessed patient's knowledge of disease and drug therapy.

4. Assessed patient's ability to handle inhaler.

5. Checked accuracy and completeness of MAR versus medication order.

6. Assessed patient's technique in using inhaler (when applicable).

NURSING DIAGNOSIS

1. Developed appropriate nursing diagnoses based on assessment data.

PLANNING

1. Identified expected outcomes.

2. Prepared medication for instillation; compared medication label versus MAR.

3. Identified patient correctly.

4. Explained procedure to patient.

5. Provided adequate time for teaching.

IMPLEMENTATION

1. Performed hand hygiene and arranged equipment.

2. Provided patient opportunity to handle inhaler, canister, and spacer.

3. Explained metered dosage and problems of overuse, including side effects.

4. Explained each step in using *inhaler*.

   a. Removed mouthpiece cover.

   b. Shook inhaler well.

   c. Had patient take deep breath and exhale.

   d. Instructed patient about how to position inhaler correctly.

	S	U	NP	Comments

e. Had patient take deep breath and exhale completely.

f. Had patient hold inhaler.

g. Instructed patient to tilt head back, inhale slowly and deeply through the mouth, and depress medication canister fully.

h. Had patient breathe in slowly for 2 to 3 seconds and hold breath for 10 seconds.

i. Instructed patient to remove MDI from mouth and exhale slowly through nose or pursed lips.

5. Explained each step in using an inhaler with a *spacer device*.

a. Removed mouthpiece covers and inserted metered-dose inhaler into end of spacer device.

b. Shook inhaler well.

c. Had patient place spacer device mouthpiece in mouth and close lips tightly.

d. Instructed patient to breathe normally through spacer device mouthpiece.

e. Had patient depress medication canister, spraying one puff into spacer.

f. Instructed patient to breathe in slowly and fully for 5 seconds. Had patient hold breath for 10 seconds.

6. Instructed patient on the correct interval between inhalations.

7. Warned patient against increasing the frequency of inhalations.

8. Described common sensations after use of inhaler.

9. Instructed patient to perform oral hygiene after each use.

10. Instructed patient in technique for cleansing inhaler.

11. Asked if patient had questions.

12. Performed hand hygiene and assisted patient to comfortable position.

EVALUATION

1. Had patient demonstrate use of inhaler.

2. Asked patient to explain drug schedule.

220

	S	U	NP	Comments

3. Asked patient to explain medication side effects and criteria for calling physician.
___ ___ ___ _____

4. Assessed respirations and lung sounds after medication instillation.
___ ___ ___ _____

5. Identified unexpected outcomes.
___ ___ ___ _____

RECORDING AND REPORTING

1. Recorded description of teaching session and patient's response.
___ ___ ___ _____

2. Recorded times used and amounts. Reported if drug was withheld.
___ ___ ___ _____

3. Recorded patient assessment and response to medication.
___ ___ ___ _____

4. Reported any undesirable effects from medication.
___ ___ ___ _____

PE: Kyla VanderWeele

Student *Darcy Brenneman*   Date *10/26/12*

Instructor _____   Date _____

PERFORMANCE CHECKLIST FOR PROCEDURAL GUIDELINE 21-1   **USING DRY POWDER INHALED MEDICATIONS**

	S	U	NP	Comments
STEPS				
1. Assessed respiratory status.	___	___	___	_____
2. Assessed patient's readiness and ability to learn.	___	___	___	_____
3. Assessed patient's knowledge and understanding of disease, purpose and action of medication.	___	___	___	_____
4. Determined patient's ability to hold, manipulate, and activate inhaler.	___	___	___	_____
5. Checked accuracy and completeness of MAR versus medication order.	___	___	___	_____
6. Assessed patient's technique if previously instructed.	___	___	___	_____
7. Prepared medication and compared label on inhaler versus MAR.	___	___	___	_____
8. Correctly identified the patient.	___	___	___	_____
9. Instructed patient to place lips around mouthpiece and quickly and deeply inhale as medication is delivered.	___	___	___	_____
10. Instructed patient to hold breath for 10 seconds and exhale slowly.	___	___	___	_____
11. Return DPI to closed position or removed loaded capsule or disk.	___	___	___	_____
12. Instructed patient on oral hygiene after every treatment.	___	___	___	_____
13. Assessed for therapeutic effect.	___	___	___	_____

Student _____ Date _____

Instructor _____ Date _____

PERFORMANCE CHECKLIST SKILL 21-8 **ADMINISTERING NEBULIZED MEDICATIONS**

	S	U	NP	Comments

ASSESSMENT

1. Assessed patient's medical, medication, nutrition, and diet history.

2. Assessed patient's ability to manipulate nebulizer equipment.

3. Checked accuracy and completeness of MAR versus medication order.

4. Assessed patient's vital signs and respiratory status.

NURSING DIAGNOSIS

1. Developed appropriate nursing diagnoses based on assessment data.

PLANNING

1. Identified expected outcomes.

2. Prepared medication; compared label on medication versus MAR.

3. Identified patient correctly.

4. Explained procedure to patient.

IMPLEMENTATION

1. Performed hand hygiene and arranged equipment.

2. Explained use of nebulizer and possible side effects.

3. Assembled equipment according to the manufacturer's instructions.

4. Added prescribed medication and diluent to nebulizer.

5. Had patient hold mouthpiece between lips with gentle pressure. Used mask or special adapter, if necessary.

6. Turned on the nebulizer machine and ensured that sufficient mist formed.

7. Had patient take a slow, deep breath, pause, and then exhale passively.

8. Reminded patient to repeat breathing pattern until medication completely nebulized or as ordered.

	S	U	NP	Comments
9. Tapped nebulizer cup periodically.	___	___	___	_____
10. Monitored patient's pulse during procedure.	___	___	___	_____
11. Turned off machine and stored tubing according to agency policy.	___	___	___	_____
12. Shook nebulizer bottle to remove remaining solution. Did not rinse with tap water.	___	___	___	_____
13. Encouraged patient to rinse mouth if steroids were used.	___	___	___	_____
14. Performed hand hygiene and assisted patient to comfortable position.	___	___	___	_____

EVALUATION

	S	U	NP	Comments
1. Assessed patient's pulse, respiratory rate, and lung sounds.	___	___	___	_____
2. Had patient explain and demonstrate steps.	___	___	___	_____
3. Asked patient to explain drug schedule, side effects, and criteria for calling physician.	___	___	___	_____
4. Identified unexpected outcomes.	___	___	___	_____

RECORDING AND REPORTING

	S	U	NP	Comments
1. Recorded drug dosage and concentration, and time and date of administration.	___	___	___	_____
2. Recorded patient's response to medication and respiratory assessment.	___	___	___	_____
3. Documented instruction provided and patient's ability to perform treatment.	___	___	___	_____
4. Recorded and reported if drug was withheld.	___	___	___	_____
5. Reported adverse effects to nurse in charge or physician.	___	___	___	_____

Student _____ Date _____

Instructor _____ Date _____

PERFORMANCE CHECKLIST SKILL 21-9 **ADMINISTERING VAGINAL INSTILLATIONS**

	S	U	NP	Comments
ASSESSMENT				
1. Checked accuracy and completeness of MAR with medication order.	___	___	___	_____
2. Reviewed pertinent drug information.	___	___	___	_____
3. Asked if patient is experiencing any symptoms.	___	___	___	_____
4. Had patient void.	___	___	___	_____
5. Determined patient's ability to self-administer medication.	___	___	___	_____
6. Reviewed patient's knowledge of drug therapy.	___	___	___	_____
NURSING DIAGNOSIS				
1. Developed appropriate nursing diagnoses based on assessment data.	___	___	___	_____
PLANNING				
1. Identified expected outcomes.	___	___	___	_____
2. Compared MAR versus order and medication label.	___	___	___	_____
3. Identified patient correctly.	___	___	___	_____
4. Explained procedure to patient.	___	___	___	_____
IMPLEMENTATION				
1. Provided privacy.	___	___	___	_____
2. Performed hand hygiene, arranged supplies at bedside, and applied clean gloves.	___	___	___	_____
3. Assisted patient to dorsal recumbent position or position of comfort.	___	___	___	_____
4. Draped abdomen and lower extremities.	___	___	___	_____
5. Illuminated vaginal orifice properly.	___	___	___	_____
6. Inspected condition of external genitalia and vaginal canal.	___	___	___	_____
7. For *suppository* insertion:				
a. Removed suppository from wrapper and applied water-soluble lubricant to smooth or rounded end. Lubricated gloved index finger of dominant hand.	___	___	___	_____
b. Separated labia with nondominant gloved hand.	___	___	___	_____

	S	U	NP	Comments

c. Inserted suppository the entire length of finger along posterior wall of vaginal canal.

d. Wiped away remaining lubricant.

8. For application of *cream* or *foam:*

a. Filled applicator according to directions.

b. Separated labial folds with nondominant gloved hand.

c. Inserted applicators 5 to 7.5 cm (2 to 3 inches) and pushed on plunger to deposit medication.

d. Withdrew applicator and wiped off residual cream or foam.

9. For *irrigation* and *douche:*

a. Placed patient on bedpan with absorbent pad underneath.

b. Made sure fluid was at body temperature and primed tubing.

c. Separated labial folds and directed nozzle toward sacrum, along the floor of the vagina.

d. Raised container to 30 to 50 cm (12 to 20 inches) above the vagina. Inserted nozzle 7 to 10 cm (3 to 4 inches) and allowed solution to flow while rotating nozzle.

e. Withdrew nozzle after all solution administered. Assisted patient to comfortable sitting position.

f. Allowed patient to remain on bedpan and cleansed perineum with soap and water.

g. Assisted patient off bedpan and dried perineum.

10. Instructed patient to lie flat for at least 10 minutes after suppository, cream, or foam insertion.

11. If applicator was used, washed it with soap and water, rinsed, and stored.

12. Offered patient perineal pad.

13. Disposed of soiled supplies and equipment. Removed gloves properly and discarded. Performed hand hygiene.

	S	U	NP	Comments

EVALUATION

1. Applied clean gloves and inspected condition of vaginal canal and external genitalia between applications. ___ ___ ___ _____

2. Evaluated patient for symptoms of vaginal irritation. ___ ___ ___ _____

3. Evaluated patient's understanding of medication therapy. ___ ___ ___ _____

4. Had patient demonstrate self-administration. ___ ___ ___ _____

5. Identified unexpected outcomes. ___ ___ ___ _____

RECORDING AND REPORTING

1. Recorded medication on medication record. ___ ___ ___ _____

2. Recorded appearance of vaginal canal and genitalia and reported any unusual findings to nurse in charge or physician. ___ ___ ___ _____

3. Recorded and reported if drug was withheld. ___ ___ ___ _____

4. Reported adverse effects to nurse in charge or physician. ___ ___ ___ _____

Student _____ Date _____

Instructor _____ Date _____

PERFORMANCE CHECKLIST SKILL 21-10   **ADMINISTERING RECTAL SUPPOSITORIES**

	S	U	NP	Comments
ASSESSMENT				
1. Reviewed accuracy and completeness of MAR versus medication order.	___	___	___	_____
2. Reviewed pertinent drug information.	___	___	___	_____
3. Determined whether patient had history of rectal surgery or bleeding.	___	___	___	_____
4. Assessed for signs and symptoms of gastrointestinal alterations.	___	___	___	_____
5. Assessed patient's ability to self-administer suppository.	___	___	___	_____
6. Reviewed patient's knowledge of drug therapy.	___	___	___	_____
NURSING DIAGNOSIS				
1. Developed appropriate nursing diagnoses based on assessment data.	___	___	___	_____
PLANNING				
1. Identified expected outcomes.	___	___	___	_____
2. Compared MAR versus order and medication label.	___	___	___	_____
3. Identified patient correctly.	___	___	___	_____
4. Explained procedure to patient.	___	___	___	_____
IMPLEMENTATION				
1. Provided privacy.	___	___	___	_____
2. Performed hand hygiene. Arranged supplies at bedside and applied gloves.	___	___	___	_____
3. Assisted patient to side-lying Sims' position with upper leg flexed; applied clean gloves.	___	___	___	_____
4. Kept patient properly draped.	___	___	___	_____
5. Examined condition of anus externally and palpated rectal wall as needed; disposed of gloves properly.	___	___	___	_____
6. Applied new gloves.	___	___	___	_____
7. Removed suppository from wrapper and lubricated rounded end of suppository and gloved finger.	___	___	___	_____

	S	U	NP	Comments

8. Instructed patient to breathe slowly through mouth and relax anal sphincter. ___ ___ ___ _____

9. Retracted buttocks and inserted suppository gently through anus for proper distance. ___ ___ ___ _____

10. Removed finger and cleaned excess lubricant from anal area. ___ ___ ___ _____

11. Properly disposed of gloves and soiled supplies. Performed hand hygiene. ___ ___ ___ _____

12. Asked patient to remain flat or on side for 5 minutes. ___ ___ ___ _____

13. Placed call light within patient's reach after administration of laxative or stool softener. ___ ___ ___ _____

14. Asked patient not to flush toilet if suppository is given for constipation. ___ ___ ___ _____

EVALUATION

1. Determined after 5 minutes whether suppository was expelled prematurely. ___ ___ ___ _____

2. Determined whether there was any discomfort during insertion. ___ ___ ___ _____

3. Evaluated effect of medication. ___ ___ ___ _____

4. Determined patient's understanding of purpose of medication. ___ ___ ___ _____

5. Had patient demonstrate self-administration. ___ ___ ___ _____

6. Identified unexpected outcomes. ___ ___ ___ _____

RECORDING AND REPORTING

1. Recorded medication correctly on medication record. ___ ___ ___ _____

2. Recorded and reported patient's response to medication and if drug was withheld. ___ ___ ___ _____

3. Reported unexpected reactions to nurse in charge or physician. ___ ___ ___ _____

Student __Darcy Brenneman__   Date __10/24/12__

Instructor _____   Date __10/25/12__

PERFORMANCE CHECKLIST SKILL 22-1   **PREPARING INJECTIONS FROM AMPULES AND VIALS**

	S	U	NP	Comments
ASSESSMENT				
1. Checked accuracy of MAR versus prescriber's medication order.				
2. Assessed patient's medical history and medication history.				
3. Assessed patient's allergy history.				
4. Reviewed medication reference information before administering medication.				
5. Assessed patient's body build, muscle size, and weight.				
PLANNING				
1. Identified expected outcomes.				
IMPLEMENTATION				
1. Performed hand hygiene and prepared supplies.				
2. Checked expiration date on medication label.				
3. Prepared medications for one patient at a time.				
4. *Preparing an Ampule*				
a. Tapped top of ampule to dislodge fluid in neck.				
b. Placed gauze pad around ampule neck.				
c. Snapped neck of ampule away from hands.				
d. Drew up medication quickly with a filter needle.				
e. Inserted filter needle through opening in center of ampule, while holding ampule on a flat surface or upside down.				
f. Aspirated medication into syringe.				
g. Kept needle tip below fluid level.				
h. Did not expel air into ampule.				
i. Expelled air from syringe correctly.				

	S	U	NP	Comments

j. Correctly expelled excess fluid within syringe into sink. ___ ___ ___ _____

k. Covered needle with sheath or cap after preparation and replaced filter needle with appropriate-size needle. ___ ___ ___ _____

5. *Preparing a Vial Containing a Solution*

a. Removed cap from vial to expose rubber seal. Wiped off surface of seal with alcohol swab and allowed to dry if a multidose vial was used. ___ ___ ___ _____

b. Drew up air in syringe equivalent to volume of medication desired. ___ ___ ___ _____

c. Inserted needle tip, bevel up, or needleless access device through center of rubber seal. ___ ___ ___ _____

d. Injected air into airspace of vial while holding on to plunger. ___ ___ ___ _____

e. With vial inverted, held vial and syringe properly. ___ ___ ___ _____

f. Kept needle tip in the fluid while withdrawing. ___ ___ ___ _____

g. Allowed air pressure to fill syringe with fluid. ___ ___ ___ _____

h. Correctly dislodged and expelled air that accumulated in syringe barrel. ___ ___ ___ _____

i. Removed needle/needleless access device from vial. ___ ___ ___ _____

j. Correctly expelled any remaining air in syringe barrel. ___ ___ ___ _____

k. Changed filter needle or needleless access device to correct needle for injection and placed cover on syringe. ___ ___ ___ _____

l. Labeled multidose vial with date of mixing, drug concentration, and nurse's initials. ___ ___ ___ _____

6. *Vial Containing a Powder (reconstituting medications)*

a. Removed cap covering vial containing powder and vial containing diluent. Wiped surfaces of seals with alcohol and allowed to dry. ___ ___ ___ _____

b. Drew up diluent according to manufacturer's instructions. ___ ___ ___ _____

234

	S	U	NP	Comments

c. Correctly injected diluent into vial with powder. Removed needle or access device.

d. Mixed medication thoroughly. Rolled vial to mix.

e. Prepared to draw correct dosage of reconstituted solution into new syringe. Compared label with MAR.

f. Drew up reconstituted medication in syringe.

7. Compared medication label with MAR.

8. Verified reconstitution with second nurse per agency policy.

9. Disposed of soiled supplies properly. Performed hand hygiene.

EVALUATION

1. Compared MAR versus label of prepared drug.

2. Checked dosage level in syringe.

3. Identified unexpected outcomes.

PE: Kyla VanDerWeen   10/24/12

Student _____ Date _____

Instructor _____ Date _____

PERFORMANCE CHECKLIST PROCEDURAL GUIDELINE 22-1 **MIXING PARENTERAL MEDICATIONS IN ONE SYRINGE**

STEPS	S	U	NP	Comments
1. Checked accuracy and completeness of MAR versus medication order.	____	____	____	_____
2. Reviewed medication reference information.	____	____	____	_____
3. Assessed patient's body build, muscle size, and weight.	____	____	____	_____
4. Considered medications to be mixed, compatibility, and type of injection.	____	____	____	_____
5. Performed hand hygiene.	____	____	____	_____
6. Checked expiration date of medication.	____	____	____	_____
7. Prepared medication for one patient at a time.	____	____	____	_____
8. *Mixing Medication From Two Vials*				
a. Took syringe and aspirated volume of air equal to first medication's dosage (vial A).	____	____	____	_____
b. Injected air into vial A without allowing filter needle or access device to touch solution.	____	____	____	_____
c. Withdrew filter needle or needleless vial access device and syringe and aspirated air equal to second medication's dosage (vial B).	____	____	____	_____
d. Inserted needle or access device into vial B, injected air, and filled syringe with proper volume of medication from vial.	____	____	____	_____
e. Withdrew needle/access device and syringe from vial and checked dose.	____	____	____	_____
f. Determined point on syringe scale for correct dosage of combined medications.	____	____	____	_____
g. Inserted filter needle/access device into vial A and allowed solution to fill syringe to desired level.	____	____	____	_____
h. Withdrew needle/access device and expelled excess air. Checked fluid level in syringe.	____	____	____	_____
i. Replaced filter needle or needleless access device with appropriate-size needle for injection.	____	____	____	_____

	S	U	NP	Comments

9. *Mixing Insulin*

a. Appropriately chose insulin vial and rolled between the hands to resuspend insulin, if needed.

b. Wiped off tops of insulin vials and allowed to dry.

c. Verified insulin dose against MAR a second time.

d. Took insulin syringe and aspirated volume of air equal to dosage to be withdrawn from intermediate or long acting.

e. Injected air into vial of intermediate or long acting without needle touching solution.

f. Withdrew needle and syringe from vial without aspirating medication.

g. Inserted needle into vial of rapid or short-acting insulin, and withdrew the correct dose.

h. Withdrew needle and syringe from vial and checked dose. Removed air bubbles as needed.

i. Verified insulin dose with MAR a third time. Had second nurse verify dose as per agency policy.

j. Inserted needle into vial of intermediate or long acting, and correctly withdrew desired amount of insulin.

k. Withdrew needle and checked fluid level in syringe. Capped until administration.

10. *Mixing Medications From a Vial and an Ampule*

a. Prepared medication from vial first.

b. Determined point on syringe scale where combined medication should measure.

c. Prepared medication from ampule.

d. Withdrew filter needle from ampule and verified fluid level in syringe. Changed filter needle to appropriate needle gauge or needleless access device for administration. Kept needle or access device sheathed or capped until administration.

238

	S	U	NP	Comments
11. Compared MAR versus prepared medication and labels from vials/ampules.	___	___	___	_____
12. Disposed of soiled supplies properly.	___	___	___	_____
13. Cleaned work area and performed hand hygiene.	___	___	___	_____
14. Checked syringe for total combined dose of medication.	___	___	___	_____
15. Performed final check of medication labels versus MAR at patient's bedside.	___	___	___	_____

Student _Darcy Brenneman_ Date _11/2/12_

Instructor _Kendall_ Date _11/2/12_

PERFORMANCE CHECKLIST SKILL 22-2 **ADMINISTERING INTRADERMAL INJECTIONS**

	S	U	NP	Comments
ASSESSMENT				
1. Checked accuracy of MAR or computer print-out versus medication order.				
2. Reviewed drug reference information.				
3. Assessed patient's history of allergies.				
4. Assessed patient's knowledge regarding procedure.				
NURSING DIAGNOSIS				
1. Developed appropriate nursing diagnoses based on assessment data.				
PLANNING				
1. Identified expected outcomes.				
IMPLEMENTATION				
1. Performed hand hygiene. Prepared medication for one patient at a time.				
2. After preparation, compared label on medication versus MAR.				
3. Provided for patient privacy.				
4. Verified patient's identity correctly.				
5. Compared label on medication versus MAR.				
6. Explained procedure and expected sensations.				
7. Applied clean gloves.				
8. Chose appropriate injection site and inspected skin surface for lesions or discoloration.				
9. Positioned patient appropriately. Had patient flex elbow and support it on flat surface.				
10. Cleaned injection site. Allowed to dry.				
11. Held swab correctly.				
12. Removed needle cap correctly.				
13. Held syringe comfortably with bevel of needle pointing up.				
14. Stretched skin over injection site.				
15. With needle at 5-through 15-degree angle, injected slowly through epidermis just below skin surface.				

	S	U	NP	Comments

16. Injected medication slowly and felt normal resistance.

17. Noticed appearance of small bleb on skin.

18. Withdrew needle slowly with swab supporting site.

19. Did not massage site.

20. Assisted patient to comfortable position.

21. Properly discarded uncapped needle or needle enclosed in safety shield and syringe.

22. Removed gloves and performed hand hygiene.

23. Stayed with patient and observed for allergic reaction.

EVALUATION

1. Returned to room in 15 to 30 minutes to reassess.

2. Encouraged patient to discuss implications of skin testing.

3. Identified unexpected outcomes.

RECORDING AND REPORTING

1. Recorded test substance data correctly on medication record.

2. Recorded area of injection and appearance of skin.

3. Reported to nurse in charge or physician any undesirable effects from medication.

4. Recorded adverse reactions, treatments, patient status, and tolerance to interventions.

PE: Kyla Vanderwell

Student _Darcy Brenneman_   Date _11/2/12_

Instructor _Kendall_   Date _11/2/12_

PERFORMANCE CHECKLIST SKILL 22-3   **ADMINISTERING SUBCUTANEOUS INJECTIONS**

	S	U	NP	Comments
ASSESSMENT				
1. Checked accuracy of MAR or computer print-out versus prescriber's order.				
2. Assessed patient's medical and medication history.				
3. Reviewed medication reference information. Checked expiration date of medication.				
4. Assessed patient's allergy history. Observed patient's verbal and nonverbal responses toward injection.				
5. Assessed indications and contraindications for subcutaneous injections.				
6. Assessed patient's symptoms.				
7. Considered adequacy of patient's adipose tissue.				
8. Assessed patient's medication knowledge.				
NURSING DIAGNOSIS				
1. Developed appropriate nursing diagnoses based on assessment data.				
PLANNING				
1. Identified expected outcomes.				
IMPLEMENTATION				
1. Performed hand hygiene. Prepared medication for one patient at a time. Compared label of medication versus MAR or computer printout twice.				
2. Took medication to patient at correct time. Performed hand hygiene.				
3. Provided for patient's privacy.				
4. Verified patient's identity correctly.				
5. Compared medication label versus MAR.				
6. Explained procedure to patient.				
7. Selected appropriate injection site.				
8. Exposed site for injection only. Applied clean gloves.				
9. Accurately determined correct needle size.				

	S	U	NP	Comments

10. Assisted patient to comfortable position.

11. Relocated site using anatomical landmarks. Had patient relax area of site selection.

12. Cleansed site with antiseptic swab. Allowed to dry.

13. Held swab between third and fourth fingers of nondominant hand.

14. Removed needle cap correctly.

15. Held syringe between thumb and index finger of dominant hand (as a dart) with palm down.

16. *Administered injection.*

    a. Spread or pinched skin as indicated.

    b. Injected needle quickly at 45- to 90-degree angle.

    c. Grasped lower end of syringe barrel with nondominant hand to secure and moved dominant hand to plunger and injected slowly. 30 sec.

    d. Withdrew needle quickly while placing swab on skin above injection site.

17. Applied gentle pressure to site. Did not massage site.

18. Assisted patient to comfortable position.

19. Properly disposed of uncapped needle and syringe.

20. Removed gloves and performed hand hygiene.

21. Remained with patient and observed for allergic reactions.

EVALUATION

1. Returned to room and evaluated for discomfort at injection site.

2. Evaluated patient's response to medication.

3. Evaluated patient's understanding of purpose and effects of medication.

4. Identified unexpected outcomes.

RECORDING AND REPORTING

1. Documented administration correctly on medication record.

2. Recorded patient's response to medication.

3. Reported to nurse in charge or physician undesirable effects from medication.

244   PE: Kyla VanderWelle

Student <u>Darcy Brenneman</u>　　　　　　　　Date <u>10/24/12</u>

Instructor <u>Becks Da</u>　　　　　　　　　Date <u>✓</u>

	S	U	NP	Comments

ASSESSMENT

1. Checked accuracy of MAR or computer print-out versus medication order.

2. Assessed patient's medical, medication, and allergy histories.

3. Reviewed medication reference information.

4. Observed patient's response toward receiving injections.

5. Assessed indications/contraindications for intramuscular injection.

6. Assessed patient's symptoms.

7. Assessed patient's medication knowledge.

NURSING DIAGNOSIS

1. Developed appropriate nursing diagnoses based on assessment data.

PLANNING

1. Identified expected outcomes.

IMPLEMENTATION

1. Performed hand hygiene. Prepared medication for one patient at a time. Compared label of medication versus MAR twice.

2. Took mediation to patient at the correct time. Performed hand hygiene.

3. Provided for patient's privacy.

4. Verified patient's identity correctly.

5. Compared label on medication versus MAR.

6. Explained procedure to patient.

7. Applied clean gloves.

8. Exposed injection site only.

9. Assessed integrity of muscle while selecting injection site.

10. Assisted patient to comfortable position according to injection site.

11. Relocated site using anatomical landmarks.

	S	U	NP	Comments

12. Cleaned injection site. Used a vapocoolant if needed. Allowed to dry. ___ ___ ___ _____

13. Held swab correctly between third and fourth fingers. ___ ___ ___ _____

14. Removed needle cap by pulling it straight off. ___ ___ ___ _____

15. Held syringe between thumb and index finger (as a dart), palm down. ___ ___ ___ _____

16. *Administered Injection*

   a. With nondominant hand, spread skin tightly and grasped muscle, or used Z-track method and administered injection at 90-degree angle. ___ ___ ___ _____

   b. With nondominant hand, grasped lower end of syringe barrel (with Z-track method, continued to spread skin taut), then moved dominant hand to plunger. ___ ___ ___ _____

   c. Aspirated to check for blood return. If blood aspirated, withdrew needle; if not, injected medication slowly. ___ ___ ___ _____

   d. Withdrew needle quickly while placing antiseptic swab on skin above injection site (with Z-track method, kept needle inserted for 10 seconds, then withdrew and released skin). ___ ___ ___ _____

17. Applied gentle pressure. Did not massage site. ___ ___ ___ _____

18. Assisted patient to comfortable position. ___ ___ ___ _____

19. Discarded in proper receptacle uncapped needle or needle enclosed in safety shield and syringe. ___ ___ ___ _____

20. Removed gloves and performed hand hygiene. ___ ___ ___ _____

21. Remained with patient. Observed for allergic reaction. ___ ___ ___ _____

EVALUATION

1. Returned to room. Reevaluated patient for discomfort at injection site. ___ ___ ___ _____

2. Inspected injection site. ___ ___ ___ _____

3. Evaluated patient's response to medication. ___ ___ ___ _____

4. Evaluated patient's understanding of purpose and effects of medication. ___ ___ ___ _____

5. Identified unexpected outcomes. ___ ___ ___ _____

RECORDING AND REPORTING

1. Documented administration correctly on medication record. ___ ___ ___ _____

2. Reported to nurse in charge or physician undesirable effects from medication. ___ ___ ___ _____

3. Recorded patient's response to drugs, if indicated. ___ ___ ___ _____

246

PE: Kyla VanderWall 10/24/12   Renee Struwe 10/24

Student _____   Date _____

Instructor _____   Date _____

PERFORMANCE CHECKLIST SKILL 22-5 **ADDING MEDICATIONS TO INTRAVENOUS FLUID CONTAINERS**

	S	U	NP	Comments
ASSESSMENT				
1. Compared accuracy and completeness of MAR versus medication order.	___	___	___	_____
2. Assessed patient's medical and medication history.	___	___	___	_____
3. Reviewed medication reference information.	___	___	___	_____
4. Assessed for drug incompatibility if more than one was mixed.	___	___	___	_____
5. Assessed patient's fluid balance.	___	___	___	_____
6. Assessed patient for drug allergies.	___	___	___	_____
7. Assessed patient's symptoms.	___	___	___	_____
8. Performed hand hygiene.	___	___	___	_____
9. Assessed condition of IV insertion site.	___	___	___	_____
10. Assessed patient's knowledge regarding medication.	___	___	___	_____
NURSING DIAGNOSIS				
1. Developed appropriate nursing diagnoses based on assessment data.	___	___	___	_____
PLANNING				
1. Identified expected outcomes.	___	___	___	_____
IMPLEMENTATION				
1. Performed hand hygiene.	___	___	___	_____
2. *Added Medication to New Container*				
a. Located injection port on IV bag.	___	___	___	_____
b. Removed cap and seal from IV bottle and located injection site.	___	___	___	_____
c. Cleaned injection port or site.	___	___	___	_____
d. Inserted needle/adapter of syringe through injection port or site and injected medication.	___	___	___	_____
e. Withdrew syringe.	___	___	___	_____
f. Mixed medications in IV solution container.	___	___	___	_____
g. Labeled container correctly; applied flow strip (optional).	___	___	___	_____

	S	U	NP	Comments

h. Spiked IV container and hung container correctly, regulating IV infusion at ordered rate. ___ ___ ___ _____

i. Brought assembled items to patient at correct time. Performed hand hygiene. ___ ___ ___ _____

j. Correctly verified patient's identity. ___ ___ ___ _____

k. Compared medication label versus MAR. ___ ___ ___ _____

l. Explained procedure to patient. ___ ___ ___ _____

m. Correctly connected bag to infusion. Regulated infusions as prescribed. ___ ___ ___ _____

3. Discarded needle appropriately. Disposed of used equipment and supplies. ___ ___ ___ _____

4. Performed hand hygiene. ___ ___ ___ _____

EVALUATION

1. Observed patient for drug reaction. ___ ___ ___ _____

2. Assessed patient for signs and symptoms of fluid volume excess. ___ ___ ___ _____

3. Evaluated condition of IV site and rate of infusion. ___ ___ ___ _____

4. Assessed for signs and symptoms of IV infiltration or phlebitis. ___ ___ ___ _____

5. Evaluated patient's understanding of drug therapy. ___ ___ ___ _____

6. Identified unexpected outcomes. ___ ___ ___ _____

RECORDING AND REPORTING

1. Recorded IV solution and medication on appropriate form. ___ ___ ___ _____

2. Reported any drug reactions to nurse in charge or physician. ___ ___ ___ _____

Student _____   Date _____

Instructor _____   Date _____

PERFORMANCE CHECKLIST SKILL 22-6 **ADMINISTERING INTRAVENOUS MEDICATIONS BY INTERMITTENT INFUSION SETS AND MINIINFUSION PUMPS**

	S	U	NP	Comments
ASSESSMENT				
1. Checked accuracy and completeness of MAR versus medication order.	___	___	___	_____
2. Assessed patient's medical and medication history.	___	___	___	_____
3. Reviewed medication reference information.	___	___	___	_____
4. Determined compatibility of drug with existing IV solution.	___	___	___	_____
5. Assessed patency and infusion rate of main IV line.	___	___	___	_____
6. Performed hand hygiene.	___	___	___	_____
7. Assessed condition of IV insertion site.	___	___	___	_____
8. Assessed patient's history of drug allergies.	___	___	___	_____
9. Assessed patient's symptoms.	___	___	___	_____
10. Assessed patient's understanding of drug therapy.	___	___	___	_____
NURSING DIAGNOSIS				
1. Developed appropriate nursing diagnoses based on assessment data.	___	___	___	_____
PLANNING				
1. Identified expected outcomes.	___	___	___	_____
IMPLEMENTATION				
1. Performed hand hygiene.	___	___	___	_____
2. Prepared medication for one patient at a time. Compared drug label versus MAR twice.	___	___	___	_____
3. Assembled medications and supplies at bedside.	___	___	___	_____
4. Performed hand hygiene.	___	___	___	_____
5. Correctly verified patient's identify.	___	___	___	_____
6. Explained purpose of medication and encouraged patient to report signs of discomfort at site.	___	___	___	_____
7. Compared medication label versus MAR one more time.	___	___	___	_____

	S	U	NP	Comments

8. Administer Infusion

  a. *Piggyback or Tandem Infusion*

    (1) Connected infusion tubing to medication bag and filled tubing.

    (2) Hung medication bag at proper level.

    (3) Connected tubing to appropriate connector or primary infusion line.

    (4) Correctly regulated flow rate or medication solution.

    (5) Checked flow regulator on primary infusion after medication infused.

    (6) Regulated main infusion line to desired rate, if necessary.

    (7) Cared for equipment or disposed of properly after administration.

  b. *Volume-Control Administration Set*

    (1) Filled Volutrol with proper volume of solution.

    (2) Closed clamp and assessed that clamp in air vent of Volutrol chamber was open.

    (3) Cleaned injection port.

    (4) Injected medication into Volutrol and mixed gently.

    (5) Regulated IV infusion.

    (6) Labeled Volutrol with name of medication, dosage, total volume, and time of administration.

    (7) Disposed of needle and syringe in proper container. Disposed of other supplies correctly. Performed hand hygiene.

  c. *Miniinfusor Administration*

    (1) Connected prefilled syringe to miniinfusion tubing.

    (2) Filled syringe with medication, avoiding air bubbles.

    (3) Placed syringe into miniinfusor pump, securing syringe.

    (4) Correctly connected miniinfusion tubing to main IV line.

    (5) Hung infusion pump with syringe on IV pole and initiated infusion.

250

	S	U	NP	Comments
(6) Assessed flow rate and patency of primary IV infusion.	___	___	___	_____
(7) Correctly disposed of supplies. Performed hand hygiene.	___	___	___	_____

EVALUATION

	S	U	NP	Comments
1. Evaluated patient's response to medication.	___	___	___	_____
2. Periodically checked infusion rate and IV site.	___	___	___	_____
3. Evaluated patient's knowledge of purpose and side effects of medication.	___	___	___	_____
4. Identified unexpected outcomes.	___	___	___	_____

RECORDING AND REPORTING

	S	U	NP	Comments
1. Correctly recorded medication data on medication form.	___	___	___	_____
2. Recorded solution on I&O form.	___	___	___	_____
3. Reported any adverse drug reactions to nurse in charge or physician.	___	___	___	_____

Student _____   Date _____

Instructor _____   Date _____

PERFORMANCE CHECKLIST SKILL 22-7   **ADMINISTERING MEDICATIONS BY INTRAVENOUS BOLUS**

	S	U	NP	Comments

ASSESSMENT

1. Checked accuracy of MAR versus medication order. Prepared medication for one patient at a time.   ___ ___ ___   _____

2. Reviewed medication reference information related to drug to be given.   ___ ___ ___   _____

3. Assessed for compatibility of medication with existing IV fluid infusion.   ___ ___ ___   _____

4. Performed hand hygiene and assessed condition of IV insertion site.   ___ ___ ___   _____

5. Assessed patency of existing IV infusion line.   ___ ___ ___   _____

6. Checked patient's medical history and medication allergies.   ___ ___ ___   _____

7. Checked expiration date of medication.   ___ ___ ___   _____

8. Assessed patient's symptoms.   ___ ___ ___   _____

9. Assessed patient's understanding of purpose of drug therapy.   ___ ___ ___   _____

NURSING DIAGNOSIS

1. Developed appropriate nursing diagnoses based on assessment data.   ___ ___ ___   _____

PLANNING

1. Identified expected outcomes.   ___ ___ ___   _____

IMPLEMENTATION

1. Performed hand hygiene. Prepared medication for one patient at a time. Compared label of medication versus MAR.   ___ ___ ___   _____

2. Took medication to patient at right time. Performed hand hygiene.   ___ ___ ___   _____

3. Correctly verified patient's identity.   ___ ___ ___   _____

4. Compared medication label versus MAR before administration.   ___ ___ ___   _____

5. Explained purpose of medication to patient.   ___ ___ ___   _____

6. Applied clean gloves.   ___ ___ ___   _____

7. Administered medications:

	S	U	NP	Comments

a. *IV Push (existing line)*

(1) Selected injection port of IV closest to patient.

(2) Cleaned injection port with antiseptic. Allowed to dry.

(3) Inserted needleless tip or small-gauge needle of syringe correctly through port.

(4) Aspirated for blood return while occluding infusion tubing. Released tubing.

(5) Slowly injected medication over appropriate time. Used watch to time administration as per institutional policy when required.

(6) Released tubing, withdrew syringe, and checked infusion rate.

b. *IV Push (intravenous lock)*

(1) Correctly prepared flush solutions.

(2) Administered medication.

   (a) Cleaned injection port with antiseptic. Allowed to dry.

   (b) Attached syringe with saline flush.

   (c) Checked for blood return.

   (d) Correctly injected saline flush.

   (e) Removed flush syringe.

   (f) Cleaned injection port with antiseptic.

   (g) Inserted syringe containing medication through injection port.

   (h) Injected medication over appropriate time interval. Used a watch to time administration.

   (i) Withdrew syringe after administering medication.

   (j) Cleaned injection site with antiseptic.

   (k) Flushed injection port with saline flush or heparin flush per agency policy.

8. Disposed of uncapped needles and syringes in proper container.

9. Removed gloves and performed hand hygiene.

254

	S	U	NP	Comments

EVALUATION

1. Observed patient for adverse reactions during and after administration of medication. ____ ____ ____ _____

2. Observed patency of IV site during injection and at recommended intervals. ____ ____ ____ _____

3. Assessed patient's tolerance and response to medication. ____ ____ ____ _____

4. Evaluated patient's knowledge of drug's purpose and side effects. ____ ____ ____ _____

5. Identified unexpected outcomes. ____ ____ ____ _____

RECORDING AND REPORTING

1. Correctly recorded drug data on medication record. ____ ____ ____ _____

2. Reported any adverse reactions to nurse in charge or physician. ____ ____ ____ _____

3. Recorded patient's medication response in nurses' notes. ____ ____ ____ _____

Student _____   Date _____

Instructor _____   Date _____

	S	U	NP	Comments
ASSESSMENT				
1. Checked accuracy of MAR versus medication order.	___	___	___	_____
2. Reviewed medication reference information.	___	___	___	_____
3. Assessed patient's medical, medication, and allergy histories.	___	___	___	_____
4. Assessed patient's verbal/nonverbal response to injections.	___	___	___	_____
5. Assessed for contraindications to continuous subcutaneous injection (CSQI).	___	___	___	_____
6. Assessed adequacy of patient's adipose tissue to determine site.	___	___	___	_____
7. Assessed patient's knowledge regarding medication.	___	___	___	_____
8. Assessed patient's symptoms.	___	___	___	_____
NURSING DIAGNOSIS				
1. Developed appropriate nursing diagnoses based on assessment data.	___	___	___	_____
PLANNING				
1. Identified expected outcomes.	___	___	___	_____
IMPLEMENTATION				
1. Reviewed manufacturer's instructions.	___	___	___	_____
2. Performed hand hygiene and arranged equipment. Prepared medication for one patient at a time. Compared label versus MAR twice.	___	___	___	_____
3. Primed tubing and programmed pump.	___	___	___	_____
4. Took medication to patient at correct time. Performed hand hygiene. Placed syringe in pump.	___	___	___	_____
5. Correctly verified patient's identity.	___	___	___	_____
6. Compared label of medication versus MAR one more time.	___	___	___	_____
7. Explained steps of procedure to patient.	___	___	___	_____
8. Provided privacy for patient.	___	___	___	_____

	S	U	NP	Comments

9. *Initiating CSQI*

   a. Assisted patient to a comfortable position. ___ ___ ___ _____

   b. Selected appropriate injection site. ___ ___ ___ _____

   c. Applied gloves. ___ ___ ___ _____

   d. Cleaned injection site with alcohol and antiseptic. Allowed to dry. ___ ___ ___ _____

   e. Held needle in dominant hand and removed needle guard. ___ ___ ___ _____

   f. Gently pinched or lifted up skin with non-dominant hand. ___ ___ ___ _____

   g. Inserted needle at 45- to 90-degree angle, as suggested by manufacturer. ___ ___ ___ _____

   h. Released skinfold and secured wings of needle with tape. ___ ___ ___ _____

   i. Placed occlusive transparent dressing over insertion site. ___ ___ ___ _____

   j. Attached tubing from needle to tubing from infusion pump. Turned pump on. ___ ___ ___ _____

   k. Disposed of sharps in appropriate container. Discarded used supplies, removed gloves, and performed hand hygiene. ___ ___ ___ _____

   l. Assessed site and instructed patient to report any alterations. ___ ___ ___ _____

10. *Discontinuing CSQI*

   a. Verified order for discontinuation, established alternate method of administration if indicated. ___ ___ ___ _____

   b. Stopped infusion pump. ___ ___ ___ _____

   c. Performed hand hygiene and applied gloves. ___ ___ ___ _____

   d. Carefully removed dressing. ___ ___ ___ _____

   e. Removed tape from wings of needle and pulled needle out along insertion line. ___ ___ ___ _____

   f. Applied pressure at site. Assessed insertion site and surrounding tissues. ___ ___ ___ _____

   g. Applied sterile gauze dressing or bandage. ___ ___ ___ _____

   h. Discarded used supplies, removed gloves, and performed hand hygiene. ___ ___ ___ _____

	S	U	NP	Comments

EVALUATION

1. Evaluated patient's response to medication. ___ ___ ___ _____

2. Observed site at least every 4 hours. ___ ___ ___ _____

3. Asked patient to verbalize understanding of medication and procedure. ___ ___ ___ _____

4. Identified unexpected outcomes. ___ ___ ___ _____

RECORDING AND REPORTING

1. Recorded medication administration and pertinent information about procedure. ___ ___ ___ _____

2. Recorded patient's response to medication and assessment of infusion site. ___ ___ ___ _____

3. Reported unexpected outcomes to the nurse in charge or physician. ___ ___ ___ _____

4. If medication is a narcotic, followed institutional policy for recording and discarding as needed. ___ ___ ___ _____

Student _____ Date _____

Instructor _____ Date _____

PERFORMANCE CHECKLIST SKILL 23-1   **APPLYING A NASAL CANNULA OR OXYGEN MASK**

	S	U	NP	Comments
ASSESSMENT				
1. Assessed respiratory status. Observed for signs and symptoms associated with hypoxia.	___	___	___	_____
2. Observed for patent airway and removed airway secretions.	___	___	___	_____
3. Obtained results of patient's most recent arterial blood gases (ABGs) or pulse oximetry (SpO_2) values.	___	___	___	_____
4. Reviewed patient's medical record for medical order for oxygen therapy; noted method, flow rate, and duration of oxygen therapy.	___	___	___	_____
NURSING DIAGNOSIS				
1. Developed appropriate nursing diagnoses based on assessment data.	___	___	___	_____
PLANNING				
1. Identified expected outcomes.	___	___	___	_____
2. Explained procedure and its purpose to patient and family.	___	___	___	_____
IMPLEMENTATION				
1. Performed hand hygiene.	___	___	___	_____
2. Attached nasal cannula/mask to oxygen tubing and attached oxygen tubing to humidified oxygen source. Adjusted oxygen flow rate to prescribed dosage.	___	___	___	_____
3. Applied oxygen delivery device properly and adjusted to patient's comfort.	___	___	___	_____
4. Allowed sufficient slack on oxygen tubing and secured to patient's clothing.	___	___	___	_____
5. Observed proper function of oxygen delivery device.	___	___	___	_____
6. Verified setting on flow meter and oxygen source for proper setup.	___	___	___	_____
7. Checked patient as needed. Kept humidification container filled.	___	___	___	_____
8. Performed hand hygiene.	___	___	___	_____

	S	U	NP	Comments

EVALUATION

1. Reassessed patient to determine response to oxygen administration. ___ ___ ___ _____

2. Monitored ABGs or pulse oximetry as ordered. ___ ___ ___ _____

3. Assessed adequacy of oxygen flow. ___ ___ ___ _____

4. Observed patient's mucous membrane and face for skin breakdown. ___ ___ ___ _____

5. Identified unexpected outcomes. ___ ___ ___ _____

RECORDING AND REPORTING

1. Recorded respiratory assessment findings before and during oxygen therapy; method of oxygen delivery, flow rate, patency, patient's response; any adverse reactions or side effects; and any change in physician's orders. ___ ___ ___ _____

2. Reported unexpected findings to nurse in charge or physician. ___ ___ ___ _____

Student _____ Date _____

Instructor _____ Date _____

PERFORMANCE CHECKLIST SKILL 23-2 **ADMINISTERING OXYGEN THERAPY TO A PATIENT WITH AN ARTIFICIAL AIRWAY**

	S	U	NP	Comments
ASSESSMENT				
1. Assessed patient's respiratory system. Observed for signs and symptoms associated with hypoxia.	___	___		_____
2. Observed for patent airway and removed airway secretions.	___	___		_____
3. Monitored pulse oximetry (SpO_2). Noted patient's most recent ABG results.	___	___		_____
4. Reviewed patient's medical order for oxygen therapy.	___	___		_____
NURSING DIAGNOSIS				
1. Developed appropriate nursing diagnoses based on assessment data.	___	___	___	_____
PLANNING				
1. Identified expected outcomes.	___	___	___	_____
2. Explained to patient and family purpose of T tube or tracheostomy collar.	___	___	___	_____
IMPLEMENTATION				
1. Performed hand hygiene. Applied gloves and goggles. Considered need for barrier gown.	___	___		_____
2. Attached T tube or tracheostomy collar to large-bore oxygen tubing and to humidified oxygen source.	___	___		_____
3. Adjusted oxygen flow rate to 10 L/min or as ordered and adjusted nebulizer to proper FiO_2 setting. Attached T tube or tracheostomy collar to endotracheal or tracheostomy tube.	___	___	___	_____
4. Observed for T tube pulling on endotracheal or tracheostomy tube. Suctioned secretions in T tube or tracheostomy collar if necessary.	___	___	___	_____
5. Observed oxygen tubing frequently for accumulation of fluid, and drained tubing correctly.	___	___	___	_____
6. Set up suction equipment at patient's bedside.	___	___	___	_____
7. Removed gloves and goggles; performed hand hygiene.	___	___	___	_____

	S	U	NP	Comments

EVALUATION

1. Assessed patient's response to procedure, including respiratory status, level of consciousness, etc. ___ ___ ___ _____

2. Determined that oxygen delivery device was not pulling on artificial airway. ___ ___ ___ _____

3. Monitored ABG levels and SpO_2 ___ ___ ___ _____

4. Identified unexpected outcomes. ___ ___ ___ _____

RECORDING AND REPORTING

1. Recorded and reported respiratory assessment findings, method of oxygen delivery, and patient's response before and during oxygen therapy. ___ ___ ___ _____

2. Reported unexpected findings to nurse in charge or physician. ___ ___ ___ _____

264

Student _____ Date _____

Instructor _____ Date _____

PERFORMANCE CHECKLIST SKILL 23-3 **USING INCENTIVE SPIROMETRY**

	S	U	NP	Comments
ASSESSMENT				
1. Identified patient as one who would benefit from incentive spirometry.	___	___	___	_____
2. Assessed patient's level of awareness, nutrition status, and motor skills.	___	___	___	_____
3. Assessed patient's respiratory status and pain level.	___	___	___	_____
4. Reviewed health care provider's order for incentive spirometry.	___	___	___	_____
NURSING DIAGNOSIS				
1. Developed appropriate nursing diagnoses based on assessment data.	___	___	___	_____
PLANNING				
1. Identified expected outcomes.	___	___	___	_____
2. Explained procedure to patient and family.	___	___	___	_____
3. Indicated target volume for patient.	___	___	___	_____
IMPLEMENTATION				
1. Performed hand hygiene.	___	___	___	_____
2 Assisted patient to the most tolerable Fowler's position.	___	___	___	_____
3. Demonstrated how to place mouthpiece correctly.	___	___	___	_____
4. Instructed patient to inhale slowly and maintain a constant flow through the unit, then hold breath for at least 3 seconds and exhale slowly.	___	___	___	_____
5. Had patient repeat maneuver 5 to 10 times per hour as tolerated.	___	___	___	_____
6. Performed hand hygiene.	___	___	___	_____
EVALUATION				
1. Reassessed patient to determine response and ability to use incentive spirometry.	___	___	___	_____
2. Assessed ability of patient to reach target volume or frequency.	___	___	___	_____
3. Auscultated chest before and during respiratory cycle.	___	___	___	_____
4. Identified unexpected outcomes.	___	___	___	_____

	S	U	NP	Comments

RECORDING AND REPORTING

1. Recorded respiratory assessment before and after incentive spirometry, frequency of use, volumes achieved, and any adverse effects.   ___ ___ ___ _____

2. Reported to health care provider changes in respiratory status or inability to use equipment.   ___ ___ ___ _____

Student _____ Date _____

Instructor _____ Date _____

PERFORMANCE CHECKLIST SKILL 23-4 **CARE OF THE PATIENT RECEIVING NONINVASIVE VENTILATION**

	S	U	NP	Comments

ASSESSMENT

1. Assessed patient's respiratory status. Observed for signs and symptoms associated with hypoxia. ___ ___ ___ _____

2. Observed patient's skin for signs of irritation on bridge of nose, around ears, and back of head. ___ ___ ___ _____

3. Observed patient's ability to clear and remove airway secretions. Assessed skin integrity. ___ ___ ___ _____

4. Noted patient's most recent ABG results or SpO_2 value. ___ ___ ___ _____

5. Obtained vital signs before initiation of therapy. ___ ___ ___ _____

6. Reviewed patient's medical order for oxygen therapy. ___ ___ ___ _____

NURSING DIAGNOSIS

1. Developed appropriate nursing diagnoses based on assessment data. ___ ___ ___ _____

PLANNING

1. Identified expected outcomes. ___ ___ ___ _____

2. Explained purpose of CPAP/BiPAP to patient and family. ___ ___ ___ _____

IMPLEMENTATION

1. Performed hand hygiene. Applied gloves and goggles. Considered need for barrier gown. ___ ___ ___ _____

2. Determined correct mask size. ___ ___ ___ _____

3. Connected CPAP/BiPAP device delivery tubing to pressure generator. ___ ___ ___ _____

4. Connected patient to pulse oximeter. ___ ___ ___ _____

5. Set CPAP-BiPAP initial settings. ___ ___ ___ _____

6. Performed frequent skin assessment. ___ ___ ___ _____

7. Disposed of supplies and performed hand hygiene. ___ ___ ___ _____

	S	U	NP	Comments

EVALUATION

1. Assessed patient's response to procedure, including respiratory status, LOC, etc.   ___ ___ ___ _____

2. Monitored ABG levels or SpO_2.   ___ ___ ___ _____

3. Observed skin integrity over the bridge of the patient's nose.   ___ ___ ___ _____

4. Determined patient's and family's ability to manipulate device and face mask.   ___ ___ ___ _____

5. Identified unexpected outcomes.   ___ ___ ___ _____

RECORDING AND REPORTING

1. Recorded respiratory assessment findings, CPAP/BiPAP settings, pulse oximetry, and patient's response.   ___ ___ ___ _____

2. Reported unexpected outcomes to nurse in charge or health care provider.   ___ ___ ___ _____

268

Student _____ Date _____

Instructor _____ Date _____

PERFORMANCE CHECKLIST PROCEDURAL GUIDELINE 23-1 **USE OF A PEAK FLOW METER**

STEPS	S	U	NP	Comments
1. Instructed patient about the procedure	___	___	___	_____
2. Positioned patient correctly, standing if possible, otherwise in high-Fowler's position.	___	___	___	_____
3. Slid mouthpiece into base of scale at the zero position.	___	___	___	_____
4. Instructed patient to take a deep breath.	___	___	___	_____
5. Instructed patient to place mouthpiece in mouth and close lips around it, making a firm seal.	___	___	___	_____
6. Instructed patient to blow out as hard and fast as possible through the mouth, in one breath.	___	___	___	_____
7. Repeated procedure two more times. Record the highest reading in the patient's diary.	___	___	___	_____
8. Had patient perform a return demonstration and indicate understanding of correct record keeping, if patient is to continue procedure at home.	___	___	___	_____
9. Verified that patient knows when to call health care provider based "red zone" reading.	___	___	___	_____
10. Assisted patient in creating action plan as prescribed.	___	___	___	_____
12. Instructed patient to clean unit weekly, following manufacturers recommendations.	___	___	___	_____

Student _____ Date _____

Instructor _____ Date _____

	S	U	NP	Comments

ASSESSMENT

1. Assessed patient's level of consciousness and ability to cooperate. ____ ____ ____ _____

2. Assessed patient's need for sedation. ____ ____ ____ _____

3. Assessed patient's respiratory status. ____ ____ ____ _____

4. Checked ventilator and alarms at beginning of shift and regularly throughout shift. ____ ____ ____ _____

5. Verified placement of artificial airway. ____ ____ ____ _____

6. Observed for patent airway and suctioned as needed. ____ ____ ____ _____

7. Noted patient's most recent ABG results or SpO_2. ____ ____ ____ _____

8. Assessed communication preference. ____ ____ ____ _____

9. Reviewed medical order for mechanical ventilation and ventilation settings. ____ ____ ____ _____

NURSING DIAGNOSIS

1. Developed appropriate nursing diagnoses based on assessment data. ____ ____ ____ _____

PLANNING

1. Identified expected outcomes. ____ ____ ____ _____

2. Explained to patient and family purpose of mechanical ventilation. ____ ____ ____ _____

3. Elevated head of bed at least 30 degrees. ____ ____ ____ _____

IMPLEMENTATION

1. Performed hand hygiene and applied gloves and goggles. Considered need for barrier gown. ____ ____ ____ _____

2. Attached mechanical ventilator to endotracheal or tracheostomy tube. Observed for proper functioning of mechanical ventilator. ____ ____ ____ _____

3. Verified that endotracheal or tracheostomy tube is positioned properly. ____ ____ ____ _____

4. Observed for patient respiration in synchronization with mechanical ventilation and response to therapy. ____ ____ ____ _____

	S	U	NP	Comments
5. Monitored vital signs and cardiac rhythm.	——	——	——	_____
6. Marked level of endotracheal tube at lips/nares.	——	——	——	_____
7. Set up suction equipment.	——	——	——	_____
8. Positioned patient to promote best oxygenation.	——	——	——	_____
9. Frequently followed up with health care provider about patient status and response to therapy.	——	——	——	_____
10. Conducted hourly safety checks on patient and ventilator system.	——	——	——	_____
11. Performed frequent mouth care.	——	——	——	_____
12. Implemented actions to prevent hazards of immobility.	——	——	——	_____
13. Kept patient and family informed of progress.	——	——	——	_____
14. Removed gloves and goggles; performed hand hygiene.	——	——	——	_____

EVALUATION

	S	U	NP	Comments
1. Evaluated patient's response to mechanical ventilation.	——	——	——	_____
2. Monitored ABG levels and/or SpO_2.	——	——	——	_____
3. Assessed integrity of patient's ventilator system.	——	——	——	_____
4. Determined effectiveness of communication methods.	——	——	——	_____
5. Identified unexpected outcomes.	——	——	——	_____

RECORDING AND REPORTING

	S	U	NP	Comments
1. Recorded respiratory assessment, method of oxygen delivery, flow rate, and patient's response.	——	——	——	_____
2. Reported unexpected findings to nurse in charge or health care provider.	——	——	——	_____

Student _____ Date _____

Instructor _____ Date _____

PERFORMANCE CHECKLIST SKILL 24-1 **PERFORMING POSTURAL DRAINAGE**

	S	U	NP	Comments

ASSESSMENT

1. Assessed patient for conditions that pose a risk for implementation of chest physiotherapy (CPT). ___ ___ ___ _____

2. Reviewed medical record and assessed patient for signs and symptoms indicating need for CPT. ___ ___ ___ _____

3. Reviewed laboratory reports and auscultated lungs. ___ ___ ___ _____

4. Assessed vital signs and pulse oximetry. ___ ___ ___ _____

5. Determined patient's understanding of and ability to perform home postural drainage. ___ ___ ___ _____

NURSING DIAGNOSIS

1. Developed appropriate nursing diagnoses based on assessment data. ___ ___ ___ _____

PLANNING

1. Identified expected outcomes. ___ ___ ___ _____

2. Explained purpose of procedure. Prepared patient for procedure, and instructed patient to remove any tight or restrictive clothing. ___ ___ ___ _____

IMPLEMENTATION

1. Provided for patient privacy. ___ ___ ___ _____

2. Performed hand hygiene and applied gloves. ___ ___ ___ _____

3. Selected areas to be drained. ___ ___ ___ _____

4. Correctly positioned patient to drain congested areas. Instructed patient on proper positioning. ___ ___ ___ _____

5. Had patient maintain position for 10 to 15 minutes. ___ ___ ___ _____

6. Performed percussion, vibration, or rib shaking with patient in each position for 10 to 15 minutes. ___ ___ ___ _____

7. After drainage in first position, had patient sit up and cough; saved expectorated secretions; suctioned if necessary. ___ ___ ___ _____

8. Allowed patient to rest. ___ ___ ___ _____

9. Had patient sip water. ___ ___ ___ _____

	S	U	NP	Comments
10. Repeated Steps 3 through 8 for all congested areas in accepted time frame.	____	____	____	_____
11. Performed hand hygiene.	____	____	____	_____

EVALUATION

	S	U	NP	Comments
1. Auscultated lung fields before and after treatment.	____	____	____	_____
2. Assessed character of sputum.	____	____	____	_____
3. Reviewed diagnostic reports on patient's pulmonary function.	____	____	____	_____
4. Monitored vital signs and pulse oximetry (if used).	____	____	____	_____
5. Identified unexpected outcomes.	____	____	____	_____

RECORDING AND REPORTING

	S	U	NP	Comments
1. Recorded preprocedure and postprocedure assessment and response.	____	____	____	_____
2. Recorded patient education for home care and referrals.	____	____	____	_____
3. Reported unexpected findings to nurse in charge or health care provider.	____	____	____	_____

Student _____ Date _____

Instructor _____ Date _____

PERFORMANCE CHECKLIST PROCEDURAL GUIDELINE 24-1 **USING AN ACAPELLA DEVICE**

	S	U	NP	Comments

STEPS

1. Verified need for physician's order per agency policy. ___ ___ ___ _____

2. Assessed patient's respiratory status. ___ ___ ___ _____

3. Explained procedure to patient and family. ___ ___ ___ _____

4. Prepared acapella device, attached nebulizer if ordered. ___ ___ ___ _____

5. Instructed patient to sit comfortably.

   a. Had patient take a deep breath, place mouthpiece in mouth, and maintain a tight seal with lips. ___ ___ ___ _____

   b. Had patient hold breath for 2 to 3 seconds, exhale slowly into device while it vibrates. ___ ___ ___ _____

   c. Had patient repeat cycle 5 to 10 times. ___ ___ ___ _____

   d. Had patient remove mouthpiece from mouth and perform 2 forceful exhalations and "huff" cough. ___ ___ ___ _____

   e. Repeated as ordered. ___ ___ ___ _____

6. Auscultated lungs. ___ ___ ___ _____

7. Obtained vital signs and SpO_2 reading. ___ ___ ___ _____

Student _____ Date _____

Instructor _____ Date _____

PERFORMANCE CHECKLIST PROCEDURAL GUIDELINE 24-2 **PERFORMING PERCUSSION, VIBRATION, AND SHAKING**

	S	U	NP	Comments

STEPS

1. Assessed patient's breathing patterns. ___ ___ ___ _____

2. Identified signs, symptoms, and conditions that indicated the need to perform skills. ___ ___ ___ _____

3. Assessed patient's rib cage and the bronchial segment being drained. ___ ___ ___ _____

4. Assessed patient's understanding and ability to perform procedure in the hospital and at home. ___ ___ ___ _____

5. Explained procedure to patient and family. ___ ___ ___ _____

6. Instructed patient in relaxation and breathing techniques. ___ ___ ___ _____

7. Performed hand hygiene and applied gloves. ___ ___ ___ _____

8. Elevated bed to good working height. ___ ___ ___ _____

9. Positioned patient appropriately. ___ ___ ___ _____

10. Performed percussion for 3 to 5 minutes in each position as tolerated.

    a. Placed hands side by side over the area to be drained. Cupped hands with fingers and thumbs held tightly together. ___ ___ ___ _____

    b. Clapped rhythmically over area for 5 minutes or for 2 to 3 minutes, alternating with vibration and shaking. ___ ___ ___ _____

    c. Alternated hands to create rhythmical popping sound. ___ ___ ___ _____

    d. Assessed patient's level of comfort and tolerance to procedure. ___ ___ ___ _____

11. Performed chest wall vibration and shaking over each affected area.

    a. Placed hands over area and had patient take a slow, deep breath through nose. ___ ___ ___ _____

    b. Gently resisted rise of chest wall during inhalation. ___ ___ ___ _____

    c. Had patient hold breath, then exhale through pursed lips while contracting abdominal muscles and relaxing chest wall muscles. ___ ___ ___ _____

	S	U	NP	Comments

d. Gently pushed down and vibrated as patient exhaled.

e. Repeated vibration 3 times, then had patient cough. Vibrated chest as patient coughed.

f. Monitored patient's tolerance of vibration and ability to cooperate with instructions.

12. Performed rib shaking with vibration.

 a. Placed flat palm of hand over area as patient inhaled slowly through nose.

 b. Applied light pressure on ribs and stretched skin during inhalation.

 c. Had patient hold breath for 2 seconds.

 d. Increased pressure as patient exhaled through pursed lips and relaxed chest wall muscles.

 e. Repeated shaking 3 times.

13. Performed three or four sets of vibration, shaking, and coughing in each posture.

14. Suctioned if unable to bring up mucus.

15. Assisted with oral hygiene.

16. Removed gloves and performed hand hygiene.

17. Instructed patient and family on procedures to be continued at home.

18. Assessed respiratory status.

19. Obtained vital signs and pulse oximetry reading.

20. Inspected characteristics of sputum.

Student _____ Date _____

Instructor _____ Date _____

PERFORMANCE CHECKLIST SKILL 25-1 **OROPHARYNGEAL SUCTIONING**

	S	U	NP	Comments

ASSESSMENT

1. Observed for signs and symptoms of upper airway obstruction requiring oropharyngeal suctioning.   ___ ___ ___ _____

2. Assessed for signs and symptoms of hypoxia.   ___ ___ ___ _____

3. Obtained baseline oxygen saturation via SpO_2.   ___ ___ ___ _____

4. Assessed patient's knowledge of catheter use.   ___ ___ ___ _____

5. Identified risk factors.   ___ ___ ___ _____

6. Assessed for presence of lower airway obstruction.   ___ ___ ___ _____

NURSING DIAGNOSIS

1. Developed appropriate nursing diagnoses based on assessment data.   ___ ___ ___ _____

PLANNING

1. Identified expected outcomes.   ___ ___ ___ _____

2. Explained procedure and expected sensations to patient.   ___ ___ ___ _____

3. Positioned patient correctly; placed towel across patient's chest.   ___ ___ ___ _____

IMPLEMENTATION

1. Performed hand hygiene and applied clean gloves. Applied mask or face shield, if indicated.   ___ ___ ___ _____

2. Filled cup or basin with approximately 100 mL of water.   ___ ___ ___ _____

3. Connected tubing properly and turned suction device to appropriate pressure.   ___ ___ ___ _____

4. Checked that apparatus was functioning properly.   ___ ___ ___ _____

5. Removed oxygen mask, if present.   ___ ___ ___ _____

6. Inserted catheter into patient's mouth and suctioned correctly. Encouraged patient to cough. Replaced oxygen mask.   ___ ___ ___ _____

7. Rinsed catheter. Turned off suction. Wiped patient's face, if needed.   ___ ___ ___ _____

8. Assessed patient's respiratory status. Repeated procedure, if indicated.   ___ ___ ___ _____

	S	U	NP	Comments

9. Disposed of chest drape and repositioned patient. ___ ___ ___ _____

10. Discarded water and cup, washed and dried basin, and placed catheter in clean, dry area. ___ ___ ___ _____

11. Removed and disposed of gloves, mask, and face shield. Performed hand hygiene. ___ ___ ___ _____

12. Provided oral hygiene as needed. ___ ___ ___ _____

EVALUATION

1. Compared assessments before and after procedure. ___ ___ ___ _____

2. Auscultated chest and airways for adventitious sounds. ___ ___ ___ _____

3. Obtained postsuction oxygen saturation levels. ___ ___ ___ _____

4. Observed patient or caregiver performing procedure. ___ ___ ___ _____

5. Identified unexpected outcomes. ___ ___ ___ _____

RECORDING AND REPORTING

1. Recorded procedure, patient's respiratory status preprocedure and postprocedure, character and amount of secretions, and education provided. ___ ___ ___ _____

2. Reported changes in patient's respiratory status. ___ ___ ___ _____

Student _____   Date _____

Instructor _____   Date _____

PERFORMANCE CHECKLIST SKILL 25-2 **AIRWAY SUCTIONING**

	S	U	NP	Comments

ASSESSMENT

1. Identified signs and symptoms of upper and lower airway obstruction requiring nasal and oral tracheal suctioning.

2. Assessed for signs and symptoms of hypoxia.

3. Assessed for risk factors for airway obstruction.

4. Determined factors that normally influence lower airway functioning.

5. Identified contraindications to nasotracheal suctioning.

6. Reviewed sputum microbiology data.

7. Assessed patient's understanding of procedure.

NURSING DIAGNOSIS

1. Developed appropriate nursing diagnoses based on assessment data.

PLANNING

1. Identified expected outcomes.

2. Explained purpose of procedure, expected sensations, and importance of coughing to patient.

3. Positioned patient.

4. Noted pulse oximetry reading. Placed towel across patient's chest.

IMPLEMENTATION

1. Performed hand hygiene and applied mask, goggles, or face shield.

2. Connected tubing to suction machine, turned suction device on, and set vacuum regulator to appropriate pressure.

3. Increased supplemental oxygen as indicated or ordered by physician. Encouraged deep breathing.

4. Prepared suction catheter correctly.

5. Applied sterile gloves properly.

6. Attached catheter to tubing; maintained sterility.

	S	U	NP	Comments

7. Verified catheter was working by suctioning small amount of normal saline from basin. ___ ___ ___ _____

8. Suctioned airway.

   a. *Nasopharyngeal and Nasotracheal Suctioning*

      (1) Coated distal end of catheter (6 to 8 cm [2 to 3 inches]) with water-soluble lubricant. ___ ___ ___ _____

      (2) Removed oxygen delivery device, if present. Inserted catheter gently and the appropriate distance into the nares on inhalation. ___ ___ ___ _____

      (3) Applied intermittent suction for up to 10 seconds while withdrawing catheter, encouraging patient to cough as appropriate. (Performed tracheal suctioning first.) Replaced oxygen device, if applicable. ___ ___ ___ _____

      (4) Rinsed catheter and connecting tubing with saline. ___ ___ ___ _____

      (5) Reassessed need to repeat suctioning. Allowed time between suction passes for oxygenation. Asked patient to breathe deeply and cough. ___ ___ ___ _____

   b. *Artificial Airway Suctioning*

      (1) Hyperoxygenated/hyperinflated patient. ___ ___ ___ _____

      (2) Opened swivel adapter or removed oxygen or humidity device with non-dominant hand. ___ ___ ___ _____

      (3) Without applying suction, inserted catheter gently and pulled catheter back 1 cm when resistance was met. ___ ___ ___ _____

      (4) Applied intermittent suction, encouraging patient to cough as appropriate. Observed for respiratory distress. ___ ___ ___ _____

      (5) Closed swivel adapter or replaced oxygen delivery device if patient is on mechanical ventilation. ___ ___ ___ _____

      (6) Encouraged patient to breathe deeply. ___ ___ ___ _____

      (7) Rinsed catheter and connecting tubing with normal saline. ___ ___ ___ _____

      (8) Assessed patient's cardiopulmonary status. Repeated suctioning if needed. ___ ___ ___ _____

      (9) Performed nasal and oral pharyngeal suctioning when tracheobronchial tree was clear. ___ ___ ___ _____

	S	U	NP	Comments
9. Disconnected catheter. Discarded gloves and catheter correctly.	___	___	___	_____
10. Discarded towel; repositioned patient.	___	___	___	_____
11. Adjusted oxygen as needed.	___	___	___	_____
12. Discarded saline and basin (washed and stored reusable basin).	___	___	___	_____
13. Removed and discarded face shield and gloves. Performed hand hygiene.	___	___	___	_____
14. Placed unopened suction kit at head of bed.	___	___	___	_____
15. Assisted patient to comfortable position and provided oral hygiene.	___	___	___	_____

EVALUATION

	S	U	NP	Comments
1. Compared assessments before and after suctioning.	___	___	___	_____
2. Asked patient if breathing is easier.	___	___	___	_____
3. Observed airway secretions.	___	___	___	_____
4. Identified unexpected outcomes.	___	___	___	_____

RECORDING AND REPORTING

	S	U	NP	Comments
1. Recorded procedure, character and amount of secretions, and patient assessments.	___	___	___	_____
2. Reported changes in patient's respiratory status.	___	___	___	_____

Student _____ Date _____

Instructor _____ Date _____

PERFORMANCE CHECKLIST PROCEDURAL GUIDELINE 25-1   **CLOSED (IN-LINE) SUCTION CATHETER**

	S	U	NP	Comments
STEPS				
1. Performed necessary assessments (refer to Skill 25-2).	___	___	___	_____
2. Explained to patient procedure and importance of coughing.	___	___	___	_____
3. Positioned patient comfortably. Placed towel across patient's chest.	___	___	___	_____
4. Performed hand hygiene. Applied sterile gloves. Attached suction according to agency policy and prepared suction apparatus correctly.	___	___	___	_____
5. Hyperinflated and/or hyperoxygenated patient according to institutional protocol and clinical status.	___	___	___	_____
6. Unlocked suction control mechanism, if required. Opened saline port and attached saline.	___	___	___	_____
7. Picked up enclosed suction catheter with dominant hand.	___	___	___	_____
8. Inserted catheter without applying suction until resistance felt.	___	___	___	_____
9. Encouraged patient to cough, applied suction correctly, and withdrew catheter.	___	___	___	_____
10. Assessed need for repeated suctioning and performed suctioning, if needed. Reassessed cardiopulmonary status.	___	___	___	_____
11. Completely withdrew catheter and rinsed properly.	___	___	___	_____
12. Performed oral or nasal suctioning, if indicated.	___	___	___	_____
13. Repositioned patient.	___	___	___	_____
14. Removed and disposed of gloves and face shield. Performed hand hygiene.	___	___	___	_____
15. Compared patient's respiratory assessments before and after suctioning.	___	___	___	_____

Student _____ Date _____

Instructor _____ Date _____

PERFORMANCE CHECKLIST SKILL 25-3 **ENDOTRACHEAL TUBE CARE**

	S	U	NP	Comments

ASSESSMENT

1. Established baseline measure of ventilation. ___ ___ ___ _____

2. Observed for signs and symptoms of need to perform endotracheal (ET) tube care and oral hygiene. ___ ___ ___ _____

3. Identified factors that place patient at greater risk. ___ ___ ___ _____

4. Determined ET tube depth. ___ ___ ___ _____

5. Assessed patient's knowledge of procedure. ___ ___ ___ _____

NURSING DIAGNOSIS

1. Developed appropriate nursing diagnoses based on assessment data. ___ ___ ___ _____

PLANNING

1. Identified expected outcomes. ___ ___ ___ _____

2. Asked another nurse to assist with procedure. ___ ___ ___ _____

3. Explained procedure and patient's participation. ___ ___ ___ _____

4. Positioned patient. ___ ___ ___ _____

5. Placed towel across patient's chest. ___ ___ ___ _____

IMPLEMENTATION

1. Performed hand hygiene. Applied mask, goggles, or face shield, if indicated. ___ ___ ___ _____

2. Administered endotracheal nasopharyngeal or oropharyngeal suctioning (see Skills 25-1 and 25-2). ___ ___ ___ _____

3. Connected left suction catheter to suction source. ___ ___ ___ _____

4. Prepared method to secure ET tube—tape or commercial device. ___ ___ ___ _____

5. Applied clean gloves and instructed assistant to apply clean gloves and hold ET tube firmly. ___ ___ ___ _____

6. Removed old tape or device carefully from tube and patient's face and discarded tape properly. ___ ___ ___ _____

7. Cleaned excess adhesive from patient's face. ___ ___ ___ _____

	S	U	NP	Comments

8. Removed oral airway or bite block and placed on towel.

9. Cleaned mouth, gums, and teeth opposite ET tube.

10. For oral ET tube only, moved ET tube to opposite side of mouth with assistant's help.

11. Repeated oral cleaning as in Step 9 for second side of mouth.

12. Cleaned and dried patient's face and neck. Shaved male patient as necessary.

13. Applied small amount of skin protectant or liquid adhesive to face and allowed it to dry.

14. Secured ET tube.

   a. *Tape Method*

     (1) Positioned tape carefully under head and neck.

     (2) Secured tape from ear to nares and across upper lip if oral ET tube or across top of nose if nasal ET tube.

     (3) Secured tape to remaining side of face and secured tape to tube correctly.

   b. *Commercial Device*

     (1) Threaded ET tube through opening to secure the tube. Ensured that pilot balloon was accessible.

     (2) Placed strips of ET holder under the patient at the occipital region of the head.

     (3) Verified that ET tube was at established depth.

     (4) Attached Velcro strips at the base of the patient's head. Left 1 cm (½ inch) slack in strips.

     (5) Verified that tube was secured.

15. Cleaned and rinsed oral airway.

16. Reinserted oral airway. Secured with tape, if indicated.

17. Discarded soiled items.

18. Repositioned patient.

19. Nurse and assistant removed gloves and face shields and disposed of them correctly. Performed hand hygiene.

288

	S	U	NP	Comments

EVALUATION

1. Compared assessments before and after procedure. ___ ___ ___ _____

2. Observed depth and position of ET tube. ___ ___ ___ _____

3. Assessed security of tape or commercial device. ___ ___ ___ _____

4. Assessed skin around mouth and oral mucous membranes. ___ ___ ___ _____

5. Identified unexpected outcomes. ___ ___ ___ _____

RECORDING AND REPORTING

1. Recorded appropriate depth of ET tube, frequency of care, procedure, and patient assessments. ___ ___ ___ _____

2. Reported unexpected findings. ___ ___ ___ _____

Student _____ Date _____

Instructor _____ Date _____

PERFORMANCE CHECKLIST SKILL 25-4 **TRACHEOSTOMY CARE**

	S	U	NP	Comments

ASSESSMENT

1. Observed for signs and symptoms of need to perform tracheostomy care. ___ ___ ___ _____

2. Observed for factors influencing tracheostomy airway function. ___ ___ ___ _____

3. Assessed patient's understanding and ability to perform own tracheostomy care. ___ ___ ___ _____

4. Checked when tracheostomy care was last performed. ___ ___ ___ _____

NURSING DIAGNOSIS

1. Developed appropriate nursing diagnoses based on assessment data. ___ ___ ___ _____

PLANNING

1. Identified expected outcomes. ___ ___ ___ _____

2. Asked another nurse or family member to assist with procedure. ___ ___ ___ _____

3. Explained procedure to patient and family. ___ ___ ___ _____

4. Positioned patient comfortably. ___ ___ ___ _____

5. Placed towel across patient's chest. ___ ___ ___ _____

IMPLEMENTATION

1. Performed hand hygiene and applied clean gloves. Applied face shield, if indicated. ___ ___ ___ _____

2. Suctioned tracheostomy. Disposed of soiled dressing and used catheter. Removed and disposed of gloves. ___ ___ ___ _____

3. Prepared equipment at bedside table. Opened sterile tracheostomy kit and dressing package. ___ ___ ___ _____

4. Applied sterile gloves. Kept dominant hand sterile throughout procedure. ___ ___ ___ _____

5. Hyperoxygenated patient, if needed. Removed oxygen source and applied oxygen loosely over tracheostomy, if needed. ___ ___ ___ _____

6. *Tracheostomy With Inner Cannula*

   a. Removed inner cannula and dropped into saline basin. ___ ___ ___ _____

	S	U	NP	Comments

b. Placed tracheostomy collar oxygen source over outer cannula. Placed T tube and ventilator oxygen sources over outer cannula.

c. Removed secretions inside and outside of inner cannula.

d. Rinsed inner cannula correctly.

e. Replaced inner cannula and secured locking mechanism. Reapplied oxygen source.

7. *Tracheostomy With Disposable Inner Cannula*

a. Removed cannula from manufacturer's packaging.

b. Withdrew inner cannula, touching only the outer aspect of the tube, and replaced with new cannula. Locked into position.

c. Disposed of contaminated cannula appropriately and applied ventilator or oxygen source.

8. Cleaned outer cannula surfaces and stoma under faceplate with saline-soaked cotton swabs.

9. Rinsed outer cannula and stoma under faceplate.

10. Lightly patted skin and outer cannula with gauze.

11. Secured tracheostomy.

a. *Trach Tie Method*

(1) Instructed assistant to apply gloves and securely hold tracheostomy tube in place. Cut ties with assistant holding tube.

(2) Inserted one end of new tie through faceplate eyelet and pulled ends even.

(3) Slid both ends of tie behind patient's head and around neck to other eyelet and inserted through other faceplate eyelet.

(4) Pulled snugly.

(5) Tied ends securely and allowed adequate space.

(6) Inserted fresh tracheostomy dressing under clean ties and faceplate.

	S	U	NP	Comments

b. *Trach Tube Holder Method*

(1) Maintained secure hold on tracheostomy tube. ___ ___ ___ _____

(2) Aligned strap under patient's neck. ___ ___ ___ _____

(3) Placed narrow end of ties under and through the faceplate eyelets. Pulled ends even and secured with Velcro holders. ___ ___ ___ _____

(4) Verified space for one loose or two snug fingers under neck strap. ___ ___ ___ _____

12. Positioned patient comfortably and assessed respiratory status. ___ ___ ___ _____

13. Replaced oxygen delivery source. ___ ___ ___ _____

14. Removed and discarded gloves and face shield. ___ ___ ___ _____

15. Stored and/or replaced supplies. ___ ___ ___ _____

16. Performed hand hygiene. ___ ___ ___ _____

EVALUATION

1. Compared assessments before and after procedure. ___ ___ ___ _____

2. Assessed comfort of new tracheostomy ties. ___ ___ ___ _____

3. Observed inner and outer cannula for secretions. ___ ___ ___ _____

4. Assessed stoma for signs of infection or skin breakdown. ___ ___ ___ _____

5. Identified unexpected outcomes. ___ ___ ___ _____

RECORDING AND REPORTING

1. Recorded type and size of tracheostomy tube, frequency of care, procedure, patient assessment, and tolerance. ___ ___ ___ _____

2. Reported unexpected findings. ___ ___ ___ _____

Student _____ Date _____

Instructor _____ Date _____

PERFORMANCE CHECKLIST SKILL 25-5 **INFLATING THE CUFF ON AN ENDOTRACHEAL OR TRACHEOSTOMY TUBE**

	S	U	NP	Comments

ASSESSMENT

1. Observed for signs and symptoms indicating need to perform cuff care. ___ ___ ___ _____

2. Determined caregiver's understanding of procedure if patient discharged with a cuffed tracheostomy tube. ___ ___ ___ _____

NURSING DIAGNOSIS

1. Developed appropriate nursing diagnoses based on assessment data. ___ ___ ___ _____

PLANNING

1. Identified expected outcomes. ___ ___ ___ _____

2. Explained procedure to patient. ___ ___ ___ _____

3. Positioned patient comfortably. ___ ___ ___ _____

IMPLEMENTATION

1. Performed hand hygiene. Applied gloves and face shield, if indicated. ___ ___ ___ _____

2. Suctioned patient using aseptic technique. ___ ___ ___ _____

3. Connected syringe to pilot balloon. ___ ___ ___ _____

4. Assessed proper cuff inflation with stethoscope. ___ ___ ___ _____

5. Removed all air from cuff if no air leak heard. ___ ___ ___ _____

6. Correctly inflated cuff per agency policy and assessed for minimum leak with stethoscope. ___ ___ ___ _____

7. Slowly reinflated cuff if excessive air was heard. ___ ___ ___ _____

8. Cleaned stethoscope with alcohol wipe after removal. ___ ___ ___ _____

9. Removed syringe and discarded in appropriate receptacle. ___ ___ ___ _____

10. Repositioned patient. ___ ___ ___ _____

11. Removed and disposed of gloves and face shield. Performed hand hygiene. ___ ___ ___ _____

	S	U	NP	Comments

EVALUATION

1. Compared assessments before and after procedure. _____ _____ _____ _____

2. Observed tidal volume exhaled from mechanical ventilator. _____ _____ _____ _____

3. Auscultated for audible air leak. _____ _____ _____ _____

4. Observed for signs of excessive cuff inflation. _____ _____ _____ _____

5. Identified unexpected outcomes. _____ _____ _____ _____

RECORDING AND REPORTING

1. Recorded presence of minimum leak at end inspiration, volume of air injected into cuff, secretions obtained when suctioning, and frequency of cuff care. _____ _____ _____ _____

Student _____ Date _____

Instructor _____ Date _____

PERFORMANCE CHECKLIST SKILL 26-1 **CARING FOR PATIENTS WITH CHEST TUBES CONNECTED TO DISPOSABLE DRAINAGE SYSTEMS**

	S	U	NP	Comments

ASSESSMENT

1. Obtained baseline vital signs, oxygen saturation (SpO_2), and level of orientation.

2. Performed pulmonary assessment. Reviewed pertinent laboratory tests.

3. Assessed patient's pulmonary status.

4. Assessed patient for known allergies.

5. Reviewed patient's medical record for anticoagulant therapy.

6. Observed insertion site dressing, patency and function of chest tube.

NURSING DIAGNOSIS

1. Developed appropriate nursing diagnoses based on assessment data.

PLANNING

1. Identified expected outcomes.

2. Determined if informed consent was obtained, if required.

3. Reviewed health care providers' roles and responsibilities for chest tube placement.

4. Explained procedure to patient.

5. Performed hand hygiene.

6. Prepared prescribed drainage system according to manufacturer's guidelines. Opened system when physician ready for insertion.

7. Provided two shodded hemostats or clamps for each tube and maintained taped to top of bed.

8. Positioned patient with insertion site accessible for placement.

IMPLEMENTATION

1. Performed hand hygiene and applied clean gloves.

2. Premedicated patient as ordered.

3. Coached and supported patient through procedure.

	S	U	NP	Comments
4. Showed local anesthetic to health care provider.	___	___	___	_____
5. Held anesthetic solution bottle upside down with label facing health care provider for withdrawal of solution.	___	___	___	_____
6. Assisted health care provider in connecting drainage system.	___	___	___	_____
7. Taped the tube connection between the chest and drainage tubes.	___	___	___	_____
8. Turned off suction source and unclamped drainage tubing before connecting patient to system.	___	___	___	_____
9. Assessed patency of drainage system.	___	___	___	_____
10. Straightened and secured excess tubing on mattress next to patient.	___	___	___	_____
11. Promoted drainage by correctly adjusting tubing to hang in a straight line from mattress to drainage chamber.	___	___	___	_____
12. Observed patency of mediastinal tubes by lifting in sections when assessing drainage.	___	___	___	_____
13. Assisted patient to comfortable position.	___	___	___	_____
14. Disposed of soiled equipment and removed gloves.	___	___	___	_____
15. Performed hand hygiene.	___	___	___	_____

EVALUATION

	S	U	NP	Comments
1. Monitored vital signs, oxygen saturation, pulmonary status, drainage, and insertion site every 15 minutes for first 2 hours.	___	___	___	_____
2. Assessed collection system for type and amount of fluid drainage.	___	___	___	_____
3. Assessed for improvement in respiratory status and vital signs.	___	___	___	_____
4. Assessed patient's level of comfort.	___	___	___	_____
5. Assessed drainage system for proper functioning.	___	___	___	_____
6. Assessed patient's physical and psychological status every 4 hours after the first 2 hours.	___	___	___	_____
7. Identified unexpected outcomes.	___	___	___	_____

RECORDING AND REPORTING

	S	U	NP	Comments
1. Recorded baseline vital signs, oxygen saturation, and level of comfort preprocedure and postprocedure.	___	___	___	_____
2. Recorded time, site, and person inserting tube.	___	___	___	_____

	S	U	NP	Comments
3. Recorded chest drainage output at appropriate time intervals.	___	___	___	_____
4. Checked chest tube insertion site and dressings at appropriate time intervals.	___	___	___	_____
5. Recorded patient's physical and psychological status at appropriate time interval.	___	___	___	_____
6. Reported changes in patient's status and/or problems with system.	___	___	___	_____

Student _____ Date _____

Instructor _____ Date _____

PERFORMANCE CHECKLIST SKILL 26-2 **ASSISTING WITH REMOVAL OF CHEST TUBES**

	S	U	NP	Comments

ASSESSMENT

1. Identified signs that reveal lung reexpansion. ___ ___ ___ _____

2. Assessed patient's comfort level. ___ ___ ___ _____

3. Determined patient's understanding of procedure. ___ ___ ___ _____

4. Clamped chest tube 12 to 24 hours before removal or as ordered by health care provider. ___ ___ ___ _____

NURSING DIAGNOSIS

1. Developed appropriate nursing diagnoses based on assessment data. ___ ___ ___ _____

PLANNING

1. Identified expected outcomes. ___ ___ ___ _____

2. Explained procedure to patient. ___ ___ ___ _____

3. Verified analgesia administration before removal. ___ ___ ___ _____

IMPLEMENTATION

1. Administered prescribed premedication approximately 30 minutes before procedure. ___ ___ ___ _____

2. Performed hand hygiene and applied gloves and face shield, if needed. ___ ___ ___ _____

3. Assisted patient to appropriate position. ___ ___ ___ _____

4. Remained with patient while health care provider or APN prepared occlusive dressing. ___ ___ ___ _____

5. Supported patient physically and emotionally while health care provider or APN removed dressing and clipped sutures. ___ ___ ___ _____

6. Assisted patient as health care provider or APN asked patient to take a deep breath and hold it or exhale completely and hold it. ___ ___ ___ _____

7. Remained with patient while health care provider or APN pulled out chest tube. ___ ___ ___ _____

8. Applied prepared occlusive dressing. ___ ___ ___ _____

9. Assisted patient to comfortable position. ___ ___ ___ _____

10. Removed used equipment from bedside. ___ ___ ___ _____

11. Removed gloves and face shield, if worn. Performed hand hygiene. ___ ___ ___ _____

	S	U	NP	Comments

EVALUATION

1. Assessed lung sounds. Observed patient for subcutaneous emphysema or respiratory distress during first few hours after removal. ___ ___ ___ _____

2. Assessed patient's vital signs, oxygen saturation, pulmonary status, and psychological status. ___ ___ ___ _____

3. Reviewed chest x-ray film. ___ ___ ___ _____

4. Asked patient about level of pain or comfort. ___ ___ ___ _____

5. Assessed chest dressing for drainage and patency. ___ ___ ___ _____

6. Identified unexpected outcomes. ___ ___ ___ _____

RECORDING AND REPORTING

1. Recorded removal of tube, amount of drainage, wound appearance, and patient assessment. ___ ___ ___ _____

2. Reported patient's response to chest tube removal. ___ ___ ___ _____

Student _____ Date _____

Instructor _____ Date _____

PERFORMANCE CHECKLIST SKILL 26-3 **REINFUSION OF CHEST TUBE DRAINAGE**

	S	U	NP	Comments
ASSESSMENT				
1. Obtained vital signs, oxygen saturation, and pulmonary status.	____	____	____	_____
2. Observed for changes in vital signs, increased apprehension, presence of active bleeding, and chest pain.	____	____	____	_____
3. Assessed patient for known allergies.	____	____	____	_____
4. Reviewed patient's medical record for anticoagulant therapy.	____	____	____	_____
5. Assessed IV site.	____	____	____	_____
6. Obtained baseline laboratory data.	____	____	____	_____
NURSING DIAGNOSIS				
1. Formulated appropriate nursing diagnoses based on assessment data.	____	____	____	_____
PLANNING				
1. Identified expected outcomes.	____	____	____	_____
2. Explained procedure to patient.	____	____	____	_____
IMPLEMENTATION				
1. Demonstrated correct technique with system setup, including proper equipment, tight connections, and maintenance of unit sterility.	____	____	____	_____
2. Performed hand hygiene and applied gloves.	____	____	____	_____
3. Correctly performed continuous collection.				
a. Opened replacement bag properly and relieved excessive negative pressure.	____	____	____	_____
b. Demonstrated proper technique, including correct clamp management, for removal of initial bag and securing replacement bag.	____	____	____	_____
4. Properly completed reinfusion process.				
a. Used new microaggregate filter for each bag.	____	____	____	_____
b. Correctly accessed bag, and, after priming filter, hung bag for reinfusion.	____	____	____	_____
c. Added any ordered anticoagulants.	____	____	____	_____
5. Correctly discontinued autotransfusion.	____	____	____	_____

	S	U	NP	Comments

6. Properly reconnected chest drainage tube to unit when autotransfusion completed.   _____ _____ _____ _____

7. Discarded used supplies and performed hand hygiene.   _____ _____ _____ _____

EVALUATION

1. Monitored vital signs, hematocrit, and hemoglobin.   _____ _____ _____ _____

2. Monitored chest drainage system and patient's lung sounds.   _____ _____ _____ _____

3. Assessed the IV infusion site for infiltration and phlebitis.   _____ _____ _____ _____

4. Identified unexpected outcomes.   _____ _____ _____ _____

RECORDING AND REPORTING

1. Recorded drainage and reinfusion, with times and amounts of each.   _____ _____ _____ _____

2. Described the condition of the IV infusion site.   _____ _____ _____ _____

3. Reported to nurse in charge or physician unusual findings and patient's responses.   _____ _____ _____ _____

Student _____ Date _____

Instructor _____ Date _____

PERFORMANCE CHECKLIST SKILL 27-1 **INSERTING AN ORAL AIRWAY**

	S	U	NP	Comments

ASSESSMENT

1. Identified signs and symptoms indicating need for insertion of an oral airway.

2. Determined factors that normally influence upper airway functioning.

3. Assessed for presence of gag reflex.

4. Assessed patient's and family's knowledge of procedure.

NURSING DIAGNOSIS

1. Developed appropriate nursing diagnoses based on assessment data.

PLANNING

1. Identified expected outcomes.

2. Correctly positioned patient.

IMPLEMENTATION

1. Performed hand hygiene. Applied clean gloves and face shield.

2. Opened patient's mouth.

3. Inserted oral airway with curved end up. Turned airway over after reaching back of throat.

4. Suctioned secretions, if needed.

5. Reassessed patient's respiratory status.

6. Provided patient hygiene after procedure.

7. Discarded used supplies into appropriate receptacle, removed gloves, and performed hand hygiene.

8. Frequently administered mouth care.

EVALUATION

1. Compared patient's respiratory assessments before and after insertion of oral airway.

2. Assessed patency of airway.

3. Reassessed need for airway if patient pushed airway out of place.

4. Identified unexpected outcomes.

	S	U	NP	Comments

RECORDING AND REPORTING

1. Recorded patient assessment, procedure, size of airway, and patient's response. ⸻ ⸻ ⸻ ⸻⸻⸻⸻⸻⸻⸻

2. Reported unexpected findings. ⸻ ⸻ ⸻ ⸻⸻⸻⸻⸻⸻⸻

Student _____ Date _____

Instructor _____ Date _____

PERFORMANCE CHECKLIST SKILL 27-2 **USE OF AN AUTOMATED EXTERNAL DEFIBRILLATOR**

	S	U	NP	Comments
ASSESSMENT				
1. Established patient's unresponsiveness and called for help.	___	___	___	_____
2. Established absence of respirations, circulation, and movement.	___	___	___	_____
NURSING DIAGNOSIS				
1. Developed appropriate nursing diagnoses based on assessment data.	___	___	___	_____
PLANNING				
1. Identified expected outcomes.	___	___	___	_____
2. Activated the code team per agency policy and procedure.	___	___	___	_____
IMPLEMENTATION				
1. Opened airway. Gave two breaths using barrier device. Watched for chest to rise and fall.	___	___	___	_____
2. Started chest compressions until AED arrived and ready to attach.	___	___	___	_____
3. Placed AED next to patient's head.	___	___	___	_____
4. Turned on power.	___	___	___	_____
5. Attached pads per device instructions.	___	___	___	_____
6. Cleared rescuers away from victim. Allowed AED time to analyze rhythm.	___	___	___	_____
7. Deliver shock(s) as indicated by AED device.	___	___	___	_____
8. Continued chest compressions for another 2 minutes.	___	___	___	_____
9. Allowed AED to resume analysis of rhythm.	___	___	___	_____
10. Repeated steps 6 through 8 until patient regained pulse or physician determined death.	___	___	___	_____
EVALUATION				
1. Inspected pad adhesion to chest wall between series of shocks.	___	___	___	_____
2. Continued resuscitative efforts until patient regained pulse or physician determined cessation.	___	___	___	_____
3. Identified unexpected outcomes.	___	___	___	_____

	S	U	NP	Comments

RECORDING AND REPORTING

1. Immediately reported arrest, including exact location of victim. _____ _____ _____ _____

2. Recorded onset of arrest, time and number of AED shocks, medications given, procedures performed, cardiac rhythm, use of CPR, and patient's response per agency protocol. _____ _____ _____ _____

Student _____ Date _____

Instructor _____ Date _____

PERFORMANCE CHECKLIST SKILL 27-3 **CODE MANAGEMENT**

	S	U	NP	Comments
ASSESSMENT				
1. Established unresponsiveness.	___	___	___	_____
NURSING DIAGNOSIS				
1. Developed appropriate nursing diagnoses based on assessment data.	___	___	___	_____
PLANNING				
1. Identified expected outcomes.	___	___	___	_____
2. Activated emergency medical services.	___	___	___	_____
IMPLEMENTATION				
PRIMARY SURVEY: ABC				
1. *Primary Survey:* A (AIRWAY)				
a. Applied clean gloves and face shield.	___	___	___	_____
b. Opened airway by using head tilt–chin lift or jaw thrust maneuver.	___	___	___	_____
2. *Primary Survey:* B (BREATHING)				
a. Attempted to ventilate using appropriate and available methods.	___	___	___	_____
b. Inserted oral airway.	___	___	___	_____
c. Gave two breaths and observed for chest rise and fall.	___	___	___	_____
d. Suctioned secretions, if necessary.	___	___	___	_____
3. *Primary Survey:* C (CIRCULATION)				
a. Correctly assessed for presence of pulse after restoring breathing.	___	___	___	_____
b. Placed victim on hard surface.	___	___	___	_____
c. Applied AE in absence of pulse.	___	___	___	_____
d. Began chest compressions, if pulse was absent, in a manner appropriate to victim's age.	___	___	___	_____
e. Continued CPR for 2 minutes in absence of carotid pulse.	___	___	___	_____
SECONDARY SURVEY: ABCD				
1. Delegated appropriate tasks to personnel upon their arrival.	___	___	___	_____

	S	U	NP	Comments

2. *Secondary Survey:* A (INTUBATION OF AIR-WAY)

   a. Assisted code team with endotracheal intubation in the absence of respirations.   ____ ____ ____ _____

3. *Secondary Survey:* B (CONFIRMATION OF AIRWAY AND VENTILATION)

   a. Assisted in confirmation of ET tube placement by auscultating lung sounds.   ____ ____ ____ _____

   b. Ventilated using a bag-valve mask.   ____ ____ ____ _____

4. *Secondary Survey:* C (ANALYSIS OF CARDIAC RHYTHM)

   a. Attached manual defibrillator/monitor to patient.   ____ ____ ____ _____

   b. Assisted code team with manual defibrillation, if appropriate rhythm identified.   ____ ____ ____ _____

   c. Established IV access and began infusion of normal saline.   ____ ____ ____ _____

   d. Assisted with procedures as needed.   ____ ____ ____ _____

   e. Continued CPR until relieved, victim responded, rescuer exhausted, or physician discontinued.   ____ ____ ____ _____

5. *Secondary Survey:* D (DIFFERENTIAL DIAGNOSIS)

   a. Assisted physician with differential diagnosis.   ____ ____ ____ _____

EVALUATION

1. Reassessed the primary and secondary survey ABCDs throughout the code event.   ____ ____ ____ _____

2. Palpated carotid pulse at least every 5 minutes after first minute of CPR.   ____ ____ ____ _____

3. Observed for spontaneous return of respirations or heart rate.   ____ ____ ____ _____

4. Ensured that interruptions in CPR were minimal.   ____ ____ ____ _____

5. Identified unexpected outcomes.   ____ ____ ____ _____

RECORDING AND REPORTING

1. Reported location of respiratory or cardiopulmonary arrest.   ____ ____ ____ _____

2. Recorded onset of arrest, assistance given, and victim's response per agency policy.   ____ ____ ____ _____

Student _____ Date _____

Instructor _____ Date _____

PERFORMANCE CHECKLIST SKILL 28-1 **INITIATING INTRAVENOUS THERAPY**

	S	U	NP	Comments
ASSESSMENT				
1. Reviewed accuracy and completeness of health care provider's order for IV therapy.	___	___	___	_____
2. Assessed for clinical factors and conditions that are affected by IV fluid administration.	___	___	___	_____
3. Assessed patient's previous experience with IV therapy.	___	___	___	_____
4. Collected information about the IV solution, any medications the patient is taking, and possible incompatibility.	___	___	___	_____
5. Determined if patient is to have surgery or receive blood.	___	___	___	_____
6. Assessed for risk factors associated with IV therapy.	___	___	___	_____
7. Assessed laboratory values and history of allergies.	___	___	___	_____
8. Assessed patient's understanding of IV therapy.	___	___	___	_____
NURSING DIAGNOSIS				
1. Developed appropriate nursing diagnoses based on assessment data.	___	___	___	_____
PLANNING				
1. Identified expected outcomes.	___	___	___	_____
IMPLEMENTATION				
1. Explained procedure to the patient.	___	___	___	_____
2. Assisted patient to a comfortable position. Provided adequate lighting.	___	___	___	_____
3. Correctly verified patient's identity.	___	___	___	_____
4. Performed hand hygiene. Organized equipment at bedside.	___	___	___	_____
5. Assisted patient to a gown with snaps on the shoulders, if available.	___	___	___	_____
6. Used sterile technique to open sterile packages.	___	___	___	_____
7. Prepared IV infusion tubing and solution:				
a. Verified IV solution correctly prepared and labeled. Checked expiration date.	___	___	___	_____
b. Opened infusion set.	___	___	___	_____

	S	U	NP	Comments

c. Placed roller clamp about 2 to 5 cm (1 to 2 inches) below drip chamber in the off position. _____ _____ _____ _____

d. Removed protective sheath over IV tubing port on IV solution bag. _____ _____ _____ _____

e. Inserted infusion set spike (sterile) into fluid bag or bottle. _____ _____ _____ _____

f. Primed infusion tubing by compressing drip chamber and filling to ⅓ to ½ full. _____ _____ _____ _____

g. Removed protector cap on end of tubing (if necessary), released roller clamp, and allowed fluid to fill tubing. Added extension tubing. _____ _____ _____ _____

h. Removed air bubbles. _____ _____ _____ _____

i. Replaced protector cap on end of infusion tubing. _____ _____ _____ _____

8. Prepared heparin or normal saline lock for infusion. _____ _____ _____ _____

9. Applied gloves. Applied face shield and mask, if indicated. _____ _____ _____ _____

10. Identified accessible vein. Applied flat tourniquet over gown sleeve above proposed insertion site. _____ _____ _____ _____

11. Selected appropriate well-dilated vein for IV insertion.

a. Avoided undesirable locations. _____ _____ _____ _____

b. Used nondominant extremity. _____ _____ _____ _____

c. Fostered venous distention.

(1) Placed extremity in dependent position. _____ _____ _____ _____

(2) Stroked extremity from distal to proximal below site. _____ _____ _____ _____

(3) Applied warmth to area for several minutes. _____ _____ _____ _____

(4) Avoided tapping or vigorous friction to vein. _____ _____ _____ _____

12. Temporarily released tourniquet. Applied topical anesthetic as needed. _____ _____ _____ _____

13. Placed connection of infusion set or saline lock nearby on sterile surface. _____ _____ _____ _____

14. Reviewed patient's allergies. Cleaned site with appropriate antiseptic and allowed to dry. _____ _____ _____ _____

	S	U	NP	Comments

15. Replaced tourniquet 4 to 5 inches above selected insertion site and checked patient's distal pulse.

16. Performed venipuncture:

   a. Anchored vein by placing thumb over vein and stretching skin distal to the selected site.

   b. Advised patient to remain still. Warned patient of sharp, quick stick.

   c. Inserted over-the-needle catheter (ONC), IV catheter safety device, or winged (butterfly) needle with bevel up at a 10- to 30-degree angle slightly distal to the actual site in the direction of the vein.

17. Observed for blood return. Lowered needle until almost flush with skin. Advanced catheter approximately ⅛ to ¼ inch. Continued to hold skin taut and advanced catheter until hub rested at insertion site.

18. Stabilized catheter/needle with one hand and released tourniquet with the other hand. Removed stylet of ONC; did not recap stylet. Glided protective guard over stylet of IV safety device.

19. Connected end of infusion tubing set of heparin/saline lock adapter to end of catheter.

20. Flushed injection cap of saline lock, if needed. Slowly slid clamp open to begin infusion.

21. Secured catheter. Followed agency policy. Used recommended dressing to secure the site.

22. Observed site for swelling.

23. Applied sterile dressing over site.

24. Looped tubing alongside arm and secured.

25. Rechecked flow rates of IV fluid infusions.

26. Wrote date and time, VAD gauge and length, and personal initials on dressing.

27. Disposed of sharps in appropriate container. Removed gloves and performed hand hygiene.

28. Instructed patient how to move around without dislodging the IV.

	S	U	NP	Comments

EVALUATION

1. Observed patient every 1 to 2 hours to determine condition of IV site and status of infusion. Changed IV site per policy or as needed.   ___ ___ ___ _____

2. Observed patient's response to IV therapy.   ___ ___ ___ _____

3. Identified unexpected outcomes.   ___ ___ ___ _____

RECORDING AND REPORTING

1. Recorded and reported IV insertion and information about infusion and insertion site.   ___ ___ ___ _____

2. Recorded patient's response to IV infusion and assessment of infusion site.   ___ ___ ___ _____

3. Documented use of electronic infusion device (EID).   ___ ___ ___ _____

4. Reported unexpected outcomes to the nurse in charge or physician.   ___ ___ ___ _____

Student _____ Date _____

Instructor _____ Date _____

PERFORMANCE CHECKLIST SKILL 28-2 **REGULATING INTRAVENOUS FLOW**

	S	U	NP	Comments
ASSESSMENT				
1. Reviewed accuracy and completeness of health care provider's orders for IV therapy.	___	___	___	_____
2. Performed hand hygiene.	___	___	___	_____
3. Assessed patient's knowledge of how positioning affects flow rate.	___	___	___	_____
4. Observed IV site and patency of VAD and IV flow rate.	___	___	___	_____
5. Identified patient risk for fluid imbalance.	___	___	___	_____
NURSING DIAGNOSIS				
1. Developed appropriate nursing diagnoses based on assessment data.	___	___	___	_____
PLANNING				
1. Identified expected outcomes.	___	___	___	_____
IMPLEMENTATION				
1. Correctly verified patient identity.	___	___	___	_____
2. Calculated hourly rate in milliliters per hour (ml/hr) to be used with EID.	___	___	___	_____
3. Placed adhesive tape on IV bottle or bag next to volume markings and timed as per order.	___	___	___	_____
4. Calculated drops per minute (gtt/min) for gravity flowing IV.	___	___	___	_____
5. Timed flow rate by watch.	___	___	___	_____
6. Followed correct procedure for using infusion controller or pump.	___	___	___	_____
7. Followed correct procedure for using gravity volume control device.	___	___	___	_____
8. Smart pump configured to specific patient care unit:				
a. Provided for patient privacy. Inserted tubing into the pump and selected patient care unit.	___	___	___	_____
b. Selected medication and concentration of drug.	___	___	___	_____
c. Programmed dose and rate. Initiated infusion.	___	___	___	_____
d. Reconfirmed ordered rate if alarm sounded.	___	___	___	_____

	S	U	NP	Comments

9. Placed volumetric device between IV container and spike using aseptic technique.

   a. Filled with 2 hours of fluid volume. ____ ____ ____ _____

   b. Assessed hourly and refilled as needed. ____ ____ ____ _____

10. Instructed patient on how to move safely with IV and purpose of alarms. Advised patient to report any discomfort or alterations and alarms, and not to touch settings. ____ ____ ____ _____

EVALUATION

1. Monitored infusion hourly, and patency of site. ____ ____ ____ _____

2. Observed patient to determine effect of IV therapy. ____ ____ ____ _____

3. Assessed for signs of infiltration or phlebitis. ____ ____ ____ _____

4. Identified unexpected outcomes. ____ ____ ____ _____

RECORDING AND REPORTING

1. Recorded appropriate information pertaining to IV therapy. ____ ____ ____ _____

2. Recorded new fluid rates. ____ ____ ____ _____

3. Documented use and type of infusion device. ____ ____ ____ _____

4. Reported appropriate IV information to nursing personnel. ____ ____ ____ _____

Student _____ Date _____

Instructor _____ Date _____

PERFORMANCE CHECKLIST SKILL 28-3 **CHANGING INTRAVENOUS SOLUTIONS**

	S	U	NP	Comments
ASSESSMENT				
1. Reviewed accuracy and completeness of health care provider's order for IV therapy.	___	___	___	_____
2. Noted date and time when solution and tubing was last changed.	___	___	___	_____
3. Determined the compatibility of all IV fluids and additives.	___	___	___	_____
4. Determined patient's understanding of need for continued IV therapy.	___	___	___	_____
5. Determined patency of IV site and tubing.	___	___	___	_____
NURSING DIAGNOSIS				
1. Developed appropriate nursing diagnoses based on assessment data.	___	___	___	_____
PLANNING				
1. Identified expected outcomes.	___	___	___	_____
IMPLEMENTATION				
1. Collected equipment, ordered solution for correct time, verified solution was correct and properly labeled. Checked expiration date.	___	___	___	_____
2. Correctly verified patient's identity.	___	___	___	_____
3. Confirmed 50 mL of fluid remained in bottle or bag, and drip chamber half full.	___	___	___	_____
4. Explained procedure to patient and family.	___	___	___	_____
5. Performed hand hygiene.	___	___	___	_____
6. Prepared solution bag/bottle for changing.	___	___	___	_____
7. Moved roller clamp to stop flow rate.	___	___	___	_____
8. Removed old solution from IV pole.	___	___	___	_____
9. Removed spike from old solution and correctly inserted spike into new solution.	___	___	___	_____
10. Hung new bag/bottle of solution on IV pole.	___	___	___	_____
11. Checked for air in IV tubing.	___	___	___	_____
12. Ensured drip chamber 1/3 to 1/2 full.	___	___	___	_____
13. Regulated flow rate to prescribed rate.	___	___	___	_____
14. Placed time label on container.	___	___	___	_____

	S	U	NP	Comments

EVALUATION

1. Evaluated flow rate hourly and observed connection site for signs of leaking. _____ _____ _____ _____

2. Reassessed patient's status to determine response to IV fluid therapy. _____ _____ _____ _____

3. Identified unexpected outcomes. _____ _____ _____ _____

RECORDING AND REPORTING

1. Recorded and reported amount and type of fluid infused and amount and type of new fluid. _____ _____ _____ _____

2. Recorded solution and tubing change; used IV flow sheet if available. _____ _____ _____ _____

Student _____ Date _____

Instructor _____ Date _____

PERFORMANCE CHECKLIST SKILL 28-4 **CHANGING INFUSION TUBING**

	S	U	NP	Comments

ASSESSMENT
1. Determined when IV tubing was last changed. Reviewed institutional policy.

2. Assessed tubing for signs of puncture, contamination, or occlusion.

3. Determined patient's understanding of need for continued IV infusions.

NURSING DIAGNOSIS
1. Developed appropriate nursing diagnoses based on assessment data.

PLANNING
1. Identified expected outcomes.

IMPLEMENTATION
1. Correctly verified patient's identity.

2. Explained procedure to patient and family.

3. Coordinated IV tubing changes with IV bag changes whenever possible.

4. Performed hand hygiene.

5. Prepared needed supplies. Kept protective coverings on infusion spike and distal adapter.

6. Applied clean gloves.

7. Removed dressings to reveal cannula hub.

8. Prepared new tubing with bag.

9. *For Continuous IV Infusion*

   a. Moved roller clamp to "off" position.

   b. Regulated drip rate on old tubing to slow rate of infusion.

   c. Compressed drip chamber and filled it while old tubing was still in place.

   d. Inverted container and discontinued old tubing from solution. Taped drip chamber to IV pole.

   e. Placed insertion spike of new tubing into solutions container. Hung solution container on IV pole.

	S	U	NP	Comments

f. Compressed and released drip chamber on new tubing. Filled drip chamber ⅓ to ½ full.

___ ___ ___ _____

g. Slowly opened roller clamp, removed protective cap from needle adapter, and primed tubing with solution. Stopped infusion, replaced cap, and placed adapter near patient's IV site.

___ ___ ___ _____

h. Turned roller clamp on old tubing to "off" position.

___ ___ ___ _____

10. *Preparing Tubing With Intermittent Saline Lock*

a. Used sterile technique to connect new injection cap to new loop or tubing if extension tubing is needed.

___ ___ ___ _____

b. Swab injection cap with antiseptic. Inject saline solution through injection cap and into extension tubing.

___ ___ ___ _____

11. Reestablished infusion:

a. Disconnected old tubing from extension tubing and quickly inserted adapter of new tubing or saline lock into tubing connection.

___ ___ ___ _____

b. For continuous infusion, opened roller clamp on new tubing, allowed solution to run rapidly for 30 to 60 seconds, then regulated drip rate to prescribed rate.

___ ___ ___ _____

c. Correctly marked tubing with date/time of tubing change.

___ ___ ___ _____

d. Secured loop of tubing to patient's arm with tape.

___ ___ ___ _____

12. Removed and discarded old IV tubing. Applied dressings as needed.

___ ___ ___ _____

13. Removed and disposed of gloves. Performed hand hygiene.

___ ___ ___ _____

EVALUATION

1. Evaluated flow rate and observed connection site for leakage.

___ ___ ___ _____

2. Identified unexpected outcomes.

___ ___ ___ _____

RECORDING AND REPORTING

1. Recorded changing of tubing and solution on patient's record. Used flow sheet for parenteral fluids.

___ ___ ___ _____

2. Recorded date and time on tape below drip chamber.

___ ___ ___ _____

Student _____ Date _____

Instructor _____ Date _____

PERFORMANCE CHECKLIST SKILL 28-5 **CHANGING A PERIPHERAL INTRAVENOUS DRESSING**

	S	U	NP	Comments

ASSESSMENT

1. Determined time of last dressing change.

2. Performed hand hygiene. Observed present dressing for moisture and intactness.

3. Observed present IV system for proper functioning. Gently palpated catheter site. Used gloves as needed.

4. Monitored patient's temperature.

5. Determined patient's understanding of need for continued IV infusion.

NURSING DIAGNOSIS

1. Developed appropriate nursing diagnoses based on assessment data.

PLANNING

1. Identified expected outcomes.

IMPLEMENTATION

1. Explained procedure to patient and family.

2. Performed hand hygiene, set up supplies at bedside, and applied gloves.

3. Correctly verified patient's identity.

4. Removed tape carefully. Stabilized IV catheter and removed transparent dressing.

5. Observed insertion site for signs of infection.

6. Prepared new tape strips for later use. Used adhesive remover to clean skin and remove adhesive residue.

7. Cleaned venipuncture site with antiseptic solution. Allowed to dry. Applied skin protectant solution, if needed, and allowed to dry.

8. Reviewed patient allergies. Applied skin protectant solution (Skin Prep, Barrier Film). Allowed to dry.

9. Secured catheter as per agency policy.

10. Removed and discarded gloves.

11. Applied site protection device if ordered.

	S	U	NP	Comments
12. Anchored IV tubing with additional pieces of tape, if necessary.	——	——	——	_____
13. Labeled dressing as per agency policy.	——	——	——	_____
14. Discarded used equipment, and performed hand hygiene.	——	——	——	_____

EVALUATION

1. Assessed functioning and patency of IV system.	——	——	——	_____
2. Inspected condition of IV site.	——	——	——	_____
3. Monitored patient's body temperature.	——	——	——	_____
4. Identified unexpected outcomes.	——	——	——	_____

RECORDING AND REPORTING

1. Documented IV dressing change, type of dressing used, assessment of venipuncture site.	——	——	——	_____
2. Reported to oncoming nursing shift nurse information about IV and patency of site and system.	——	——	——	_____
3. Reported complications to health care provider and documented outcome and patient status.	——	——	——	_____

Student _____ Date _____

Instructor _____ Date _____

PERFORMANCE CHECKLIST PROCEDURAL GUIDELINE 28-1 **DISCONTINUING PERIPHERAL INTRAVENOUS ACCESS**

	S	U	NP	Comments
STEPS				
1. Observed IV site for signs and symptoms of infection, infiltration, and phlebitis.	___	___	___	_____
2. Reviewed accuracy and completeness of health care provider's order for discontinuation of IV.	___	___	___	_____
3. Determined patient's understanding of need for discontinuation of peripheral IV access.	___	___	___	_____
4. Correctly verified patient's identity.	___	___	___	_____
5. Explained procedure to patient, describing sensation when catheter was removed.	___	___	___	_____
6. Turned IV tubing roller clamp to "off" position or turned EID off and roller clamp to off position.	___	___	___	_____
7. Performed hand hygiene and applied gloves.	___	___	___	_____
8. Removed IV site dressing carefully and gently. Removed tape securing catheter.	___	___	___	_____
9. Cleaned site with antimicrobial swab. Allowed to dry completely.	___	___	___	_____
10. Placed sterile gauze above site and withdrew catheter carefully.	___	___	___	_____
11. Applied pressure to site for 2 to 3 minutes according to patient's medical or medication history.	___	___	___	_____
12. Inspected catheter for intactness after removal, noting tip integrity and length.	___	___	___	_____
13. Applied clean folded gauze dressing over site and secured with tape.	___	___	___	_____
14. Discarded used supplies, removed gloves, and performed hand hygiene.	___	___	___	_____
15. Observed site for evidence of bleeding, redness, pain, drainage, and swelling.	___	___	___	_____

Student _____ Date _____

Instructor _____ Date _____

PERFORMANCE CHECKLIST SKILL 28-6 **CARING FOR CENTRAL VASCULAR ACCESS DEVICES**

	S	U	NP	Comments

ASSESSMENT

1. Reviewed accuracy and completeness of health care provider's order for insertion of CVAD. ___ ___ ___ _____

2. Assessed patient's hydration status. ___ ___ ___ _____

3. Assessed patient for presence of any surgical procedures of the upper chest or anatomical irregularities. ___ ___ ___ _____

4. Assessed condition of patient's skin over supraclavicular and infraclavicular areas. ___ ___ ___ _____

5. Reviewed patient's history of medications and allergies. ___ ___ ___ _____

6. Assessed CVAD site for skin integrity and infection. ___ ___ ___ _____

7. Assessed type of CVAD device in use, reviewed manufacturer's directions for use and maintenance. ___ ___ ___ _____

8. Assessed need to use CVC for blood sampling. ___ ___ ___ _____

NURSING DIAGNOSIS

1. Developed appropriate nursing diagnoses based on assessment data. ___ ___ ___ _____

PLANNING

1. Identified expected outcomes. ___ ___ ___ _____

IMPLEMENTATION

1. Explained procedure to patient and family. Instructed patient not to move during procedure. ___ ___ ___ _____

2. Correctly verified patient's identity. ___ ___ ___ _____

3. *Catheter Insertion*

a. Positioned patient flat on bed with rolled towel or bath blanket between scapulas. Placed protected pad under shoulders. ___ ___ ___ _____

b. Removed hair around insertion site, if needed. ___ ___ ___ _____

c. Applied cap, mask, and eyewear. Performed hand hygiene. ___ ___ ___ _____

d. Soaked 4 × 4 gauze pads with recommended antiseptic for use in swabbing insertion site. ___ ___ ___ _____

	S	U	NP	Comments

e. Set up IV bag, primed tubing, and covered end of tubing with sterile cap until needed. ___ ___ ___ _____

f. Placed patient on right side in a 10-degree Trendelenburg's position and turned patient's head away from site of insertion. ___ ___ ___ _____

g. Wiped off top of 1% lidocaine bottle with alcohol swab, and held bottle upside down for physician to access. ___ ___ ___ _____

h. Adjusted IV infusion rate, once line was established, to prescribed rate. Connected to infusion pump after x-ray film confirmed location of catheter tip. ___ ___ ___ _____

4. *Insertion Site Care and Dressing Changes*

a. Positioned patient comfortably with head elevated. ___ ___ ___ _____

b. Provided dressing care on a schedule appropriate to dressing type in use. ___ ___ ___ _____

c. Performed hand hygiene and applied mask and clean gloves. ___ ___ ___ _____

d. Removed old dressing carefully and discarded in appropriate container. ___ ___ ___ _____

e. Removed catheter stabilization device, if used. ___ ___ ___ _____

f. Inspected insertion site and surrounding skin. ___ ___ ___ _____

g. Removed and discarded gloves. Performed hand hygiene and applied sterile gloves. ___ ___ ___ _____

h. Cleaned catheter and insertion site with antiseptic swab. Allowed to dry completely. ___ ___ ___ _____

i. Applied skin protectant to entire area. Allowed to dry completely. ___ ___ ___ _____

j. Applied new catheter stabilization device, if needed. ___ ___ ___ _____

k. Applied transparent dressing over insertion site. ___ ___ ___ _____

l. Applied label to dressing with date, time, and initials. ___ ___ ___ _____

m. Disposed of soiled supplies and used equipment appropriately. Discarded gloves and performed hand hygiene. ___ ___ ___ _____

5. *Blood Sampling*

a. Performed hand hygiene. Applied clean gloves. ___ ___ ___ _____

b. Turned off infusion for a minute before drawing blood. ___ ___ ___ _____

326

	S	U	NP	Comments
c. *If Using Injection Cap*	___	___	___	_____
(1) Cleansed thoroughly and allowed to dry. Used proximal red/brown lumen to draw blood.	___	___	___	_____
(2) Flushed catheter per agency policy.	___	___	___	_____
d. *If Using Catheter Hub*				
(1) Clamped catheter, removed end of IV tubing from injection hub.	___	___	___	_____
(2) Attached 10-mL syringe and flushed per agency policy.	___	___	___	_____
e. Slowly aspirated 5 mL of blood from catheter and discarded syringe in biohazard container when done.	___	___	___	_____
f. Cleansed injection cap with antiseptic swab and allowed to dry completely.	___	___	___	_____
g. Attached appropriate-size syringe and withdrew blood. Clamped catheter when done.	___	___	___	_____
h. Continued to collect blood sampling with vacutainer system.	___	___	___	_____
i. Cleansed injection cap with antiseptic. Allowed to dry.	___	___	___	_____
j. Flushed catheter with 10 mL 0.9% normal saline.	___	___	___	_____
k. Flushed port with heparinized solution as per agency policy.	___	___	___	_____
l. Removed syringe, attached IV tubing, and resumed infusion as ordered.	___	___	___	_____
m. Discarded used equipment and supplies. Removed gloves and performed hand hygiene.	___	___	___	_____
6. *Changing Injection Cap*				
a. Determined when to change injection caps.	___	___	___	_____
b. Prepared new injection cap(s).	___	___	___	_____
c. Clamped catheter lumens one at a time with slide or squeeze clamp.	___	___	___	_____
d. Removed old caps using aseptic technique.	___	___	___	_____
e. Cleaned catheter hub with antiseptic swab. Connected new cap to hub.	___	___	___	_____
f. Flushed per agency policy or initiated infusion.	___	___	___	_____
g. Disposed of used items. Removed gloves and performed hand hygiene.	___	___	___	_____

	S	U	NP	Comments

7. *Flushing a Positive-Pressure Device*

a. Performed hand hygiene and applied gloves.

b. Attached prefilled saline syringe to positive pressure device and primed.

c. Thoroughly cleaned the cap-catheter junction.

d. Clamped catheter. Removed cap and discarded.

e. Connected positive-pressure device, unclamped catheter, and flushed with saline as ordered.

f. Disposed of all used supplies. Removed gloves and performed hand hygiene.

8. *Discontinuing Nontunneled Catheters or PICCs*

a. Confirmed medical order. Checked agency policy, catheters to be discontinued by physicians or certified nurses.

b. If IV fluids are to continue, prepared to convert infusion. If not, discontinued fluids.

c. Performed hand hygiene.

d. Turned off IV fluids running through central line.

e. Placed moisture proof pad under site.

f. Applied gown, mask, goggles, and clean gloves.

g. Removed dressing gently. Discarded in biohazard container. Inspected insertion site.

h. Removed and disposed of gloves, performed hand hygiene, and applied clean gloves.

i. Cleaned site with antiseptic swabs. Allowed to dry completely.

j. Removed catheter securement device if present. Used sterile scissors to remove sutures, if present.

k. Positioned patient in 10-degree Trendelenburg's position.

l. Applied sterile 4×4 gauge to site.

m. Had patient perform Valsalva maneuver as CVAD was slowly and steadily removed.

n. Applied firm pressure on site for 5 minutes or as needed.

328

	S	U	NP	Comments

o. Applied clean sterile dressing with antiseptic solution. Labeled dressing. ⎯ ⎯ ⎯ _____

p. Inspected integrity of catheter tip and discarded in biohazard container. ⎯ ⎯ ⎯ _____

q. Returned patient to a comfortable position. Adjusted peripheral IV, if present, to prescribed rate. ⎯ ⎯ ⎯ _____

r. Disposed of equipment appropriately and performed hand hygiene. ⎯ ⎯ ⎯ _____

EVALUATION

1. Observed patient for shortness of breath and pain after CVAD insertion. ⎯ ⎯ ⎯ _____

2. Observed patient for bleeding or swelling at insertion site and occlusiveness of dressing. ⎯ ⎯ ⎯ _____

3. Monitored intake and output every 4 hours to assess fluid balance. ⎯ ⎯ ⎯ _____

4. Routinely assessed vital signs and symptoms of infection. ⎯ ⎯ ⎯ _____

5. Observed insertion site or port of exit for erythema, warmth, tenderness, edema, or drainage. ⎯ ⎯ ⎯ _____

6. Inspected catheter and connection tubing on recommended schedule. ⎯ ⎯ ⎯ _____

7. Observed for clot formation in catheter, air embolisms, extravasation, and migration. ⎯ ⎯ ⎯ _____

8. Checked x-ray film to confirm catheter placement. ⎯ ⎯ ⎯ _____

9. Evaluated ability of patient or family members to provide care and maintain catheter or infusion port. ⎯ ⎯ ⎯ _____

10. Identified unexpected outcomes. ⎯ ⎯ ⎯ _____

RECORDING AND REPORTING

1. Recorded medications, blood products, and parenteral nutrition given or samples obtained. ⎯ ⎯ ⎯ _____

2. Recorded condition of exit site or port of implantation. ⎯ ⎯ ⎯ _____

3. Recorded dressing change procedure. ⎯ ⎯ ⎯ _____

4. Recorded patency of catheter, ability to draw blood, and any difficulty with infusions. ⎯ ⎯ ⎯ _____

5. Recorded patient and family education measures. ⎯ ⎯ ⎯ _____

6. Immediately notified nursing or health care provider of any signs and symptoms of complications. ⎯ ⎯ ⎯ _____

Student _____ Date _____

Instructor _____ Date _____

PERFORMANCE CHECKLIST SKILL 29-1 **INITIATING BLOOD THERAPY**

	S	U	NP	Comments

ASSESSMENT

1. Reviewed physician's order. ___ ___ ___ _____

2. Inspected integrity and intactness of present IV line. ___ ___ ___ _____

3. Obtained patient's transfusion history. ___ ___ ___ _____

4. Verified consent forms were signed. ___ ___ ___ _____

5. Identified indication for blood product. ___ ___ ___ _____

6. Obtained vital signs before initiating transfusion. ___ ___ ___ _____

7. Assessed patient's need for IV fluids or medication before transfusion. ___ ___ ___ _____

8. Assessed patient's understanding of procedure. ___ ___ ___ _____

NURSING DIAGNOSIS

1. Developed appropriate nursing diagnoses based on assessment data. ___ ___ ___ _____

PLANNING

1. Identified expected outcomes. ___ ___ ___ _____

2. Explained procedure and its purpose to patient. ___ ___ ___ _____

IMPLEMENTATION

1. *Preadministration*

   a. Obtained blood product from blood bank per agency protocol. ___ ___ ___ _____

   b. Checked appearance of blood product. ___ ___ ___ _____

   c. Correctly verified right blood product and right patient. ___ ___ ___ _____

   d. Reviewed purpose of treatment and asked patient to report any changes felt during transfusion. ___ ___ ___ _____

   e. Had patient void or emptied urine collection container. ___ ___ ___ _____

2. *Administration*

   a. Performed hand hygiene and applied clean gloves. ___ ___ ___ _____

   b. Opened Y tubing blood administration set. ___ ___ ___ _____

	S	U	NP	Comments
c. Set roller clamp(s) to "off" position.	___	___	___	_____
d. Spiked normal saline IV bag with Y tubing spike. Primed both sides of Y tubing, filled half of drip chamber, and closed clamps.	___	___	___	_____
e. Hung on IV pole and finished priming the tubing.	___	___	___	_____
f. Prepared blood component for administration. Opened clamp of Y tubing and primed with blood.	___	___	___	_____
g. Attached primed tubing to patient's venous access device and opened common tubing clamp.	___	___	___	_____
h. Initiated infusion of blood product.	___	___	___	_____
i. Remained with patient during the first 15 minutes of transfusion.	___	___	___	_____
j. Appropriately monitored patient's vital signs.	___	___	___	_____
k. Regulated infusion according to health care provider's orders.	___	___	___	_____
l. Cleared infusion tubing with 0.9% normal saline after blood completely infused.	___	___	___	_____
m. Disposed of supplies. Removed gloves and performed hand hygiene.	___	___	___	_____

EVALUATION

	S	U	NP	Comments
1. Monitored IV site and status of infusion.	___	___	___	_____
2. Assessed patient for any changes in vital signs, or other signs of transfusion reaction.	___	___	___	_____
3. Reassessed patient and assessed laboratory values to determine response to administration of blood components.	___	___	___	_____
4. Identified unexpected outcomes.	___	___	___	_____

RECORDING AND REPORTING

	S	U	NP	Comments
1. Recorded on appropriate form type and amount of blood component administered, vital signs before, during, and after transfusion, and patient's response to blood therapy.	___	___	___	_____
2. Reported immediately signs and symptoms of a transfusion reaction or deterioration in cardiac, respiratory, and/or renal status.	___	___	___	_____

Student _____ Date _____

Instructor _____ Date _____

PERFORMANCE CHECKLIST SKILL 29-2   **MONITORING FOR ADVERSE REACTIONS TO TRANSFUSIONS**

	S	U	NP	Comments

ASSESSMENT

1. Observed patient for fever with or without chills. ___ ___ ___ _____

2. Assessed patient for tachycardia and/or tachypnea and dyspnea. ___ ___ ___ _____

3. Observed patient for hives or skin rash. ___ ___ ___ _____

4. Observed patient for flushing. ___ ___ ___ _____

5. Observed patient for GI symptoms. ___ ___ ___ _____

6. Observed patient for a fall in blood pressure. ___ ___ ___ _____

7. Observed patient for wheezing, chest pain, and possible cardiac arrest. ___ ___ ___ _____

8. Assessed patient for complaints of headache or muscle pain with fever. ___ ___ ___ _____

9. Monitored patient for DIC, renal failure, and other late signs of an acute hemolytic reaction. ___ ___ ___ _____

10. Auscultated lungs and monitored CVP, if possible. ___ ___ ___ _____

11. Observed patient for jaundice and increased liver enzymes, and decreased RBCs, WBCs, and platelets. ___ ___ ___ _____

12. Monitored patient's laboratory values. ___ ___ ___ _____

13. Observed patient receiving massive transfusions for mild hypothermia, dysrhythmias, hypotension, hypocalcemia, and hemochromatosis. ___ ___ ___ _____

NURSING DIAGNOSIS

1. Developed appropriate nursing diagnoses based on assessment data. ___ ___ ___ _____

PLANNING

1. Identified expected outcomes. ___ ___ ___ _____

2. Explained to patient and family treatment for a reaction. ___ ___ ___ _____

IMPLEMENTATION

1. Discontinued transfusion. ___ ___ ___ _____

2. Removed tubing with blood in it and replaced with new tubing. ___ ___ ___ _____

	S	U	NP	Comments

3. Maintained patent IV line using 0.9% normal saline.   ___ ___ ___ _____

4. Remained with patient. Obtained and documented vital signs, continuous monitoring, and assessment.   ___ ___ ___ _____

5. Notified physician or health care provider of reaction.   ___ ___ ___ _____

6. Notified blood bank.   ___ ___ ___ _____

7. Obtained blood samples from opposite extremity per agency policy.   ___ ___ ___ _____

8. Returned remaining blood and attached tubing to blood bank according to agency policy.   ___ ___ ___ _____

9. Monitored patient's vital signs every 15 minutes.   ___ ___ ___ _____

10. Administered prescribed medications and IV fluids according to type of reaction.   ___ ___ ___ _____

11. Initiated CPR if necessary.   ___ ___ ___ _____

12. Obtained first voided urine.   ___ ___ ___ _____

13. Completed transfusion reaction report.   ___ ___ ___ _____

EVALUATION

1. Assessed patient to determine improvement or changes in physiological status.   ___ ___ ___ _____

2. Identified unexpected outcomes.   ___ ___ ___ _____

RECORDING AND REPORTING

1. Recorded pertinent information about transfusion reaction.   ___ ___ ___ _____

2. Reported transfusion reaction immediately to nurse in charge and health care provider.   ___ ___ ___ _____

3. Recorded exact time of transfusion reaction, assessment findings, nursing and medical actions taken, and patient's response.   ___ ___ ___ _____

Student _____ Date _____

Instructor _____ Date _____

PERFORMANCE CHECKLIST SKILL 30-1 **PERFORMING NUTRITIONAL ASSESSMENT**

	S	U	NP	Comments
ASSESSMENT				
1. Assessed patient for usual body weight changes.	___	___	___	_____
2. Obtained complete history, including social, economic, and psychological factors.	___	___	___	_____
3. Performed physical assessment.	___	___	___	_____
4. Reviewed laboratory results.	___	___	___	_____
5. Determined medications and other supplements patient is taking.	___	___	___	_____
6. Measured actual height and weight.	___	___	___	_____
7. Calculated IBW and BMI.	___	___	___	_____
8. Assessed risk factors affecting adequate diet and appetite. Noted food intolerances and allergies.	___	___	___	_____
9. Assessed present nutritional intake. Asked patient to maintain a 24-hour intake diary.	___	___	___	_____
10. Determined patient's ability to manipulate eating utensils and self-feed.	___	___	___	_____
11. Explained completed assessment to patient.	___	___	___	_____
12. Notified the nutrition department of prescribed diet and patient's food (cultural) preferences.	___	___	___	_____
NURSING DIAGNOSIS				
1. Developed appropriate nursing diagnoses based on assessment data.	___	___	___	_____
EVALUATION				
1. Reviewed history and physical examination.	___	___	___	_____
2. Compared patient's height and weight versus ideal height and weight for age-group.	___	___	___	_____
3. Compared patient's laboratory data versus expected values.	___	___	___	_____
4. Identified unexpected outcomes.	___	___	___	_____
RECORDING AND REPORTING				
1. Documented findings and made recommendations on nutritional assessment form.	___	___	___	_____

PERFORMANCE CHECKLIST SKILL 30-2 **ASSISTING AN ADULT PATIENT WITH ORAL NUTRITION**

	S	U	NP	Comments
ASSESSMENT				
1. Assessed that GI tract is functioning and types of diet patient can tolerate.	___	___	___	_____
2. Reviewed prescribed diet.	___	___	___	_____
3. Assessed patient's ability to swallow and gag reflex.	___	___	___	_____
4. Assessed oral cavity and proper fit and availability of dentures.	___	___	___	_____
5. Assessed patient's energy level and appetite.	___	___	___	_____
6. Assessed patient's cognitive and sensory status, motor skills, and ability to feed self.	___	___	___	_____
7. Determined patient's food preferences and tolerance.	___	___	___	_____
NURSING DIAGNOSIS				
1. Developed appropriate nursing diagnoses based on assessment data.	___	___	___	_____
PLANNING				
1. Identified expected outcomes.	___	___	___	_____
2. Collaborated with dietitian on meal plans.	___	___	___	_____
3. Prepared patient's room.	___	___	___	_____
4. Prepared patient for meal—provided mouth care, dentures, positioning, and sensory aids.	___	___	___	_____
IMPLEMENTATION				
1. *Prepared Patient's Tray*				
a. Performed hand hygiene.	___	___	___	_____
b. Assessed tray for completeness and correct diet.	___	___	___	_____
c. Prepared tray to meet patient's needs.	___	___	___	_____
d. Determined how well patient was eating independently.	___	___	___	_____
2. *Assisted Patient Who Could Not Eat Independently*				
a. Established comfortable position from which to offer assistance.	___	___	___	_____

	S	U	NP	Comments

b. Asked in what order the patient would like the food, and cut food into bite-size pieces. ___ ___ ___ _____

c. Identified food by location on the plate. ___ ___ ___ _____

d. Fed patient small amounts at a time and assessed ability to chew and swallow.

   (1) Older adult: Fed small amounts, observed ability to chew and swallow. Observed for fatigue. Allowed rest periods. ___ ___ ___ _____

   (2) Neurologically impaired patient: Fed small amounts, assessed ability to chew and properly swallow. Provided small amounts of thickened fluids as requested. ___ ___ ___ _____

   (3) Oncology patient: Assessed for presence of nausea, and premedicated as ordered. Asked about food aversions. ___ ___ ___ _____

e. Monitored fluid intake throughout meal, not all liquid at the beginning of meal. ___ ___ ___ _____

f. Conversed with patient during meal. Provided patient education as appropriate. ___ ___ ___ _____

g. Assisted patient with oral and hand hygiene. ___ ___ ___ _____

h. Assisted patient to resting position, with head properly elevated. ___ ___ ___ _____

i. Returned patient's tray and washed hands. ___ ___ ___ _____

EVALUATION

1. Observed patient's ability to swallow. ___ ___ ___ _____

2. Monitored patient's weight if ordered. ___ ___ ___ _____

3. Assessed patient's tolerance to diet. ___ ___ ___ _____

4. Monitored patient's fluid and food intake. ___ ___ ___ _____

5. Assessed patient's ability to assist with feeding. ___ ___ ___ _____

6. Identified unexpected outcomes. ___ ___ ___ _____

RECORDING AND REPORTING

1. Documented tolerance of diet, amount eaten, and intake and output. ___ ___ ___ _____

2. Documented calorie count, nutritional supplements taken, I&O, weight and elimination pattern. ___ ___ ___ _____

3. Report nutritional alterations to nurse in charge and/or physician. ___ ___ ___ _____

338

Student _____ Date _____

Instructor _____ Date _____

PERFORMANCE CHECKLIST SKILL 30-3 **ASPIRATION PRECAUTIONS**

	S	U	NP	Comments

ASSESSMENT

1. Performed nutritional assessment. ____ ____ ____ _____

2. Assessed patient for dysphagia. ____ ____ ____ _____

3. Assessed patient for abnormal eating patterns. ____ ____ ____ _____

4. Noted evidence of dysphagia on patient's record and notified physician. ____ ____ ____ _____

5. Placed identification of risk on patient's chart or Kardex. ____ ____ ____ _____

NURSING DIAGNOSIS

1. Developed appropriate nursing diagnoses based on assessment data. ____ ____ ____ _____

PLANNING

1. Identified expected outcomes. ____ ____ ____ _____

IMPLEMENTATION

1. Performed hand hygiene. ____ ____ ____ _____

2. Provided oral hygiene before meal. ____ ____ ____ _____

3. Applied pulse oximeter to patient's finger. ____ ____ ____ _____

4. Positioned patient to facilitate eating and swallowing. ____ ____ ____ _____

5. Inspected mouth for pockets of food. ____ ____ ____ _____

6. Discussed and demonstrated chin-tuck position. Observed return demonstration. ____ ____ ____ _____

7. Added thickener to liquids as needed. ____ ____ ____ _____

8. Offered small amounts of food, touching utensil to patient's mouth or tongue to provide tactile cue to begin eating. ____ ____ ____ _____

9. Provided verbal cueing while feeding and observed for coughing, choking, gagging, and drooling. Suctioned airway as necessary. ____ ____ ____ _____

10. Advised patient to remain sitting upright for at least 30 to 60 minutes after the meal. ____ ____ ____ _____

11. Assisted patient hand hygiene and oral care. ____ ____ ____ _____

12. Returned patient's tray to appropriate place and washed hands. ____ ____ ____ _____

	S	U	NP	Comments

EVALUATION

1. Assessed patient's ability to ingest foods of various textures and consistencies.

2. Assessed patient's food and fluid intake.

3. Monitored pulse oximetry during meal.

4. Weighed patient weekly.

5. Identified unexpected outcomes.

RECORDING AND REPORTING

1. Documented tolerance of various food textures, amount of assistance required, position during meal, absence or presence of dysphagia, and amount eaten.

2. Reported dysphagia to nurse in charge or physician.

340

Student _____ Date _____

Instructor _____ Date _____

PERFORMANCE CHECKLIST SKILL 31-1 **INSERTING A NASOGASTRIC OR NASOENTERIC FEEDING TUBE**

	S	U	NP	Comments
ASSESSMENT				
1. Verified physician's orders.	___	___	___	_____
2. Assessed patient's need for tube feedings. Consulted with nutritionist.	___	___	___	_____
3. Assessed patency of nares.	___	___	___	_____
4. Reviewed past medical history.	___	___	___	_____
5. Assessed patient's mental status. Evaluated gag reflex.	___	___	___	_____
6. Assessed for bowel sounds.	___	___	___	_____
7. Determined if prokinetic agent to be administered.	___	___	___	_____
NURSING DIAGNOSIS				
1. Developed appropriate nursing diagnoses based on assessment data.	___	___	___	_____
PLANNING				
1. Identified expected outcomes.	___	___	___	_____
2. Explained procedure to patient.	___	___	___	_____
3. Explained to patient how to communicate during procedure.	___	___	___	_____
IMPLEMENTATION				
1. Performed hand hygiene.	___	___	___	_____
2. Positioned patient properly per medical condition.	___	___	___	_____
3. Determined length of tube to be inserted.	___	___	___	_____
4. Prepared tube for insertion:				
a. Injected 10 mL water into tube.	___	___	___	_____
b. Verified stylet securely positioned and connections secure.	___	___	___	_____
5. Prepared tape and dressings.	___	___	___	_____
6. Applied clean gloves.	___	___	___	_____
7. Dipped tube with surface lubricant into glass of room temperature water or applied water-soluble lubricant.	___	___	___	_____

	S	U	NP	Comments

8. Provided patient with a glass of water and straw or ice chips, if alert. ___ ___ ___ _____

9. Explained next step to patient, then gently inserted tube through nostril following natural contour of posterior nasopharynx. ___ ___ ___ _____

10. Instructed/assisted patient to flex head toward chest after tube had passed through nasopharynx. ___ ___ ___ _____

11. Encouraged patient to swallow small sips of water as allowed. ___ ___ ___ _____

12. Advanced tube each time patient swallowed until desired length was passed. ___ ___ ___ _____

13. Checked for position of tube in back of throat. ___ ___ ___ _____

14. Temporarily secured tube and checked placement. ___ ___ ___ _____

15. Applied tube fixation device. If tape used, applied tincture of benzoin on tip of patient's nose and tube, allowed to dry, and secured tube. ___ ___ ___ _____

16. Secured tube with membrane dressing to cheek. ___ ___ ___ _____

17. Fastened end of nasogastric tube (NGT) to patient's gown. ___ ___ ___ _____

18. Positioned patient comfortably. ___ ___ ___ _____

19. Obtained x-ray examination of chest/abdomen, if ordered. ___ ___ ___ _____

20. Applied clean gloves and administered oral hygiene. ___ ___ ___ _____

21. Removed gloves, disposed of equipment, and performed hand hygiene. ___ ___ ___ _____

EVALUATION

1. Assessed patient for reaction to procedure, including vital signs and oxygen saturation. ___ ___ ___ _____

2. Confirmed x-ray examination results. ___ ___ ___ _____

3. Removed guidewire or stylet after x-ray verification. ___ ___ ___ _____

4. Checked external marking on tube. ___ ___ ___ _____

5. Identified unexpected outcomes. ___ ___ ___ _____

RECORDING AND REPORTING

1. Recorded and reported tube size/length, patient's tolerance of procedure, and confirmation of placement by x-ray examination. ___ ___ ___ _____

2. Reported unexpected outcomes to nurse in charge and/or physician. ___ ___ ___ _____

342

Student _Darcy Brenneman_   Date _9/28/12_

Instructor _____   Date _9/28/12_

PERFORMANCE CHECKLIST SKILL 31-2   **VERIFYING FEEDING TUBE PLACEMENT**

	S	U	NP	Comments
ASSESSMENT				
1. Reviewed agency policy and procedures for checking tube placement.	✓			
2. Identified signs and symptoms of inadvertent respiratory placement.	✓			
3. Identified conditions that increase risk for tube dislocation.	✓			
4. Observed external portion of tube for a change in length.	✓			
5. Reviewed medication record for gastric acid inhibitor or proton pump inhibitor.	✓	Excellent		
6. Reviewed patient's record for history of previous tube placement.				
NURSING DIAGNOSIS				
1. Developed appropriate nursing diagnoses based on assessment data.				
PLANNING				
1. Identified expected outcomes.				
2. Explained procedure to patient.				
IMPLEMENTATION				
1. Prepared equipment at bedside. Performed hand hygiene and applied clean gloves.	✓			
2. Verified placement of tube according to feeding and medication schedule.	✓			
3. Drew up 30 mL of air into 60 mL syringe and attached to end of feeding tube. Flushed tube with air before fluid was aspirated. Repeated as necessary.	✓			
4. Drew back on syringe and obtained 5 to 10 mL of gastric aspirate. Observed characteristics of aspirate.	✓			
5. Mixed gastric aspirate in syringe and measured pH.	✓			
6. If unable to obtain aspirate after tube positioning, confirmed by x-ray film; if patient not experiencing any distress, tube assumed to be placed correctly.	✓			

	S	U	NP	Comments

7. Irrigated tube.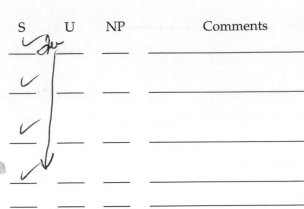

8. Removed and disposed of gloves and used supplies; performed hand hygiene.

EVALUATION

1. Observed patient for respiratory distress.

2. Verified results of aspirate analysis consistent with initial tube placement.

3. Identified unexpected outcomes.

RECORDING AND REPORTING

1. Recorded and reported information about tube, results of verification, and patient's response.

9-27-12

Student _____ Date _____

Instructor _____ Date _____

PERFORMANCE CHECKLIST SKILL 31-3 **IRRIGATING A FEEDING TUBE**

	S	U	NP	Comments
ASSESSMENT				
1. Checked character of gastric aspirates.	___	___	___	_____
2. Assessed bowel sounds and determined ease of infusion through tubing.	___	___	___	_____
3. Monitored volume of tube feeding administered and compared versus amount ordered.	___	___	___	_____
4. Referred to agency policy regarding routine irrigations or followed physician's orders.	___	___	___	_____
NURSING DIAGNOSIS				
1. Developed appropriate nursing diagnoses based on assessment data.	___	___	___	_____
PLANNING				
1. Identified expected outcomes.	___	___	___	_____
2. Explained procedure to patient.	___	___	___	_____
3. Assisted patient to high-Fowler's or semi-Fowler's position.	___	___	___	_____
IMPLEMENTATION				
1. Performed hand hygiene.	___	___	___	_____
2. Prepared equipment at bedside and applied clean gloves.	___	___	___	_____
3. Checked tube placement.	___	___	___	_____
4. Drew up 30 mL saline or tap water in syringe.	___	___	___	_____
5. Kinked feeding tube while disconnecting from feeding bag or plug and placed end of tubing on towel.	___	___	___	_____
6. Inserted tip of syringe into end of feeding tube. Released kink of tubing and slowly instilled irrigating solution into tube.	___	___	___	_____
7. Repositioned patient if unable to instill solution and tried again.	___	___	___	_____
8. Removed syringe after fluid instilled and reinstituted tube feeding or medication as ordered. Irrigated before administering medication, between medications, and after final medication.	___	___	___	_____
9. Disposed of supplies, removed gloves, and performed hand hygiene.	___	___	___	_____

	S	U	NP	Comments

EVALUATION

1. Observed ease of tube feeding infusion.   ____ ____ ____ _____

2. Identified unexpected outcomes.   ____ ____ ____ _____

RECORDING AND REPORTING

1. Recorded time of irrigation, fluid instilled, and results.   ____ ____ ____ _____

2. Reported unexpected outcomes to the nurse in charge or physician.   ____ ____ ____ _____

Student _Darcy Brenneman_   Date _9/27/12_

Instructor _Kendell Re_   Date _9/08/12_

PERFORMANCE CHECKLIST SKILL 31-4   **ADMINISTERING ENTERAL NUTRITION: NASOENTERIC, GASTROSTOMY, OR JEJUNOSTOMY TUBE**

	S	U	NP	Comments
ASSESSMENT				
1. Assessed patient's needs for enteral feedings. Referred to nutritionist.				
2. Assessed patient for food sensitivities and allergies.	✓			
3. Auscultated for bowel sounds.	✓			
4. Obtained baseline weight and laboratory values.	✓			
5. Verified health care provider's order.	✓			
NURSING DIAGNOSIS				
1. Developed appropriate nursing diagnoses based on assessment data.				
PLANNING				
1. Identified expected outcomes.				
2. Explained procedure to patient.	✓			
IMPLEMENTATION				
1. Performed hand hygiene.	✓			
2. Prepared feeding container:				
a. Checked expiration date on formula and integrity of container.	✓			
b. Ensured room temperature of solution.	✓			
c. Connected tubing to prepared container. Applied clean gloves, if needed.	✓			
d. Shook formula and filled container bag. Primed tubing.	✓			
3. Had syringe ready for intermittent feedings.	✓			
4. Placed patient in appropriate position.	✓			
5. Applied clean gloves, if not already applied.	✓			
6. Checked placement of tube.	✓			
7. Checked gastric residual by connecting syringe to tube and checking pH of aspirate.	✓			
8. Flushed tubing with 30 mL of water.	✓			

	S	U	NP	Comments

9. Initiated Feeding

   a. Initiated *intermittent feeding:*

     (1) Pinched proximal end of feeding tube. ✓

     (2) Attached administration tubing to end of feeding tube. ✓

     (3) Set rate by adjusting roller clamp on tubing, and allowed bag to empty gradually over 30 to 60 minutes. ✓

     (4) Labeled bag and changed every 24 hours. ✓

   b. *Continuous drip method:*

     (1) Connected distal end of tubing to proximal end of feeding tube.

     (2) Connected tubing through infusion pump and set prescribed rate.

10. Advanced rate of concentration of tube feeding gradually.

11. Irrigated tube per agency policy following feeding.

12. Capped or clamped the proximal end of feeding tube when not administering feedings.

13. Rinsed bag and tubing with warm water between feedings. Used a new administration set every 24 hours.

14. Disposed of supplies and performed hand hygiene.

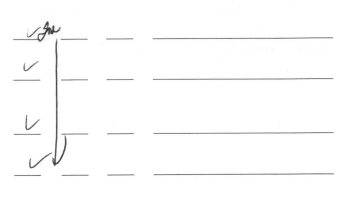

EVALUATION

1. Measured amount of residual volume every 4 to 6 hours. ✓

2. Monitored blood glucose as ordered. ✓

3. Monitored I&O every 8 hours. ✓

4. Weighed patient daily. ✓

5. Observed laboratory values. ✓

6. Observed respiratory status. ✓

7. Observed patient's level of comfort. ✓

8. Auscultated bowel sounds. ✓

9. Inspected site for signs of impaired skin integrity. ✓

10. Identified unexpected outcomes. ✓

	S	U	NP	Comments

RECORDING AND REPORTING

1. Recorded amount, type of feeding, and any additional water taken.   ___ ___ ___ _____

2. Recorded patient's response to feeding.   ___ ___ ___ _____

3. Reported unexpected outcomes to nurse in charge or physician.   ___ ___ ___ _____

Bero Pratt

9-27-12

Student _____ Date _____

Instructor _____ Date _____

PERFORMANCE CHECKLIST PROCEDURAL GUIDELINE 31-1 **CARE OF A GASTROSTOMY OR JEJUNOSTOMY TUBE**

	S	U	NP	Comments
STEPS				
1. Determined whether exit site was left open to air or covered with drain sponge.	___	___	___	_____
2. Performed hand hygiene and applied clean gloves.	___	___	___	_____
3. Removed and discarded old dressings if present.	___	___	___	_____
4. Assessed exit site for excoriation, drainage, infection, or bleeding.	___	___	___	_____
5. Cleaned skin around site with warm water and mild soap.	___	___	___	_____
6. Rotated external bumper 90 degrees.	___	___	___	_____
7. Dried site completely.	___	___	___	_____
8. Applied thin layer of protective skin barrier to site, if needed.	___	___	___	_____
9. Placed drain-gauze dressing over external bar, if ordered.	___	___	___	_____
10. Secured dressing with tape.	___	___	___	_____
11. Placed date, time, and initials on dressing.	___	___	___	_____
12. Removed gloves, disposed of supplies, and performed hand hygiene.	___	___	___	_____
13. Documented appearance of site, drainage, and dressing application.	___	___	___	_____
14. Reported any complications to health care provider.	___	___	___	_____

Student _____ Date _____

Instructor _____ Date _____

PERFORMANCE CHECKLIST SKILL 32-1   **ADMINISTERING CENTRAL PARENTERAL NUTRITION**

	S	U	NP	Comments
ASSESSMENT				
1. Assessed indications and risks for protein-calorie malnutrition.	—	—	—	_____
2. Inspected condition of central vein access site. Inspected tubing of access device for patency.	—	—	—	_____
3. Assessed patient's nutritional status, caloric intake, and laboratory tests (blood glucose level).	—	—	—	_____
4. Assessed patient's medical history for factors influencing CPN administration and history of allergies.	—	—	—	_____
5. Assessed vital signs, respiratory status, and weight.	—	—	—	_____
6. Consulted with physician and dietitian on patient requirements.	—	—	—	_____
7. Verified physician's orders. Checked for compatibility of added medication.	—	—	—	_____
NURSING DIAGNOSIS				
1. Developed appropriate nursing diagnoses based on assessment data.	—	—	—	_____
PLANNING				
1. Identified expected outcomes.	—	—	—	_____
2. Explained to patient need for CPN and follow-up care.	—	—	—	_____
3. Removed CPN solution from refrigerator 1 hour before infusion, if refrigerated.	—	—	—	_____
IMPLEMENTATION				
1. Performed hand hygiene and applied gloves.	—	—	—	_____
2. Inspected parenteral nutrition solution for solution, additives, and label.	—	—	—	_____
3. Inspected solution for particulate matter or separation, and expiration date.	—	—	—	_____
4. Correctly verified patient's identification.	—	—	—	_____
5. Connected CPN solution to IV tubing with filter and primed tubing.	—	—	—	_____

	S	U	NP	Comments
6. Placed IV tubing into intravenous infusion pump and regulated prescribed flow rate or connected to appropriate tubing.	——	——	——	———————————
7. Infused all other IV medications through alternate IV line.	——	——	——	———————————
8. Did not interrupt CPN infusion. Used a different line/site for blood sampling.	——	——	——	———————————
9. Changed infusion tubing and filter using strict aseptic technique every 24 hours.	——	——	——	———————————
10. Discarded used supplies and performed hand hygiene.	——	——	——	———————————

EVALUATION

	S	U	NP	Comments
1. Monitored infusion rate.	——	——	——	———————————
2. Monitored fluid intake every 8 hours.	——	——	——	———————————
3. Obtained daily weights, as ordered.	——	——	——	———————————
4. Assessed for fluid retention.	——	——	——	———————————
5. Monitored patient's glucose and laboratory parameters to determine response to CPN.	——	——	——	———————————
6. Inspected central venous access site.	——	——	——	———————————
7. Monitored for signs of systemic infection.	——	——	——	———————————
8. Identified unexpected outcomes.	——	——	——	———————————

RECORDING AND REPORTING

	S	U	NP	Comments
1. Recorded condition of central venous access device, rate of infusion, I&O, vital signs, and weight as per agency policy.	——	——	——	———————————
2. Reported complications to nurse in charge or physician.	——	——	——	———————————

Student _____ Date _____

Instructor _____ Date _____

	S	U	NP	Comments
ASSESSMENT				
1. Assessed patient for potential lipid intolerance.	___	___	___	_____
2. Selected appropriate IV site and initiated IV with 18-gauge catheter for fat emulsion administration.	___	___	___	_____
3. Checked physician's order for volume of fat emulsion and PPN solution against MAR.	___	___	___	_____
4. Assessed appropriate infusion time to administer fat emulsion.	___	___	___	_____
5. Carefully selected correct fat emulsion from supply area.	___	___		_____
6. Assessed blood glucose levels by finger-stick.	___	___		_____
NURSING DIAGNOSIS				
1. Developed appropriate nursing diagnoses based on assessment data.	___	___	___	_____
PLANNING				
1. Identified expected outcomes.	___	___	___	_____
2. Explained to patient the reason for PPN and fat emulsion infusion.	___	___	___	_____
3. Placed patient in comfortable position for IV insertion or initiation of infusion.	___	___	___	_____
4. Removed PPN solution from the refrigerator an hour before infusion.	___	___	___	_____
IMPLEMENTATION				
1. Performed hand hygiene and applied gloves.	___	___	___	_____
2. Compared label of PPN solution versus prescriber's order.	___	___	___	_____
3. Inspected PPN and fat emulsion for patency.	___	___	___	_____
4. Checked patient's identification correctly.	___	___	___	_____
5. Performed vital sign and respiratory assessment.	___	___	___	_____
6. Properly prepared IV tubing for PPN administration and set prescribed infusion rate on IV pump. Initiated infusion checking patency of peripheral IV insertion site.	___	___	___	_____
7. Cleaned peripheral line tubing injection port.	___	___	___	_____

	S	U	NP	Comments

8. Inserted fat emulsion infusion into injection port using a needleless access device. ___ ___ ___ _____

9. Set flow rate on infusion pump. Initiated fat emulsion infusion. ___ ___ ___ _____

10. Discarded supplies and performed hand hygiene. ___ ___ ___ _____

EVALUATION

1. Monitored flow rate as per agency policy. ___ ___ ___ _____

2. Assessed vital signs, respiratory status, IV site, and general comfort level to determine response to fat emulsion. ___ ___ ___ _____

3. Monitored laboratory values. ___ ___ ___ _____

4. Assessed patient's response to fluid volume. ___ ___ ___ _____

5. Identified unexpected outcomes. ___ ___ ___ _____

RECORDING AND REPORTING

1. Recorded at every shift type of PPN and fat emulsion, rate, status of IV site, vital signs, finger-stick blood glucose levels, and I&O. ___ ___ ___ _____

2. Reported complications to nurse in charge or physician. ___ ___ ___ _____

Student _____ Date _____

Instructor _____ Date _____

All

PERFORMANCE CHECKLIST PROCEDURAL GUIDELINE 33-1   **ASSISTING A PATIENT IN USING A URINAL**

STEPS

1. Assessed patient's normal urinary elimination pattern. ✓ ___ ___ _____

2. Assessed for incontinence or any other urinary alteration. ✓ ___ ___ _____

3. Palpated patient for distended bladder. ✓ ___ ___ _____

4. Assessed patient's cognitive and physical status. ✓ ___ ___ _____

5. Assessed patient's knowledge regarding urinal use. ✓ ___ ___ _____

6. Performed hand hygiene and applied clean gloves. ✓ ___ ___ _____

7. Provided privacy. ✓ ___ ___ _____

8. Assisted patient into appropriate position. ✓ ___ ___ _____

9. Assisted patient with urinal as needed. ✓ ___ ___ _____

10. Removed urinal when finished. Assisted with perineal hygiene, if applicable. ✓ ___ ___ _____

11. Assessed output. Emptied, cleaned, and returned urinal. ✓ ___ ___ _____

12. Allowed/assisted patient to perform hand hygiene. ✓ ___ ___ _____

13. Removed and disposed of gloves; performed hand hygiene. ✓ ___ ___ _____

PE: Kyla Vanderwall 9/10/12

Student Darcy Brenneman   Date 11/16/12

Instructor _____ _Kimball Ga_____   Date 11/30/12

PERFORMANCE CHECKLIST SKILL 33-1   **INSERTING A STRAIGHT OR INDWELLING URINARY CATHETER**

	S	U	NP	Comments
ASSESSMENT				
1. Reviewed patient's medical record and physician's order.	KV			
2. Assessed patient's general status.				
3. Assessed for distended bladder.				
4. Performed hand hygiene and applied clean gloves.				
5. Inspected perineal area. Removed gloves and performed hand hygiene.				
6. Reviewed medial records for presence of conditions that may impair passage of catheter.				
7. Assessed patient's knowledge of purpose for catheterization.				
NURSING DIAGNOSIS				
1. Developed appropriate nursing diagnoses based on assessment data.				
PLANNING				
1. Identified expected outcomes.				
2. Explained procedure to patient.				
3. Arranged for extra personnel to assist, if necessary.				
IMPLEMENTATION				
1. Performed hand hygiene.	KV			
2. Provided privacy.				
3. Raised bed to appropriate height.				
4. Positioned self correctly and arranged equipment.				
5. Raised appropriate side rail.				
6. Placed pad under patient.				
7. Correctly positioned male or female patient.				
8. Draped patient.				
9. Applied clean gloves, then cleansed and dried perineal area using clean technique.				
10. Positioned lamp.				

	S	U	NP	Comments

11. Removed and disposed of gloves. Performed hand hygiene. _____ _____ _____ _____

12. Prepared urinary drainage container. _____ _____ _____ _____

13. Maintained sterile asepsis while opening catheter kit. _____ _____ _____ _____

14. Placed kit within reach. _____ _____ _____ _____

15. Applied sterile gloves. _____ _____ _____ _____

16. Placed sterile drape under patient. _____ _____ _____ _____

17. Placed fenestrated sterile drape over patient, if available. _____ _____ _____ _____

18. Organized supplies on sterile field. _____ _____ _____ _____

19. Checked integrity of inflatable balloon of indwelling catheter. _____ _____ _____ _____

20. Loosened lid on specimen container, if needed. Poured sterile antiseptic solution over cotton balls/opened package of sterile swabs. Opened package of lubricant and spread proper amount on sterile tray. _____ _____ _____ _____

21. Coiled catheter in hand and applied lubricant to catheter tip. _____ _____ _____ _____

22. Correctly cleansed urethral meatus.

   a. *Female Patient*

     (1) With nondominant hand, carefully retracted labia to expose urethral meatus. Maintained position of nondominant hand throughout procedure. _____ _____ _____ _____

     (2) With forceps in sterile dominant hand, picked up cotton ball saturated with antiseptic solution and cleansed perineal area, wiping front to back from clitoris toward anus. Used a new cotton ball for each area, wiped along the far labial fold, near labial fold, and directly over center of urethral meatus. _____ _____ _____ _____

   b. *Male Patient*

     (1) If patient not circumcised, retracted foreskin with nondominant hand. Grasped penis at shaft just below glans. Retracted urethral meatus between thumb and forefinger. Maintained nondominant hand in this position throughout procedure. _____ _____ _____ _____

     (2) With dominant hand, picked up cotton ball with forceps and cleansed penis. Moved in circular motion from urethral meatus down to base of glans. Repeated cleansing 3 more times, using clean cotton ball each time. _____ _____ _____ _____

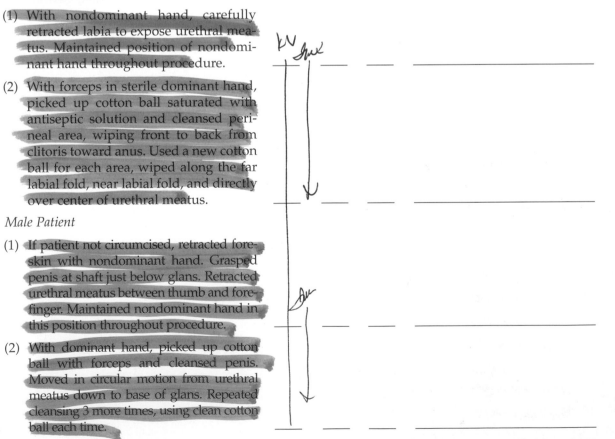

360

	S	U	NP	Comments

23. Handled catheter properly.

24. Inserted catheter correctly.

   a. *Female Patient*

     (1) Asked patient to bear down gently as if to void and slowly inserted catheter through urethral meatus.

     (2) Advanced catheter a total of 5 to 7.5 cm (2 to 3 inches) in adult or until urine flowed out catheter's end. As soon as urine appeared, advanced catheter another 2.5 to 5 cm (1 to 2 inches). Did not force against resistance. Placed end of catheter in urine tray receptacle.

     (3) Released labia and held catheter securely with nondominant hand.

   b. *Male Patient*

     (1) Lifted penis to position perpendicular to patient's body and applied light traction.

     (2) Asked patient to bear down as if to void and slowly inserted catheter through urethral meatus.

25. Collected urine specimen, if needed.

26. Allowed bladder to empty fully. If using straight single-use catheter, withdrew it slowly and smoothly. If using indwelling catheter, correctly inflated balloon.

27. Attached end of catheter to collecting tube, and placed drainage bag below level of bladder.

28. Taped catheter or applied Velcro tube holder.

29. Assisted patient to comfortable position. Washed and dried perineal area as needed.

30. Removed gloves and properly disposed of equipment.

31. Performed hand hygiene.

EVALUATION

1. Palpated patient's bladder.

2. Assessed patient's comfort.

3. Observed character and amount of urine.

4. Determined that no urine was leaking from catheter or tubing.

5. Identified unexpected outcomes.

RECORDING AND REPORTING

1. Reported and recorded pertinent data: catheter description, assessment of urine, specimen collection, and patient's response to procedure.

   ___   ___   ___   _____

2. Initiated I&O records.

   ___   ___   ___   _____

PE: Kyla VanDerWeele

Renee S.
11/14   1hr.

Student _Darcy Brenneman_   Date _____

Instructor _____ _Kendee_ _____   Date _11/30/12_

PERFORMANCE CHECKLIST SKILL 33-2   **CARE AND REMOVAL OF THE INDWELLING CATHETER**

	S	U	NP	Comments

ASSESSMENT

1. *For Catheter Care*

   a. Observed urinary output and characteristics.

   b. Assessed for history or presence of bowel incontinence.

   c. Assessed patient's knowledge of catheter care.

   d. Assessed urethral meatus for redness and drainage.

2. *For Catheter Removal*

   a. Determined how long catheter was in place.

   b. Determine size of catheter inflation balloon.

   c. Reviewed chart for physician's order.

NURSING DIAGNOSIS

1. Developed appropriate nursing diagnoses based on assessment data.

PLANNING

1. Identified expected outcomes.

2. Explained procedure to patient.

IMPLEMENTATION

1. Provided privacy.

2. Performed hand hygiene.

3. Raised bed to appropriate height.

4. Organized equipment.

5. Correctly positioned and draped patient.

6. Placed waterproof pad under patient.

7. Applied clean gloves.

8. Removed anchor device and freed tubing.

9. Assessed urethral meatus.

10. Performed perineal care.

	S	U	NP	Comments

11. Cleansed catheter.

   a. Cleansed approximately 10-cm (4-inch) length of catheter.

   b. Replaced adhesive tape or tube holder, if needed.

   c. Avoided placing tension on catheter.

12. Catheter removal: Followed Steps 1 through 5 before catheter removal.

   a. Placed waterproof pad correctly.

   b. Obtained sterile urine specimen as required.

   c. Removed tape or Velcro tube holder.

   d. Aspirated fluid used to inflate catheter balloon.

   e. Gently removed catheter and wrapped in waterproof pad.

   f. Unhooked bag and tubing from bed.

   g. Repositioned patient. Provided perineal care, if necessary. Measured contents and emptied collection bag.

13. Disposed of contaminated gloves and supplies; performed hand hygiene.

EVALUATION

1. Inspected urethra and surrounding tissue.

2. Observed time and amount of first voiding.

3. Noted character of urine.

4. Identified unexpected outcomes.

RECORDING AND REPORTING

1. Recorded when care was given and when urethral meatus and urine were assessed. Documented removal of catheter.

2. Reported pertinent data to appropriate health care team member(s).

3. Recorded urinary output on I&O form.

PE: Kyla vanDerWeen

Renee S
11/14

Student _____ Date _____

Instructor _____ Date _____

PERFORMANCE CHECKLIST PROCEDURAL GUIDELINE 33-2 **BLADDER SCAN AND CATHETERIZATION TO DETERMINE RESIDUAL URINE**

	S	U	NP	Comments
STEPS				
1. Determined patient's urine output trends and reviewed I&O.	___	___	___	_____
2. Palpated and percussed for signs of bladder distention.	___	___	___	_____
3. Reviewed physician's order.	___	___	___	_____
4. Assessed patient's knowledge regarding urinary retention and purpose of bladder scanner procedure or intermittent/straight catheterization.	___	___	___	_____
5. Checked time of last voiding and measured amount voided before catheterization.	___	___	___	_____
6. Used bladder scanner or straight catheterized patient 15 minutes post void.	___	___	___	_____
7. *Assessed PVR With Bladder Scanner*				
a. Assisted patient to a supine position.	___	___	___	_____
b. Exposed patient's lower abdomen.	___	___	___	_____
c. Turned on the scanner machine and screen.	___	___	___	_____
d. Selected male or female setting.				
(1) Use the FEMALE option only for female patients who have *not* had a hysterectomy.	___	___	___	_____
(2) Use the MALE option when scanning female patients who *have had* a hysterectomy.	___	___	___	_____
e. Wiped the scan head with an alcohol pad.	___	___	___	_____
f. Applied a generous amount of transmission/conductivity gel midline on abdomen above symphysis pubis.	___	___	___	_____
g. Placed the scan head on the gel with the directional icon toward the bladder.	___	___	___	_____
h. Light pressure applied and kept scan head steady for accuracy. Pressed and released the scan button.	___	___	___	_____
i. Checked manufacturer's directions for details to verify aim. Pressed the "Done" button to display the volume measurements. Results may be printed.	___	___	___	_____

	S	U	NP	Comments

8. *Straight or Intermittent Catheterization to Assess for PVR*

   a. Performed hand hygiene.   ——— ——— ——— ————————————

   b. Proceeded as for inserting straight/intermittent catheter (Skill 33-1).   ——— ——— ——— ————————————

   c. Removed catheter slowly to ensure complete urine drainage from bladder.   ——— ——— ——— ————————————

   d. Discarded used supplies, removed gloves, performed hand hygiene.   ——— ——— ——— ————————————

   e. Recorded and reported amount of urine voided, amount obtained from catheterization, and the patient's response.   ——— ——— ——— ————————————

Student _____ Date _____

Instructor _____ Date _____

PERFORMANCE CHECKLIST SKILL 33-3 **PERFORMING CATHETER IRRIGATION**

	S	U	NP	Comments
ASSESSMENT				
1. Reviewed patient's medical record.	___	___	___	_____
2. Assessed characteristics of urine, patency of tubing, and status of existing closed system.	___	___	___	_____
3. Reviewed I&O record.	___	___	___	_____
4. Assessed patient for presence of bladder spasms and discomfort. Palpated bladder.	___	___	___	_____
5. Assessed patient's knowledge of procedure.	___	___	___	_____
NURSING DIAGNOSIS				
1. Developed appropriate nursing diagnoses based on assessment data.	___	___	___	_____
PLANNING				
1. Identified expected outcomes.	___	___	___	_____
2. Explained procedure to patient.	___	___	___	_____
IMPLEMENTATION				
1. Performed hand hygiene.	___	___	___	_____
2. Provided privacy. Covered patient's upper body with blanket.	___	___	___	_____
3. Correctly positioned patient and removed tape or Velcro tube holder.	___	___	___	_____
4. Organized necessary supplies.	___	___	___	_____
5. *Performed Closed Intermittent Irrigation*				
a. Poured prescribed, room temperature solution into sterile container.	___	___	___	_____
b. Applied gloves.	___	___	___	_____
c. Drew solution into syringe.	___	___	___	_____
d. Clamped indwelling retention catheter below injection port on drainage tubing.	___	___	___	_____
e. Cleansed injection port with antiseptic.	___	___	___	_____
f. Inserted needle/needleless device of syringe into injection port at 30-degree angle.	___	___	___	_____
g. Slowly injected fluid into catheter. If medicated fluid was injected, left fluid in bladder for prescribed time.	___	___	___	_____
h. Withdrew syringe and removed clamp.	___	___	___	_____

	S	U	NP	Comments

6. *Performed Closed Continuous Irrigation*

   a. Applied clean gloves.

   b. Closed clamp on tubing and placed bag of solution on IV pole. Filled drip chamber to ½ full.

   c. Inserted tip of tubing into bag containing solution.

   d. Opened clamp and allowed solution to flow.

   e. Connected tubing to catheter.

   f. Calculated drip rate and adjusted roller clamp on tubing accordingly. Checked volume of drainage in output bag.

7. *Performed Open Intermittent Irrigation*

   a. Applied gloves.

   b. Opened sterile irrigation tray and set up sterile field. Poured required amount of sterile solution into sterile container.

   c. Positioned sterile waterproof pad under catheter.

   d. Aspirated prescribed amount of solution into syringe.

   e. Moved sterile collection basin close to patient's thigh.

   f. Wiped connection point between catheter and drainage tubing with antiseptic before disconnecting.

   g. Disconnected catheter from drainage tubing, allowing urine to flow into sterile collection basin.

   h. Inserted tip of syringe into catheter lumen and gently instilled solution.

   i. Withdrew syringe, lowered catheter, and allowed solution to drain into basin. Repeated instillation until drainage clear.

   j. Had patient turn onto side and gently aspirated solution if solution did not return.

   k. Cleansed and aseptically replaced drainage tubing adapter.

8. Reanchored catheter to patient.

9. Assisted patient to comfortable position.

10. Lowered bed and side rails, if appropriate.

11. Disposed of contaminated supplies and gloves. Performed hand hygiene.

	S	U	NP	Comments

EVALUATION

1. Accurately calculated the difference between the amount of irrigating solution instilled and the amount of drainage returned.

2. Assessed characteristics of output and urine.

3. Observed patency of catheter.

4. Observed patient for pain or fever.

5. Identified unexpected outcomes.

RECORDING AND REPORTING

1. Recorded in nurse's notes and on I&O form amount of solution used to irrigate and amount and consistency of drainage returned.

2. Reported to physician occlusion, sudden bleeding, infection, or pain.

Student _Darcy_____ Date _____

Instructor _____ Date _____

PERFORMANCE CHECKLIST SKILL 33-4 **APPLYING A CONDOM CATHETER**

	S	U	NP	Comments

ASSESSMENT

1. Determined patient's urinary pattern and degree of incontinence. ___ ___ ___ _____

2. Assessed condition of penis. ___ ___ ___ _____

3. Assessed patient's knowledge of purpose of condom catheter. ___ ___ ___ _____

4. Assessed patient's ability to self-apply device. ___ ___ ___ _____

NURSING DIAGNOSIS

1. Developed appropriate nursing diagnoses based on assessment data. ___ ___ ___ _____

PLANNING

1. Identified expected outcomes. ___ ___ ___ _____

2. Explained procedure to patient. ___ ___ ___ _____

IMPLEMENTATION

1. Performed hand hygiene. ___ ___ ___ _____

2. Provided privacy. ___ ___ ___ _____

3. Raised bed to working height. Lowered appropriate side rail. ___ ___ ___ _____

4. Assisted patient to a comfortable position. ___ ___ ___ _____

5. Prepared urinary drainage collection bag and tubing. ___ ___ ___ _____

6. Put on gloves and provided perineal care. ___ ___ ___ _____

7. Applied skin barrier preparation to penis and allowed to dry. ___ ___ ___ _____

8. Clipped hair at base of penis, if necessary. ___ ___ ___ _____

9. Put condom catheter on patient's penis. Allowed space between glans and end of condom catheter. ___ ___ ___ _____

10. Attached Velcro or elastic adhesive to condom. ___ ___ ___ _____

11. Connected drainage tubing to end of condom. ___ ___ ___ _____

12. Secured excess tubing. ___ ___ ___ _____

13. Positioned patient comfortably. Raised side rail and lowered bed. ___ ___ ___ _____

	S	U	NP	Comments

14. Disposed of contaminated supplies and gloves. Performed hand hygiene.   ___ ___ ___ _____

15. Replaced daily and reassessed skin of penis.   ___ ___ ___ _____

EVALUATION

1. Observed urinary drainage.   ___ ___ ___ _____

2. Inspected penis within 30 minutes after application of catheter.   ___ ___ ___ _____

3. Removed and changed condom and assessed skin of penis and color of glans penis at least once daily.   ___ ___ ___ _____

4. Identified unexpected outcomes.   ___ ___ ___ _____

RECORDING AND REPORTING

1. Recorded and reported pertinent information related to procedure and assessment.   ___ ___ ___ _____

2. Monitored I&O as indicated.   ___ ___ ___ _____

Student _____ Date _____

Instructor _____ Date _____

PERFORMANCE CHECKLIST SKILL 33-5   **CARE OF A SUPRAPUBIC CATHETER**

	S	U	NP	Comments
ASSESSMENT				
1. Assessed urine amount in bag and characteristics in drainage tube.	___	___	___	_____
2. Assessed dressing for drainage and intactness.	___	___	___	_____
3. Assessed catheter insertion site for signs of inflammation. Asked patient if there was discomfort or tenderness at the site.	___	___	___	_____
4. Monitored vital signs and signs and symptoms of systemic infection.	___	___	___	_____
5. Assessed patient's knowledge of catheter and its care.	___	___	___	_____
NURSING DIAGNOSIS				
1. Developed appropriate nursing diagnoses based on assessment data.	___	___	___	_____
PLANNING				
1. Identified expected outcomes.	___	___	___	_____
2. Explained procedure to patient.	___	___	___	_____
IMPLEMENTATION				
1. Performed hand hygiene.	___	___	___	_____
2. Provided privacy.	___	___	___	_____
3. *Site Care for a Newly Inserted Suprapubic Catheter*				
a. Prepared supplies as for a dry sterile dressing	___	___	___	_____
b. Applied gloves and gently removed existing dressing. Disposed of soiled dressing.	___	___	___	_____
c. Removed gloves, performed hand hygiene, and applied clean gloves.	___	___	___	_____
d. Cleansed site around drain with a sterile gauze moistened in sterile saline.	___	___	___	_____
e. Cleansed base of catheter, moving up and away from insertion site, taking care to not pull on the catheter.	___	___	___	_____
f. Applied sterile split gauze around catheter and applied tape.	___	___	___	_____

	S	U	NP	Comments

4. *Site Care for an Established Suprapubic Catheter*

   a. Applied gloves. ___ ___ ___ _____

   b. Used soap and warm water to cleanse around insertion site and catheter away from site. Dried completely. ___ ___ ___ _____

   c. Removed gloves and performed hand hygiene. ___ ___ ___ _____

5. Secured catheter to abdomen with tape or Velcro tube holder. ___ ___ ___ _____

6. Checked bag and tubing placement. ___ ___ ___ _____

7. Assessed excess tubing for kinks. ___ ___ ___ _____

EVALUATION

1. Asked patient if there was pain or discomfort from suprapubic catheter. ___ ___ ___ _____

2. Observed patient's urine for signs of infection. ___ ___ ___ _____

3. Inspected dressing, if present, at least once every shift. ___ ___ ___ _____

4. Monitored for signs and symptoms of systemic infection. ___ ___ ___ _____

5. Identified unexpected outcomes. ___ ___ ___ _____

RECORDING AND REPORTING

1. Reported and recorded dressing procedure, assessment of site, and patient's tolerance of procedure. ___ ___ ___ _____

2. Reported presence of unexpected outcomes. ___ ___ ___ _____

Student _____ Date _____

Instructor _____ Date _____

PERFORMANCE CHECKLIST PROCEDURAL GUIDELINE 33-3 **PERITONEAL DIALYSIS AND CONTINUOUS AMBULATORY PERITONEAL DIALYSIS**

STEPS

1. Reviewed physician's orders. Verified dialysis solutions and medication. Verified number and duration of exchanges.　　____　____　____　_____

2. Reviewed agency's procedure for peritoneal dialysis (PD) or continuous ambulatory peritoneal dialysis (CAPD).　　____　____　_____

3. Correctly verified patient's identity.　　____　____　____　_____

4. Assessed patient's and family's knowledge of procedure.　　____　____　_____

5. Monitored laboratory tests for fluid and electrolyte balance.　　____　____　_____

6. Obtained patient's vital signs, respiratory assessment, abdominal girth, and weight.　　____　____　_____

7. Provided privacy. Placed sign outside door indicating "Dialysis in Progress."　　____　____　_____

8. Assisted patient to a comfortable position.　　____　____　____　_____

9. Inspected dialysate bags for patency.　　____　____　____　_____

10. Applied PPE to self, patient, and family members, if present. Applied sterile gloves.　　____　____　_____

11. Followed six rights of medication administration if required to add medication to dialysate bag. Disinfected top of vial and port on bag, drew additive into syringe, and injected medication into port on bag.　　____　____　_____

12. Hung 2 bags of warmed dialysate solution from IV pole. Aseptically spiked and primed tubing.　　____　____　_____

13. Aseptically disinfected PD catheter cap, end of catheter, and adapter and connected tubing.　　____　____　____　_____

14. Opened clamp and infused dialysate as prescribed (2 liters in 10 to 15 minutes).　　____　____　____　_____

15. Clamped inflow tubing for prescribed dwell time of

　　a. IPD—30 minutes　　____　____　____　_____

　　b. CAPD—3 to 5 hours　　____　____　____　_____

16. Replaced empty dialysate bag with third warmed bag.　　____　____　____　_____

	S	U	NP	Comments

17. Unclamped outflow tubing and drained for prescribed time. ___ ___ ___ _____

18. Clamped outflow tubing when exchange was completed. ___ ___ ___ _____

19. Measured volume of effluent (1 g = 1 mL). Applied PPE and protective eye wear if effluent needed to be emptied into graduated cylinder for measurement. ___ ___ ___ _____

20. Discarded all soiled items. Removed PPE and performed hand hygiene. ___ ___ ___ _____

21. Repeated cycle of drainage-infusion-dwell until prescribed amount completed. ___ ___ ___ _____

22. When exchanges were completed,

   a. Performed hand hygiene, applied PPE to everyone present in room and self. ___ ___ ___ _____

   b. Disinfected connections, disconnected. Disconnected catheter rim and applied sterile cap. ___ ___ ___ _____

23. *PD Dressing Change*

   a. Placed "Do Not Enter" sign on door. ___ ___ ___ _____

   b. Applied PPE to everyone present. ___ ___ ___ _____

   c. Performed hand hygiene, applied gloves. Exposed patient's abdomen. Carefully removed, assessed, and discarded present dressing. ___ ___ ___ _____

   d. Removed and disposed of gloves. Performed hand hygiene. ___ ___ ___ _____

   e. Set up sterile field. Applied sterile gloves. ___ ___ ___ _____

   f. Cleansed insertion site per agency policy, considering patient's skin sensitivities and allergies. ___ ___ ___ _____

   g. Applied a sterile split gauze and taped or left OTA if ordered. ___ ___ ___ _____

   h. Disposed of contaminated supplies. Removed and disposed of gloves. ___ ___ ___ _____

   i. Performed hand hygiene. ___ ___ ___ _____

PERFORMANCE CHECKLIST SKILL 34-1 **ASSISTING A PATIENT IN USING A BEDPAN**

	S	U	NP	Comments
ASSESSMENT				
1. Assessed patient's normal bowel elimination and factors causing alterations.				
2. Reviewed patient's medical, nutritional, and medication history.				
3. Auscultated and palpated abdomen.				
4. Assessed patient's mobility status.				
5. Assessed for rectal or abdominal pain and irritation of skin surrounding anus.				
6. Determined if stool specimen needed.				
NURSING DIAGNOSIS				
1. Developed appropriate nursing diagnoses based on assessment data.				
PLANNING				
1. Identified expected outcomes.				
2. Explained procedure to patient.				
3. Obtained assistance from additional nursing personnel, if indicated.				
IMPLEMENTATION				
1. Performed hand hygiene and applied gloves.				
2. Provided privacy.				
3. Warmed bedpan before use. Applied powder to surface of bedpan.				
4. Put opposite side rail up.				
5. Positioned bed at appropriate working height.				
6. Ensured that patient was positioned properly.				
7. Mobile patient who is able to assist:				
a. Raised patient's head 30 to 60 degrees.				
b. Removed upper bed linen.				
c. Instructed patient to flex knees and lift hips.				
d. Correctly assisted patient onto bedpan (open rim of bedpan was facing toward foot of bed).				
e. Optional: Slipped fracture pan under patient.				

	S	U	NP	Comments

8. *Immobile Patient*

   a. Positioned bed flat if tolerated.

   b. Removed top bed linens.

   c. Rolled patient onto side and placed bedpan against buttocks.

   d. Correctly assisted patient to roll onto bedpan.

   e. Raised patient's head 30 to 60 degrees (unless contraindicated).

   f. Raised knee gatch on bed or had patient bend knees.

9. Ensured patient's comfort. Covered patient. Supported lumbar spine.

10. Placed call bell and toilet tissue within patient's reach.

11. Ensured that bed was in lowest position with side rails up.

12. Removed gloves and performed hand hygiene.

13. Allowed patient to be alone, but monitored status. Responded to patient's call bell immediately.

14. Performed hand hygiene. Applied new gloves.

15. Positioned patient's bedside chair near working side of bed.

16. Collected basin of warm water.

17. Raised bed to a good working height. Lowered nearest side rail.

18. Removed upper linens. Covered patient with towel.

19. Determined if patient was able to wipe perineal area.

20. Removed bedpan for mobile patient.

   a. Correctly removed bedpan while patient lifted buttocks up from bedpan.

   b. Offered patient opportunity to perform perineal and hand hygiene.

21. Removed bedpan for immobile patient.

   a. Lowered head of bed.

   b. Assisted patient to roll off bedpan.

   c. Wiped patient's anal area. Provided perineal care, as necessary.

378

	S	U	NP	Comments

22. Covered bedpan.

23. Returned patient to comfortable position.

24. Positioned bed in lowest position and returned patient's environment to former status.

25. While wearing gloves, emptied contents of bedpan and rinsed it. Obtained stool specimen, if indicated.

26. Replaced all used equipment. Disposed of soiled linens.

27. Removed gloves and performed hand hygiene.

EVALUATION

1. Assessed characteristics of urine and stool.

2. Evaluated patient's ability to use bedpan.

3. Inspected condition of patient's perineal skin.

4. Evaluated patient's overall state of well-being.

5. Identified unexpected outcomes.

RECORDING AND REPORTING

1. Documented character of stool and urinary output if patient also voided.

2. Completed laboratory requisition for stool or urine specimen.

PE: kyla vanderween 9/12/12

Student _____ Date _____

Instructor _____ Date _____

PERFORMANCE CHECKLIST SKILL 34-2 **REMOVING FECAL IMPACTION DIGITALLY**

	S	U	NP	Comments

ASSESSMENT

1. Assessed patient's nutritional and elimination status, level of mobility, and abdomen. ___ ___ ___ _____

2. Reviewed patient's medical and medication (narcotic analgesics) history. ___ ___ ___ _____

3. Obtained baseline vital signs. ___ ___ ___ _____

4. Reviewed physician's order. ___ ___ ___ _____

NURSING DIAGNOSIS

1. Developed appropriate nursing diagnoses based on assessment data. ___ ___ ___ _____

PLANNING

1. Identified expected outcomes. ___ ___ ___ _____

2. Explained procedure to patient. ___ ___ ___ _____

IMPLEMENTATION

1. Performed hand hygiene and applied gloves. ___ ___ ___ _____

2. Obtained assistance to position patient, if needed. Raised bed to working height with opposite rail up. ___ ___ ___ _____

3. Provided privacy. ___ ___ ___ _____

4. Assisted patient to a side-lying position. Draped patient. Placed waterproof pad under patient's buttocks. ___ ___ ___ _____

5. Placed bedpan next to patient. ___ ___ ___ _____

6. Lubricated index finger of glove with anesthetic lubricant. ___ ___ ___ _____

7. Instructed patient to take slow, deep breaths. Inserted index finger gradually into patient's rectum. ___ ___ ___ _____

8. Gradually advanced fingers along rectal wall. ___ ___ ___ _____

9. Gently loosened fecal mass. ___ ___ ___ _____

10. Moved mass toward end of rectum. Removed and discarded feces into bedpan. ___ ___ ___ _____

11. Checked patient's heart rate and looked for signs of fatigue. ___ ___ ___ _____

12. Allowed patient to rest at intervals during procedure. ___ ___ ___ _____

	S	U	NP	Comments
13. Washed anal area after disimpaction.	—	—	—	_____
14. Removed bedpan and inspected and disposed of feces. Removed and disposed of gloves.	—	—	—	_____
15. Assisted patient to toilet or to use a clean bedpan.	—	—	—	_____
16. Performed hand hygiene.	—	—	—	_____

EVALUATION

	S	U	NP	Comments
1. Performed rectal examination.	—	—	—	_____
2. Reassessed vital signs and compared versus baseline values.	—	—	—	_____
3. Assessed bowel sounds.	—	—	—	_____
4. Assessed for soft and nontender abdomen.	—	—	—	_____
5. Identified unexpected outcomes.	—	—	—	_____

RECORDING AND REPORTING

	S	U	NP	Comments
1. Documented and reported patient's tolerance, amount and consistency of stool, and any adverse effects.	—	—	—	_____
2. Reported adverse effects to nurse in charge or physician.	—	—	—	_____

Student Darcy Brenneman   Date 9/20/12

Instructor _____ Kendall R. _____   Date 9/21/12

PERFORMANCE CHECKLIST SKILL 34-3   **ADMINISTERING AN ENEMA**

	S	U	NP	Comments
ASSESSMENT				
1. Assessed patient's bowel status. Determined what type of enema needed.	KV Jn			
2. Reviewed medical record for history of increased intracranial pressure, glaucoma, cardiac disease, or recent rectal or prostate surgery.				
3. Inspected abdomen for distention and auscultated for bowel sounds.	Jn			
4. Determined patient's understanding of procedure.	Jn			
5. Reviewed physician's order.	Jn			
NURSING DIAGNOSIS				
1. Developed appropriate nursing diagnoses based on assessment data.				
PLANNING				
1. Identified expected outcomes.				
2. Collected equipment and arranged at patient's bedside.				
3. Correctly identified patient.	Jn			
4. Explained procedure to patient.	Jn			
5. Warmed prepared enema bottle in basin of warm water.				
IMPLEMENTATION				
1. Performed hand hygiene and applied gloves.	KV Jn			
2. Provided privacy.	Jn			
3. Raised bed to working height with opposite side rail up.	Jn			
4. Assisted patient to a side-lying position, Sims position	Jn			
5. Placed waterproof pad under patient's hips and buttocks.	Jn			
6. Draped patient exposing only rectal area.	Jn			
7. Examined perianal region for hemorrhoids/rectal prolapse	Jn			
8. Placed bedpan within easy reach.				

	S	U	NP	Comments

9. Administered enema

   a. Administered prepackaged disposable enema:

     (1) Removed plastic cap from tip of container and lubricated, if necessary.

     (2) Separated patient's buttocks and located anus. Instructed patient to relax by breathing out through the mouth.

     (3) Expelled air from container.

     (4) Inserted nozzle into anal canal, angling toward the umbilicus, to appropriate depth for age of patient.

     (5) Squeezed bottle until all solution instilled. Instructed patient to retain solution until urge to defecate occurs.

   b. Administered enema using enema bag:

     500 mL

     (1) Added warmed solution to enema bag; checked temperature of solution. Added castille soap if ordered.

     (2) Raised bag, released clamp, and allowed solution to fill tubing.

     (3) Reclamped tubing.

     (4) Lubricated 6 to 8 cm (2½ to 3 inches) of tip of tubing.

     (5) Separated patient's buttocks and located anus. Instructed patient to breathe in and out.

     (6) Inserted tip to appropriate depth (step 9a[4]).

     (7) Held tubing in patient's rectum until completion of instillation.

     (8) Opened regulating clamp and allowed solution to enter slowly.

     (9) Raised height of container to appropriate level (7.5 to 45 cm [3 to 18 inches]).

     (10) Clamped tubing after all fluid instilled.

10. Placed toilet tissue around end of tubing and withdrew tubing from patient's anus.

11. Reassured patient that feeling of distention is expected, and instructed patient to retain fluid.

12. Discarded enema containers and tubing.

13. Assisted patient to bathroom or commode or onto bedpan.

384

	S	U	NP	Comments
14. Observed character of feces and solution.				
15. Assisted patient with perineal care.				
16. Removed and discarded gloves. Performed hand hygiene.				

EVALUATION

	S	U	NP	Comments
1. Inspected character of stool and fluid.				
2. Assessed condition of abdomen.				
3. Identified unexpected outcomes.				

RECORDING AND REPORTING

	S	U	NP	Comments
1. Recorded type and volume of enema and results.				
2. Reported failure of patient to defecate or any adverse effects.				

PE: Kyla VanDerWeele 9-20-12

Student _____ Date _____

Instructor _____ Date _____

PERFORMANCE CHECKLIST SKILL 34-4 **INSERTING AND MAINTAINING A NASOGASTRIC TUBE FOR GASTRIC DECOMPRESSION**

	S	U	NP	Comments
ASSESSMENT				
1. Performed hand hygiene. Inspected condition of patient's nasal and oral cavity.	___	___	___	_____
2. Determined history of nasal surgery and noted if deviated nasal septum present.	___	___	___	_____
3. Auscultated for bowel sounds. Palpated patient's abdomen.	___	___	___	_____
4. Assessed patient's level of consciousness and ability to follow instructions.	___	___	___	_____
5. Determined if patient had a nasogastric (NG) tube in the past.	___	___	___	_____
6. Checked medical record for order.	___	___	___	_____
NURSING DIAGNOSIS				
1. Developed appropriate nursing diagnoses based on assessment data.	___	___	___	_____
PLANNING				
1. Identified expected outcomes.	___	___	___	_____
2. Prepared equipment at bedside.	___	___	___	_____
3. Identified patient and explained procedure.	___	___	___	_____
IMPLEMENTATION				
1. Performed hand hygiene and applied clean gloves.	___	___	___	_____
2. Positioned patient in high-Fowler's position with pillows behind head and shoulder. Raised bed to a comfortable working height.	___	___	___	_____
3. Provided privacy.	___	___	___	_____
4. Placed bath towel over patient's chest. Placed emesis basin within reach.	___	___	___	_____
5. Washed bridge of patient's nose.	___	___	___	_____
6. Assessed nares for most appropriate placement.	___	___	___	_____
7. Measured distance to insert tube using traditional or Hanson method.	___	___	___	_____
8. Marked length of tube to be inserted from nares to stomach.	___	___	___	_____
9. Curved tip of NG tube tightly around index finger and then released.	___	___	___	_____

	S	U	NP	Comments

10. Lubricated 7.5 to 10 cm (3 to 4 inches) of the end of the tube with water-soluble lubricating jelly. _____ _____ _____ _____

11. Alerted patient that procedure was about to begin. _____ _____ _____ _____

12. Instructed patient to extend neck, and inserted tube slowly through naris with curved end pointing downward. _____ _____ _____ _____

13. Continued to pass tube along floor of nasal passage. _____ _____ _____ _____

14. If resistance met, rotated tube or withdrew tube, allowed patient to rest, relubricated tube, and inserted into other naris. _____ _____ _____ _____

15. Continued tube insertion by gently rotating tube toward opposite naris; stopped tube advancement; allowed patient to relax; provided tissues; explained to patient that next step requires patient to swallow. _____ _____ _____ _____

16. With tube above oropharynx, instructed patient to flex head forward and take a sip of water if allowed or dry swallow or suck in air through a straw; advanced the tube 1 to 2 inches with each swallow. _____ _____ _____ _____

17. If patient began to cough, gag, or choke, stopped tube advancement; instructed patient to breathe easily and to take sips of water. _____ _____ _____ _____

18. If patient continued to cough, pulled tube back slightly. _____ _____ _____ _____

19. If patient continued to gag, checked back of oropharynx. _____ _____ _____ _____

20. After patient relaxed, continued to advance tube the desired distance. After tube had been advanced, anchored tube with prepared split tape and marked tube length. _____ _____ _____ _____

21. Verified tube placement, according to agency policy.

   a. Asked patient to talk. _____ _____ _____ _____

   b. Checked posterior pharynx for coiling of tube. _____ _____ _____ _____

   c. Aspirated gently back on syringe to obtain gastric contents. _____ _____ _____ _____

   d. Measured pH of aspirate (Gastroccult). _____ _____ _____ _____

   e. Had x-ray examination of chest and abdomen performed, if ordered. _____ _____ _____ _____

	S	U	NP	Comments

f. If tube not in stomach, advanced it 1 to 2 inches and repeated steps to check tube position. ___ ___ ___ _____

22. *Anchoring Tube*

   a. Clamped end or connected to a drainage bag or suction machine. ___ ___ ___ _____

   b. Taped tube to nose or applied commercial tube fixation device; avoided putting pressure on nares. ___ ___ ___ _____

   c. Fastened end of NG tube to patient's gown with rubber band and safety pin; provided slack for patient's movement. Maintained pigtail of Salem sump tube above level of stomach. ___ ___ ___ _____

   d. Kept head of bed elevated 30 degrees, unless contraindicated. ___ ___ ___ _____

   e. Explained that sensation of tube should decrease. ___ ___ ___ _____

   f. Removed gloves and performed hand hygiene. ___ ___ ___ _____

23. After tube placement confirmed,

   a. Placed mark on tape where tube exits nose. ___ ___ ___ _____

   b. Option: Measured tube length from nares to connector. ___ ___ ___ _____

   c. Documented tube length. ___ ___ ___ _____

24. Attached NG tube to suction as ordered. ___ ___ ___ _____

25. *Tube Irrigation*

   a. Performed hand hygiene and applied gloves. ___ ___ ___ _____

   b. Checked tube placement. ___ ___ ___ _____

   c. Drew up 30 mL normal saline into Asepto or catheter-tipped syringe. ___ ___ ___ _____

   d. Clamped NG tube. Disconnected tube and laid end on towel. ___ ___ ___ _____

   e. Inserted tip of syringe into end of NG tube; held syringe with tip pointed at the floor and slowly injected solution; did not force. ___ ___ ___ _____

   f. If resistance occurred, checked tube for kinks; turned patient onto left side. ___ ___ ___ _____

   g. After instilling saline, aspirated with syringe to withdraw fluids; measured volume returned. Cleared air vent with 10 ml of air. ___ ___ ___ _____

	S	U	NP	Comments

h. Reconnected NG tube to drainage or suction; if solution did not return, repeated irrigation. ___ ___ ___ _____

i. Removed gloves and performed hand hygiene. ___ ___ ___ _____

26. *Discontinuation of NG Tube*

a. Verified order to discontinue NG tube. ___ ___ ___ _____

b. Explained procedure to patient. ___ ___ ___ _____

c. Performed hand hygiene and applied gloves. ___ ___ ___ _____

d. Turned off suction; disconnected NG tube from drainage bag or suction. Inserted 20 mL of air into lumen of NG tube. Removed tape from nose; unpinned tube from gown. ___ ___ ___ _____

e. Stood on correct side of bed for dominant hand. ___ ___ ___ _____

f. Provided patient facial tissue and placed towel across patient's chest. ___ ___ ___ _____

g. Clamped tube securely. Pulled tube out steadily and smoothly as patient held breath. Inspected intactness of tube. ___ ___ ___ _____

h. Measured drainage. Disposed of tube and drainage unit. ___ ___ ___ _____

i. Cleaned nares and provided mouth care. ___ ___ ___ _____

j. Repositioned patient comfortably and explained fluid intake procedure. ___ ___ ___ _____

26. Cleaned and stored equipment. Properly disposed of soiled supplies. ___ ___ ___ _____

27. Removed gloves and performed hand hygiene. ___ ___ ___ _____

EVALUATION

1. Observed amount and character of NG drainage. ___ ___ ___ _____

2. Palpated patient's abdomen and auscultated bowel sounds. ___ ___ ___ _____

3. Inspected condition of nares and nose. ___ ___ ___ _____

4. Observed position of tubing. ___ ___ ___ _____

5. Asked if patient felt pharyngeal irritation. ___ ___ ___ _____

6. Identified unexpected outcomes. ___ ___ ___ _____

RECORDING AND REPORTING

1. Correctly recorded insertion procedure, patient's tolerance, and character of drainage. ___ ___ ___ _____

	S	U	NP	Comments
2. Correctly recorded tube irrigation and amount and type of aspirate.	____	____	____	_____
3. Recorded on I&O sheet balance of fluid instilled and aspirated.	____	____	____	_____
4. Recorded discontinuation of tube.	____	____	____	_____
5. Reported absence or character of drainage and onset of abdominal distention.	____	____	____	_____
6. Recorded presence or absence of bowel sounds.	____	____	____	_____

Student _____ Date _____

Instructor _____ Date _____

PERFORMANCE CHECKLIST SKILL 35-1 **POUCHING A COLOSTOMY OR AN ILEOSTOMY**

	S	U	NP	Comments
ASSESSMENT				
1. Performed hand hygiene and applied gloves. Assessed GI system. Auscultated for bowel sounds.	___	___	___	_____
2. Assessed for effectiveness of pouching system and skin condition. Avoided unnecessary changing of pouch.	___	___	___	_____
3. Assessed type of stoma. Observed stoma for color and condition.	___	___	___	_____
4. Observed abdomen to determine best type of pouching system.	___	___	___	_____
5. Determined patient's ability and readiness to learn self-care.	___	___	___	_____
NURSING DIAGNOSIS				
1. Developed appropriate nursing diagnoses based on assessment data.	___	___	___	_____
PLANNING				
1. Identified expected outcomes.	___	___	___	_____
2. Explained to patient steps of procedure.	___	___	___	_____
3. Assembled equipment at bedside and provided privacy.	___	___	___	_____
IMPLEMENTATION				
1. Positioned patient correctly and comfortably. If possible, provided mirror for observation.	___	___	___	_____
2. Performed hand hygiene and applied clean gloves.	___	___	___	_____
3. Placed towel or barrier across lower abdomen.	___	___	___	_____
4. Removed used pouch and skin barrier.	___	___	___	_____
5. Cleansed peristomal skin, patted dry.	___	___	___	_____
6. Measured stoma.	___	___	___	_____
7. Cut opening, selected and prepared pouch. Removed backing from barrier and applied without gaps.	___	___	___	_____
8. Secured clamp to open-ended pouch.	___	___	___	_____

	S	U	NP	Comments
9. Properly disposed of old pouch and soiled equipment.	——	——	——	——————
10. Removed gloves and performed hand hygiene.	——	——	——	——————

EVALUATION

	S	U	NP	Comments
1. Observed condition of skin barrier for presence of leaks.	——	——	——	——————
2. Assessed appearance of stoma, peristomal skin, and incision.	——	——	——	——————
3. Observed willingness of patient and family to view stoma and ask questions.	——	——	——	——————
4. Identified unexpected outcomes.	——	——	——	——————

RECORDING AND REPORTING

	S	U	NP	Comments
1. Documented type and size of pouch.	——	——	——	——————
2. Recorded character of effluent and appearance of stoma and peristomal skin.	——	——	——	——————
3. Documented teaching and feedback from patient/family.	——	——	——	——————
4. Reported to charge nurse or physician abnormal appearance of stoma, suture line, or peristomal skin and output.	——	——	——	——————

Student _____ Date _____

Instructor _____ Date _____

PERFORMANCE CHECKLIST SKILL 35-2 **POUCHING A UROSTOMY**

	S	U	NP	Comments

ASSESSMENT

1. Assessed effectiveness of pouching system and condition of skin to determine need to change pouch. ___ ___ ___ _____

2. Observed characteristics of output from stoma, stents, or catheters. ___ ___ ___ _____

3. Assessed characteristics of stoma. ___ ___ ___ _____

4. Assessed abdomen. ___ ___ ___ _____

5. Determined patient's emotional response, ability and readiness to learn self-care. ___ ___ ___ _____

NURSING DIAGNOSIS

1. Developed appropriate nursing diagnoses based on assessment data. ___ ___ ___ _____

PLANNING

1. Identified expected outcomes. ___ ___ ___ _____

2. Explained steps of procedure to patient and encouraged participation. ___ ___ ___ _____

3. Assembled equipment. Provided privacy. ___ ___ ___ _____

IMPLEMENTATION

1. Positioned patient correctly and comfortably. If possible, provided a mirror for observation. ___ ___ ___ _____

2. Performed hand hygiene and applied gloves. ___ ___ ___ _____

3. Placed towel across lower abdomen. Placed wick or gauze pad over stoma. ___ ___ ___ _____

4. Gently removed old pouch so as not to displace stents if present. ___ ___ ___ _____

5. Cleansed peristomal skin, patted dry. Inspected stoma and surrounding skin. ___ ___ ___ _____

6. Wicked and measured stoma. Used skin barrier or sealant as indicated. Applied pouch. ___ ___ ___ _____

7. Opened drain spout and attached to urinary bag. Placed bag at foot of bed. ___ ___ ___ _____

8. Properly disposed of used pouch and soiled equipment. ___ ___ ___ _____

9. Removed gloves and performed hand hygiene. ___ ___ ___ _____

	S	U	NP	Comments

EVALUATION

1. Noted condition of stoma, peristomal skin, and suture line. ___ ___ ___ _____

2. Evaluated character and volume of urine. ___ ___ ___ _____

3. Noted patient's and/or significant other's willingness to view stoma and ask questions. ___ ___ ___ _____

4. Identified unexpected outcomes. ___ ___ ___ _____

RECORDING AND REPORTING

1. Recorded type of pouch, time of change, appearance of stoma and peristomal skin, and character of urine. ___ ___ ___ _____

2. Recorded urinary output on I&O flowsheet. ___ ___ ___ _____

3. Noted patient's or significant other's reaction to procedure. ___ ___ ___ _____

4. Reported any abnormalities to nurse in charge or physician. ___ ___ ___ _____

Student _____   Date _____

Instructor _____   Date _____

PERFORMANCE CHECKLIST SKILL 35-3   **CATHETERIZING A URINARY DIVERSION**

	S	U	NP	Comments

ASSESSMENT

1. Assessed for signs and symptoms of a UTI. Determined need to obtain urine specimen.   ___ ___ ___ _____

2. Obtained physician's order for catheterization.   ___ ___ ___ _____

3. Assessed patient's understanding of procedure.   ___ ___ ___ _____

NURSING DIAGNOSIS

1. Developed appropriate nursing diagnoses based on assessment data.   ___ ___ ___ _____

PLANNING

1. Identified expected outcomes.   ___ ___ ___ _____

2. Assembled equipment.   ___ ___ ___ _____

3. Provided for patient's privacy.   ___ ___ ___ _____

4. Explained procedure to patient and timed procedure in accordance with pouch change.   ___ ___ ___ _____

IMPLEMENTATION

1. Positioned patient comfortably in a sitting position, if possible.   ___ ___ ___ _____

2. Performed hand hygiene and applied gloves.   ___ ___ ___ _____

3. Gently removed old pouch.   ___ ___ ___ _____

4. Removed and discarded gloves. Performed hand hygiene. Opened sterile catheterization set or needed equipment.   ___ ___ ___ _____

5. Applied sterile gloves. Had patient hold absorbent wick on stoma, if needed.   ___ ___ ___ _____

6. Cleansed surface of stoma with antiseptic swabs (checked patient's allergy history).   ___ ___ ___ _____

7. Allowed small amount of urine to flow from stoma, if specimen required.   ___ ___ ___ _____

8. Lubricated catheter tip.   ___ ___ ___ _____

9. Placed distal end of catheter in sterile specimen container.   ___ ___ ___ _____

10. Using dominant hand, gently inserted catheter 2 to 2½ inches (5 to 6.5 cm) into stoma; instructed patient to cough or turn slightly.   ___ ___ ___ _____

	S	U	NP	Comments
11. Placed specimen container below level of stoma to collect urinary drainage.	——	——	——	_____
12. Withdrew catheter and placed 4 × 4-inch gauze pad over stoma.	——	——	——	_____
13. Secured specimen container and labeled specimen.	——	——	——	_____
14. Reapplied new pouch.	——	——	——	_____
15. Disposed of soiled pouch and equipment.	——	——	——	_____
16. Removed gloves, performed hand hygiene, and sent specimen to laboratory.	——	——	——	_____

EVALUATION

	S	U	NP	Comments
1. Compared results of culture and sensitivity tests versus normal expected findings.	——	——	——	_____
2. Instructed patient about signs and symptoms of urinary tract infection.	——	——	——	_____
3. Identified unexpected outcomes.	——	——	——	_____

RECORDING AND REPORTING

	S	U	NP	Comments
1. Recorded specimen collection, patient's tolerance of procedure, and appearance of urine, peristomal skin, and stoma.	——	——	——	_____
2. Reported results of laboratory test to nurse in charge or physician.	——	——	——	_____

Student _____   Date _____

Instructor _____   Date _____

PERFORMANCE CHECKLIST SKILL 36-1   **PREPARING A PATIENT FOR SURGERY**

	S	U	NP	Comments
ASSESSMENT				
1. Correctly identified patient.	___	___	___	_____
2. Determined patient's ability to answer questions.	___	___	___	_____
3. Obtained nursing history and identified risk factors.	___	___	___	_____
4. Performed physical examination.	___	___	___	_____
5. Applied allergy/sensitivity band, if indicated.	___	___	___	_____
6. Assessed patient's and family member's expectations of surgery. Encouraged questions.	___	___	___	_____
7. Reviewed patient's preoperative orders.	___	___	___	_____
8. Validated that preoperative preps were completed.	___	___	___	_____
9. Asked patient about advance directives.	___	___	___	_____
NURSING DIAGNOSIS				
1. Developed appropriate nursing diagnoses based on assessment data.	___	___	___	_____
PLANNING				
1. Identified expected outcomes.	___	___	___	_____
2. Prepared patient's chart, and assembled necessary equipment.	___	___	___	_____
3. Explained procedures and allowed patient, family members, or significant others to ask questions.	___	___	___	_____
IMPLEMENTATION				
1. Oriented patient to room or presurgical area.	___	___	___	_____
2. Witnessed informed consent.	___	___	___	_____
3. Checked medical record, and completed preoperative checklist.	___	___	___	_____
4. Provided preoperative teaching.	___	___	___	_____
5. Confirmed that preoperative orders were completed.	___	___	___	_____
6. Provided privacy and instructed (assisted) patient to remove clothes and put on gown and cap. Performed (assisted with) personal hygiene.	___	___	___	_____

	S	U	NP	Comments

7. Instructed patient to remove hair accessories, jewelry, body piercings, and makeup. If wedding band could not be removed, taped to finger. Checked institutional policy for removal of acrylic nails. Listed all items removed and their location on preoperative clothing list. ___ ___ ___ _____

8. Assisted patient to remove prostheses. Listed all items removed and their location on preoperative checklist. ___ ___ ___ _____

9. Stored valuables per agency policy. If given to family, release form signed. ___ ___ ___ _____

10. Applied antiembolism stockings as ordered. ___ ___ ___ _____

11. Assessed patient's vital signs immediately before going to OR. ___ ___ ___ _____

12. Assisted patient to void before receiving preoperative medication. ___ ___ ___ _____

13. Administered preoperative medications as ordered. ___ ___ ___ _____

14. Placed patient on bed rest with side rails up and call light within reach. ___ ___ ___ _____

EVALUATION

1. Confirmed patient's level of knowledge about surgical procedure. ___ ___ ___ _____

2. Compared assessment data versus patient's baseline and expected normal values. ___ ___ ___ _____

3. Had patient repeat preoperative instructions and demonstrate postoperative exercises. ___ ___ ___ _____

4. Assessed patient for signs and symptoms of anxiety. ___ ___ ___ _____

5. Identified unexpected outcomes. ___ ___ ___ _____

RECORDING AND REPORTING

1. Documented all preoperative preparations. ___ ___ ___ _____

2. Documented patient condition on transfer to operating room. ___ ___ ___ _____

3. Documented allergies/sensitivities on armband, in MAR, and in medical records. ___ ___ ___ _____

4. Recorded patient's valuables and belongings that were collected. ___ ___ ___ _____

5. Reported abnormal findings, lack of signed consent form, or failure to maintain NPO status. ___ ___ ___ _____

6. Recorded and reported patient's cultural practices or religious beliefs that may necessitate modification of the care plan. ___ ___ ___ _____

PERFORMANCE CHECKLIST SKILL 36-2 **DEMONSTRATING POSTOPERATIVE EXERCISES**

	S	U	NP	Comments
ASSESSMENT				
1. Assessed patient's risk for postoperative respiratory complications.	___	___	___	_____
2. Auscultated lungs.	___	___	___	_____
3. Assessed patient's ability to cough and deep breathe.	___	___	___	_____
4. Assessed patient's risk for postoperative thrombus formation.	___	___	___	_____
5. Assessed patient's ability to move independently in bed.	___	___	___	_____
6. Assessed patient's willingness and ability to learn exercises.	___	___	___	_____
7. Assessed family members' willingness to learn and to support patient.	___	___	___	_____
8. Assessed patient's medical orders preoperatively and postoperatively.	___	___	___	_____
NURSING DIAGNOSIS				
1. Developed appropriate nursing diagnoses based on assessment data.	___	___	___	_____
PLANNING				
1. Identified expected outcomes.	___	___	___	_____
2. Prepared necessary equipment.	___	___	___	_____
3. Prepared room for teaching.	___	___	___	_____
IMPLEMENTATION				
1. *Instructed and Demonstrated Diaphragmatic Breathing*				
a. Assisted patient to comfortable sitting or standing position. In bed, repositioned to a semi-Fowler's or high-Fowler's as tolerated.	___	___	___	_____
b. Stood or sat facing patient.	___	___	___	_____
c. Correctly placed hands on anterior rib cage.	___	___	___	_____
d. Instructed patient to take slow deep breaths.	___	___	___	_____
e. Instructed patient to avoid using chest and shoulders while inhaling.	___	___	___	_____

	S	U	NP	Comments

f. Had patient hold slow, deep breath for a count of 3 and exhale through pursed lips. ____ ____ ____ _____

g. Repeated breathing exercise 3 to 5 times. ____ ____ ____ _____

h. Had patient practice the exercise. ____ ____ ____ _____

2. *Instructed and Demonstrated Positive Expiratory Pressure (PEP) Therapy and "Huff" Coughing*

   a. Set the PEP device to the setting ordered. ____ ____ ____ _____

   b. Assisted to a semi-Fowler's or high-Fowler's position and placed nose clip on nose. ____ ____ ____ _____

   c. Had patient place lips tightly around mouth piece, take a slow full breath, and exhale 2 to 3 times longer than inhalation. Repeated 10 to 20 times. ____ ____ ____ _____

   d. Had patient inhale, hold breath to count of 3, and exhale in quick, short, forced "huffs." ____ ____ ____ _____

3. *Instructed and Demonstrated Controlled Coughing*

   a. Assisted patient to a semi-Fowler's or high-Fowler's position as tolerated. ____ ____ ____ _____

   b. Demonstrated coughing by taking 2 slow, deep breaths, inhaling through nose, and exhaling through pursed lips. ____ ____ ____ _____

   c. Inhaled deeply the third time and held breath for count of 3. Fully coughed 2 to 3 consecutive coughs without inhaling in between. ____ ____ ____ _____

   d. Instructed patient to cough deeply. ____ ____ ____ _____

   e. Instructed patient to splint abdominal incision while coughing, if present. ____ ____ ____ _____

   f. Had patient cough 2 to 3 times every hour while awake. ____ ____ ____ _____

   g. Instructed patient to examine sputum regularly and to notify nurse of any changes. ____ ____ ____ _____

4. *Taught Turning*

   a. Instructed patient to assume a supine position on the right side of the bed. ____ ____ ____ _____

   b. Instructed patient to place right hand or pillow over incisional area to splint it. ____ ____ ____ _____

   c. Instructed patient to keep right leg straight and to flex left knee up and over right leg. ____ ____ ____ _____

	S	U	NP	Comments

d. Had patient grab right side rail with left hand and pull toward and roll onto right side. ___ ___ ___ _____

e. Instructed patient to turn every 2 hours while awake. ___ ___ ___ _____

5. *Taught Leg Exercises*

a. Had patient assume supine position and demonstrate passive range of motion exercises. ___ ___ ___ _____

b. Rotated each ankle 5 times. ___ ___ ___ _____

c. Alternated dorsiflexion and plantar flexion of both feet. ___ ___ ___ _____

d. Had patient flex and extend knees 5 times. ___ ___ ___ _____

e. Had patient alternately raise each leg straight up from bed, keeping legs straight, 5 times. ___ ___ ___ _____

f. Had patient continue to practice exercises at least every 2 hours. ___ ___ ___ _____

EVALUATION

1. Observed patient's ability to perform all 4 exercises independently. ___ ___ ___ _____

2. Observed family members' ability to coach patient. ___ ___ ___ _____

3. Assessed patient's chest excursion. ___ ___ ___ _____

4. Auscultated patient's lungs. ___ ___ ___ _____

5. Assessed for signs of thrombophlebitis. ___ ___ ___ _____

6. Identified unexpected outcomes. ___ ___ ___ _____

RECORDING AND REPORTING

1. Recorded physical assessment findings. ___ ___ ___ _____

2. Recorded any assessed complications and actions. ___ ___ ___ _____

3. Recorded exercises that had been demonstrated to patient and whether patient could perform exercises independently. ___ ___ ___ _____

4. Reported to the next shift any problems with patient performance of exercises. ___ ___ ___ _____

Student _____ Date _____

Instructor _____ Date _____

PERFORMANCE CHECKLIST SKILL 36-3 **PERFORMING POSTOPERATIVE CARE OF A SURGICAL PATIENT**

	S	U	NP	Comments

ASSESSMENT
1. *Phase 1: Immediate Recovery Period*

   a. Determined patient's condition during operative procedure. ___ ___ ___ _____

   b. Obtained report from surgeon and anesthesiologist. ___ ___ ___ _____

   c. Considered surgery performed. ___ ___ ___ _____

   d. Performed thorough patient assessment. ___ ___ ___ _____

2. *Phase 2: Convalescent Period*

   a. Received phone report from nurse in RR/PACU. ___ ___ ___ _____

   b. Obtained detailed report from nurse at time of patient's transfer to division. ___ ___ ___ _____

   c. Reviewed patient's medical record. ___ ___ ___ _____

   d. Reviewed surgeon's postoperative orders. ___ ___ ___ _____

   e. Assessed patient's knowledge and expectations of surgical recovery. ___ ___ ___ _____

NURSING DIAGNOSIS
1. Developed appropriate nursing diagnoses based on assessment data. ___ ___ ___ _____

PLANNING
1. Identified expected outcomes. ___ ___ ___ _____

2. Prepared equipment at bedside. ___ ___ ___ _____

3. Explained procedures to patient. ___ ___ ___ _____

IMPLEMENTATION
1. *Phase 1: Immediate Recovery Period*

   a. Performed hand hygiene. ___ ___ ___ _____

   b. Checked equipment setup in RR/PACU. ___ ___ ___ _____

   c. Immediately after patient entered RR/PACU, attached oxygen equipment and drainage tubes, and checked IV flow rates. ___ ___ ___ _____

   d. Conducted complete patient assessment. Assessed vital signs every 15 minutes and continued monitoring as needed. Provided warm blankets. ___ ___ ___ _____

	S	U	NP	Comments

e. Maintained patent airway with proper patient positioning and suctioning, and encouraged deep breathing and coughing. ____ ____ ____ _____

f. Called patient by name, and oriented patient to surroundings. ____ ____ ____ _____

g. Assessed circulatory perfusion. ____ ____ ____ _____

h. Inspected surgical dressing and drains for bright red blood.

   (1) Inspected area of surgical wound. ____ ____ ____ _____

   (2) Inspected condition of dressing. Reinforced dressing as needed. ____ ____ ____ _____

   (3) Inspected condition and contents of drainage tubes. ____ ____ ____ _____

   (4) Observed patency and intactness of urinary catheter and volume and character of urine. ____ ____ ____ _____

   (5) If nasogastric tube was present, verified placement and irrigated as ordered. ____ ____ ____ _____

   (6) Monitored IV fluid infusion. ____ ____ ____ _____

i. Provided patient mouth care. ____ ____ ____ _____

j. Assessed patient's pain and administered analgesia as ordered. ____ ____ ____ _____

k. Encouraged patient to begin deep breathing and coughing exercises. ____ ____ ____ _____

l. Encouraged leg exercises. ____ ____ ____ _____

m. Explained to patient status of recovery. ____ ____ ____ _____

n. Contacted physician for order to transfer stabilized patient. Measured I&O. ____ ____ ____ _____

2. *Phase 2: Convalescent Period*

a. Checked equipment setup in patient's room. ____ ____ ____ _____

b. Transferred patient to bed. ____ ____ ____ _____

c. Connected any existing oxygen tubing, nasogastric tube, and indwelling catheter to drainage, and regulated IV infusion. ____ ____ ____ _____

d. Assessed vital signs routinely, as ordered. ____ ____ ____ _____

e. Maintained airway correctly through patient positioning, deep breathing, and coughing. ____ ____ ____ _____

f. Ensured patency and intactness of all drainage tubes. ____ ____ ____ _____

g. Inspected condition of dressing or wound. ____ ____ ____ _____

h. Assessed patient for bladder distention. ____ ____ ____ _____

	S	U	NP	Comments
i. Measured sources of fluid intake and output.	___	___	___	_____
j. Positioned patient for comfort.	___	___	___	_____
k. Encouraged continuation of leg exercises every 1 to 2 hours.	___	___	___	_____
l. Applied elastic stockings or pneumatic compression cuffs.	___	___	___	_____
m. Explained to patient nature of observations, and allowed family into room.	___	___	___	_____
n. Explained to family activities and purpose of room equipment.	___	___	___	_____
o. Appropriately administered analgesia.	___	___	___	_____
p. Provided oral hygiene.	___	___	___	_____
q. Maintained support measures for functioning body systems:				
(1) Encouraged postoperative exercises.	___	___	___	_____
(2) Encouraged use of incentive spirometer.	___	___	___	_____
(3) Implemented activity orders.	___	___	___	_____
(4) Monitored bowel sounds.	___	___	___	_____
(5) Promoted and monitored voiding.	___	___	___	_____
(6) Monitored wound healing.	___	___	___	_____
(7) Monitored wound drainage.	___	___	___	_____
r. Increased patient's involvement in decision making.	___	___	___	_____
s. Taught patient and family signs and symptoms of complications.	___	___	___	_____
t. Included family in discussion about discharge.	___	___	___	_____
u. Prepared for referral to home health or convalescent care.	___	___	___	_____

EVALUATION

	S	U	NP	Comments
1. Compared assessment findings versus patient's baseline and expected range.	___	___	___	_____
2. Evaluated pain relief measures.	___	___	___	_____
3. Monitored changes in surgical wound.	___	___	___	_____
4. Monitored lung sounds.	___	___	___	_____
5. Auscultated patient's bowel sounds.	___	___	___	_____
6. Monitored I&O.	___	___	___	_____
7. Discussed with patient his or her feelings about recovery.	___	___	___	_____
8. Routinely conducted needed physical assessments.	___	___	___	_____
9. Identified unexpected outcomes.	___	___	___	_____

	S	U	NP	Comments

RECORDING AND REPORTING

1. Recorded patient's arrival at recovery room or nursing division, assessments made, and nursing care initiated. ____ ____ ____ _____

2. Recorded vital signs and I&O on flowsheets. ____ ____ ____ _____

3. Reported abnormal assessment findings and signs of complications to nurse in charge or physician. ____ ____ ____ _____

Student _____ Date _____

Instructor _____ Date _____

PERFORMANCE CHECKLIST SKILL 37-1 **SURGICAL HAND ANTISEPSIS**

	S	U	NP	Comments

ASSESSMENT

1. Checked institutional policy for type and length of time for hand hygiene. ___ ___ ___ _____

2. Removed watch and jewelry. ___ ___ ___ _____

3. Assessed condition of nails for length and presence of polish and artificial nails. ___ ___ ___ _____

4. Inspected skin integrity of forearms and of hands. ___ ___ ___ _____

NURSING DIAGNOSIS

1. Developed appropriate nursing diagnoses based on assessment data. ___ ___ ___ _____

PLANNING

1. Identified expected outcomes. ___ ___ ___ _____

IMPLEMENTATION

1. Applied appropriate surgical attire. ___ ___ ___ _____

2. Performed a prescrub at beginning of shift:

   a. Turned on water with knee or foot controls and adjusted temperature. ___ ___ ___ _____

   b. Wet hands thoroughly: followed manufacturer's direction for application of soap. ___ ___ ___ _____

   c. Rubbed all hand surfaces for at least 15 seconds. ___ ___ ___ _____

   d. Rinsed well; dried thoroughly with a paper towel. ___ ___ ___ _____

3. Performed a surgical hand scrub with a sponge:

   a. Turned on water with knee or foot controls and adjusted temperature. Cleaned under nails of both hands with disposable nail pick. Rinsed hands and forearms under running water. ___ ___ ___ _____

   b. Dispensed antimicrobial agent according to manufacturer's instructions; applied to wet hands and forearms using sponge. ___ ___ ___ _____

   c. Scrubbed 3 to 5 minutes; washed all 4 sides of each finger, hand, and arm. Kept hand elevated, elbow down, while scrubbing. ___ ___ ___ _____

	S	U	NP	Comments

d. Did not splash on clothing; discarded sponge in correct container. ___ ___ ___ _____

e. Thoroughly rinsed hands and arms under running water, keeping hands above elbows and away from clothing. ___ ___ ___ _____

f. Turned off water with foot/knee control; backed into OR holding hands higher than elbows and away from clothing. ___ ___ ___ _____

g. Grasped sterile towel, taking care not to drip onto sterile field. ___ ___ ___ _____

h. Kept hands and arms above waist and away from body; thoroughly dried hands from fingers to elbow. ___ ___ ___ _____

i. Used other end of towel to dry other hand. Properly disposed of towel. ___ ___ ___ _____

4. Performed a spongeless surgical hand scrub with alcohol-based hand rub product

a. After prescrub wash (step 2), turned on water using foot/knee control. Cleaned under nails of both hands using a disposable nail pick. Rinsed hands and forearms under running water. Thoroughly dried hands with a paper towel. ___ ___ ___ _____

b. Dispensed recommended amount of antimicrobial agent. Applied to hands and forearms according to instructions. ___ ___ ___ _____

c. Repeated antimicrobial application if recommended. ___ ___ ___ _____

d. Rubbed thoroughly until completely dry. Proceeded to OR to apply gloves. ___ ___ ___ _____

EVALUATION

1. Monitored patient postoperatively for signs of localized wound infection. ___ ___ ___ _____

2. Identified unexpected outcomes. ___ ___ ___ _____

RECORDING AND REPORTING

1. Recorded area and description of surgical site postoperatively. ___ ___ ___ _____

Student _____ Date _____

Instructor _____ Date _____

PERFORMANCE CHECKLIST SKILL 37-2 **DONNING A STERILE GOWN AND CLOSED GLOVING**

	S	U	NP	Comments

ASSESSMENT

1. Chose proper type and size of sterile gloves and gown. Considered patient's and personnel's sensitivity/allergy to latex. ____ ____ ____ _____

NURSING DIAGNOSIS

1. Developed appropriate nursing diagnoses based on assessment data. ____ ____ ____ _____

PLANNING

1. Identified expected outcomes. ____ ____ ____ _____

I MPLEMENTATION

1. *Gowning*

   a. Opened sterile gown pack. ____ ____ ____ _____

   b. Performed surgical hand scrub. Kept hands above waist. Dried hands. ____ ____ ____ _____

   c. Grasped gown appropriately and lifted from sterile package. ____ ____ ____ _____

   d. Lifted gown upward and stepped away from table. ____ ____ ____ _____

   e. Located neckband and grasped gown appropriately. ____ ____ ____ _____

   f. Properly allowed gown to unfold. ____ ____ ____ _____

   g. Inserted arms into gown and had circulating nurse bring gown over shoulders. Left sleeves covering hands. ____ ____ ____ _____

   h. Appropriately secured gown with assistance of circulating nurse. ____ ____ ____ _____

2. *Closed Gloving*

   a. Opened inner sterile glove package with gown covering hands. ____ ____ ____ _____

   b. With nondominant hand, grasped folded cuff of glove for dominant hand. ____ ____ ____ _____

   c. Correctly placed glove on dominant palm. ____ ____ ____ _____

   d. Had glove cuff correctly turned over end of dominant hand. ____ ____ ____ _____

	S	U	NP	Comments
e. Carefully extended fingers into glove.	——	——	——	———————————
f. Gloved nondominant hand in same manner. Made sure fingers were fully extended into both gloves.	——	——	——	———————————
10. With wrap-around sterile gown, released fasteners on front of gown. Had gown flap wrapped and tied appropriately.	——	——	——	———————————

EVALUATION

	S	U	NP	Comments
1. Observed for break in sterile technique. Observed patient postoperatively for signs and symptoms of surgical wound infection.	——	——	——	———————————
2. Identified unexpected outcomes.	——	——	——	———————————

RECORDING AND REPORTING

	S	U	NP	Comments
1. Recorded area and description of surgical site postoperatively.	——	——	——	———————————

Student _____ Date _____

Instructor _____ Date _____

PERFORMANCE CHECKLIST PROCEDURAL GUIDELINE 38-1 **PERFORMING A WOUND ASSESSMENT**

	S	U	NP	Comments
STEPS				
1. Reviewed frequency of wound assessment and examined information from last assessment.	___	___	___	_____
2. Assessed level of pain and signs of anxiety.	___	___	___	_____
3. Explained procedure to patient.	___	___	___	_____
4. Provided privacy.	___	___	___	_____
5. Positioned patient comfortably; exposed wound only.	___	___	___	_____
6. Performed hand hygiene; prepared biohazard bag and placed within reach.	___	___	___	_____
7. Applied clean gloves and removed soiled dressing.	___	___	___	_____
8. Examined dressings for quality and quantity of drainage, presence of odor. Disposed of soiled dressings in biohazard bag. Discarded gloves in biohazard bag.	___	___	___	_____
9. Performed hand hygiene; applied clean gloves.	___	___	___	_____
10. Used approved assessment tool:				
a. Assessed location of wound in body.	___	___	___	_____
b. Assessed extent of tissue loss.	___	___	___	_____
c. Assessed type and percentage of tissue present: granulation, slough, eschar.	___	___	___	_____
d. Measured length, width, and depth of wound.	___	___	___	_____
e. Noted presence and amount of exudate from wound.	___	___	___	_____
f. Noted presence/absence of odor.	___	___	___	_____
g. Assessed skin integrity around wound.	___	___	___	_____
11. Reassessed patient's pain level.	___	___	___	_____
12. Applied clean dressings per physician's order.	___	___	___	_____
13. Appropriately discarded soiled dressings, biohazard bag, and gloves.	___	___	___	_____
14. Performed hand hygiene.	___	___	___	_____
15. Recorded assessment data, compared findings versus previous assessment to evaluate healing progress.	___	___	___	_____

Student _____ Date _____

Instructor _____ Date _____

PERFORMANCE CHECKLIST SKILL 38-1 **PERFORMING WOUND IRRIGATION**

	S	U	NP	Comments
ASSESSMENT				
1. Reviewed patient's medical record for physician's order.	___	___	___	_____
2. Performed wound assessment and compared with recent records for wound progress.	___	___	___	_____
3. Assessed pain (pain scale, PQRST) and identified symptoms of anxiety.	___	___	___	_____
4. Identified history of allergies.	___	___	___	_____
NURSING DIAGNOSIS				
1. Developed appropriate nursing diagnoses based on assessment data.	___	___	___	_____
PLANNING				
1. Identified expected outcomes.	___	___	___	_____
2. Explained procedure to patient.	___	___	___	_____
3. Administered premedication.	___	___	___	_____
4. Gathered supplies.	___	___	___	_____
5. Provided privacy.	___	___	___	_____
6. Positioned patient.	___	___	___	_____
7. Protected bed linens.	___	___	___	_____
8. Exposed wound only.	___	___	___	_____
IMPLEMENTATION				
1. Prepared waterproof bag.	___	___	___	_____
2. Applied gown and goggles, if needed.	___	___	___	_____
3. Performed hand hygiene.	___	___	___	_____
4. Provided privacy.	___	___	___	_____
5. Prepared equipment and opened sterile supplies.	___	___	___	_____
6. Applied sterile gloves.	___	___	___	_____
7. *Irrigated Wound With Wide Opening*				
a. Filled 35-mL syringe with solution.	___	___	___	_____
b. Attached a 19-gauge angiocatheter or needle on syringe.	___	___	___	_____
c. Held syringe 1 inch (2.5 cm) above wound.	___	___	___	_____
d. Flushed wound until return was clear.	___	___	___	_____

	S	U	NP	Comments

8. *Irrigated Deep Wound With Small Opening*

  a. Attached soft angiocatheter to syringe. ____ ____ ____ _____

  b. Inserted tip of catheter 1 cm (½ inch). ____ ____ ____ _____

  c. Using slow continuous pressure, flushed wound. ____ ____ ____ _____

  d. Pinched off catheter. ____ ____ ____ _____

  e. Removed and refilled syringe. Flushed wound until return was clear. ____ ____ ____ _____

9. *Cleansed Wound With Handheld Shower*

  a. Seated patient comfortably in shower/tub. ____ ____ ____ _____

  b. Held shower approximately 12 inches from patient and flushed wound with water for 5 to 10 minutes. ____ ____ ____ _____

10. Obtained necessary wound cultures. ____ ____ ____ _____

11. Dried wound edges with sterile gauze. Dried patient if showered. ____ ____ ____ _____

12. Applied appropriate dressing. ____ ____ ____ _____

13. Removed gloves, mask, goggles, and gown. ____ ____ ____ _____

14. Assisted patient to comfortable position. ____ ____ ____ _____

15. Disposed of used equipment and soiled supplies. Performed hand hygiene. ____ ____ ____ _____

EVALUATION

1. Had patient rate level of comfort. ____ ____ ____ _____

2. Assessed type of tissue in wound bed. ____ ____ ____ _____

3. Periodically inspected dressing. ____ ____ ____ _____

4. Evaluated skin integrity. ____ ____ ____ _____

5. Observed for retained irrigant. ____ ____ ____ _____

6. Identified unexpected outcomes. ____ ____ ____ _____

RECORDING AND REPORTING

1. Recorded wound assessment, irrigation, dressing application, and patient's response. ____ ____ ____ _____

2. Reported to physician any evidence of fresh bleeding, increase in pain, retention of irrigant, or signs of shock. ____ ____ ____ _____

Student _____   Date _____

Instructor _____   Date _____

PERFORMANCE CHECKLIST SKILL 38-2   **PERFORMING SUTURE AND STAPLE REMOVAL**

	S	U	NP	Comments
ASSESSMENT				
1. Identified patient's need for suture/staple removal and reviewed physician's order.	___	___	___	_____
2. Assessed patient for history of allergies.	___	___	___	_____
3. Assessed patient's comfort level (pain scale, PQRST).	___	___	___	_____
4. Observed healing status of wound and associated risk factors.	___	___	___	_____
NURSING DIAGNOS				
1. Developed appropriate nursing diagnoses related to suture or staple removal.	___	___	___	_____
PLANNING				
1. Identified expected outcomes.	___	___	___	_____
2. Explained procedure to patient.	___	___	___	_____
IMPLEMENTATION				
1. Provided privacy.	___	___	___	_____
2. Correctly verified patient identity.	___	___	___	_____
3. Positioned patient.	___	___	___	_____
4. Adjusted light on suture line.	___	___	___	_____
5. Performed hand hygiene.	___	___	___	_____
6. Prepared waterprooof disposal bag.	___	___	___	_____
7. Prepared sterile field and supplies.	___	___	___	_____
8. Applied clean gloves and carefully removed dressing; discarded dressing and gloves.	___	___	___	_____
9. Inspected wound.	___	___	___	_____
10. Applied sterile gloves or clean gloves according to agency policy.	___	___	___	_____
11. Cleansed sutures or staples and incision with antiseptic swabs.	___	___	___	_____
12. *Removed Staples*				
a. Correctly applied staple extractor.	___	___	___	_____
b. Carefully controlled staple extractor.	___	___	___	_____
c. Moved staple away from skin surface.	___	___	___	_____

	S	U	NP	Comments

d. Released handles of staple extractor, allowing staple to fall into refuse bag. ____ ____ ____ _____

e. Repeated Steps a through d until all staples removed. ____ ____ ____ _____

13. *Removed Intermittent Sutures*

   a. Placed sterile gauze and correctly grasped scissors and forceps. ____ ____ ____ _____

   b. Snipped sutures close to skin surface at end distal to knot. ____ ____ ____ _____

   c. Grasped knotted end with forceps and removed suture. Placed removed suture on gauze. ____ ____ ____ _____

   d. Repeated Steps a through c until all sutures removed. ____ ____ ____ _____

   e. Observed healing level. ____ ____ ____ _____

   f. Notified physician, if necessary. ____ ____ ____ _____

14. *Removed Continuous Sutures, Including Blanket Stitch Sutures*

   a. Placed sterile gauze and correctly grasped scissors and forceps. ____ ____ ____ _____

   b. Correctly snipped first suture. ____ ____ ____ _____

   c. Snipped second suture on same side. ____ ____ ____ _____

   d. Grasped knotted end and removed suture from beneath skin in continuous smooth action. Placed removed suture on gauze compress. ____ ____ ____ _____

   e. Repeated Steps a through d until entire line removed. ____ ____ ____ _____

15. Inspected incision site. Cleansed suture line. ____ ____ ____ _____

16. Placed supportive Steri-Strips at areas of separation. ____ ____ ____ _____

17. Applied light dressing, as indicated. ____ ____ ____ _____

18. Discarded contaminated supplies, and removed and disposed of gloves. ____ ____ ____ _____

19. Routed reusable items for sterilization and performed hand hygiene. ____ ____ ____ _____

EVALUATION

1. Assessed site of suture or staple removal. ____ ____ ____ _____

2. Determined if patient had pain along incision. ____ ____ ____ _____

3. Identified unexpected outcomes. ____ ____ ____ _____

	S	U	NP	Comments

RECORDING AND REPORTING

1. Recorded time of removal, number of sutures or staples removed, wound appearance, and patient's response. ⎯ ⎯ ⎯ ⎯⎯⎯⎯⎯⎯⎯⎯⎯⎯⎯

2. Immediately notified physician of abnormal findings. ⎯ ⎯ ⎯ ⎯⎯⎯⎯⎯⎯⎯⎯⎯⎯⎯

Student _____   Date _____

Instructor _____   Date _____

PERFORMANCE CHECKLIST SKILL 38-3 **MANAGING DRAINAGE EVACUATION**

	S	U	NP	Comments
ASSESSMENT				
1. Identified presence of closed wound drain and drainage system.	___	___	___	_____
2. Identified number of wound drainage tubes.	___	___	___	_____
3. Verified physician's order to determine if suction is needed.	___	___	___	_____
4. Inspected system for straight tube or Y-tube arrangement.	___	___	___	_____
5. Inspected system for patency and proper functioning.	___	___	___	_____
6. Verified that Penrose drain, if used, is anchored correctly.	___	___	___	_____
7. Secured drainage reservoirs.	___	___	___	_____
8. Identified type of drainage container to be used.	___	___	___	_____
NURSING DIAGNOSIS				
1. Developed appropriate nursing diagnoses based on assessment data.	___	___	___	_____
PLANNING				
1. Identified expected outcomes.	___	___	___	_____
2. Explained procedure to patient.	___	___	___	_____
IMPLEMENTATION				
1. Provided privacy.	___	___	___	_____
2. Performed hand hygiene and applied gloves.	___	___	___	_____
3. Placed open sterile specimen container or graduated container on bed.	___	___	___	_____
4. Maintained asepsis while opening and emptying evacuator; followed correct procedure for Hemovac or Jackson-Pratt evacuator. Noted characteristics of drainage.	___	___	___	_____
5. Placed and secured drainage reservoirs to prevent pull on insertion sites.	___	___	___	_____
6. Routed labeled specimen to laboratory.	___	___	___	_____
7. Discarded soiled supplies, and performed hand hygiene.	___	___	___	_____

	S	U	NP	Comments
8. Applied new clean gloves. Changed dressing and inspected skin.	___	___	___	_____
9. Discarded contaminated materials, and performed hand hygiene.	___	___	___	_____

EVALUATION

	S	U	NP	Comments
1. Evaluated for presence and characteristics of drainage.	___	___	___	_____
2. Inspected wound for drainage and formation of seroma.	___	___	___	_____
3. Emptied and measured drainage.	___	___	___	_____
4. Assessed patient's comfort level (pain scale, PQRST).	___	___	___	_____
5. Identified unexpected outcomes.	___	___	___	_____

RECORDING AND REPORTING

	S	U	NP	Comments
1. Recorded procedure and patient status. Completed an I&O report.	___	___	___	_____
2. Recorded and reported to physician immediately any changes or abnormal findings.	___	___	___	_____
3. Reported procedure and findings at change of shift.	___	___	___	_____

Student _____ Date _____

Instructor _____ Date _____

PERFORMANCE CHECKLIST SKILL 39-1 **APPLYING A DRESSING (DRY AND MOIST-TO-DRY)**

	S	U	NP	Comments

ASSESSMENT

1. Accurately assessed size of wound. ____ ____ ____ _____

2. Assessed location of wound. ____ ____ ____ _____

3. Assessed patient's comfort (scale 0 to 10, PQRST). Administered prescribed analgesic 30 minutes before dressing change if needed. ____ ____ ____ _____

4. Assessed patient's knowledge about dressing. ____ ____ ____ _____

5. Assessed readiness and need for patient and family participation. ____ ____ ____ _____

6. Reviewed physician's orders. ____ ____ ____ _____

7. Identified patients at risk for wound healing problems. ____ ____ ____ _____

NURSING DIAGNOSIS

1. Developed appropriate nursing diagnoses based on assessment data. ____ ____ ____ _____

PLANNING

1. Identified expected outcomes. ____ ____ ____ _____

2. Explained procedure to patient. ____ ____ ____ _____

IMPLEMENTATION

1. Provided privacy. Performed hand hygiene. Applied PPE. ____ ____ ____ _____

2. Correctly verified patient's identity. ____ ____ ____ _____

3. Positioned patient comfortably. Exposed only wound. ____ ____ ____ _____

4. Properly placed disposable bag. Put on clean gloves. ____ ____ ____ _____

5. Removed tape, observed skin integrity. ____ ____ ____ _____

6. Removed present dressing carefully and assessed drainage on dressing. Disposed of dressing and gloves. ____ ____ ____ _____

7. Observed appearance of wound. ____ ____ ____ _____

8. Described to patient appearance of wound, if applicable. ____ ____ ____ _____

9. Prepared sterile field on over-bed table. ____ ____ ____ _____

10. Applied sterile gloves. ____ ____ ____ _____

	S	U	NP	Comments
11. Cleansed wound with single strokes from least contaminated to most contaminated area.	___	___	___	_____
12. Gently blotted wound dry.	___	___	___	_____
13. Applied antiseptic ointment if ordered.	___	___	___	_____
14. Applied dressing to incision or wound:				
a. Dry dressing:				
(1) Applied sterile gloves.	___	___	___	_____
(2) Applied loose woven gauze as contact layer.	___	___	___	_____
(3) Used a precut or drain sponge around drain.	___	___	___	_____
(4) Applied additional layers of gauze as needed.	___	___	___	_____
(5) Applied thicker woven pad if needed.	___	___	___	_____
b. Moist-to-dry dressing:				
(1) Applied sterile gloves.	___	___	___	_____
(2) Placed fine-mesh gauze in container of sterile solution or poured solution directly over gauze if container was not available. Squeezed out excess solution.	___	___	___	_____
(3) Applied moist, fluffed, woven-mesh gauze or packing strip in a single layer directly onto wound surface. Gently packed deep wound using forceps. Did not have gauze touch the surrounding (periwound) skin.	___	___	___	_____
(4) Made sure dead spaces (undermining, tunneling) were loosely packed with gauze.	___	___	___	_____
(5) Applied dry sterile gauze over wet gauze.	___	___	___	_____
(6) Covered packed wound with secondary dressing.	___	___	___	_____
15. Secured dressing appropriately.	___	___	___	_____
16. Disposed of all supplies. Removed and disposed of PPE.	___	___	___	_____
17. Wrote date, time of dressing change on tape and initialed.	___	___	___	_____
18. Positioned patient comfortably.	___	___	___	_____
19. Performed hand hygiene.	___	___	___	_____

	S	U	NP	Comments

EVALUATION

1. Assessed appearance of wound for healing progress.

2. Asked patient to rate pain.

3. Inspected condition of dressing at least once every shift.

4. Asked patient to describe steps and techniques of dressing change.

5. Identified unexpected outcomes.

RECORDING AND REPORTING

1. Recorded dressing change and wound assessment.

2. Reported unexpected outcomes to nurse in charge or physician.

Student _____ Date _____

Instructor _____ Date _____

PERFORMANCE CHECKLIST SKILL 39-2   **APPLYING A PRESSURE BANDAGE**

	S	U	NP	Comments
ASSESSMENT				
1. Identified patient's risk for unexpected bleeding.	___	___	___	_____
Phase I: Immediate Action—First Nurse				
1. Identified patient with sudden hemorrhage, and applied direct pressure to site.	___	___	___	_____
2. Called for assistance.	___	___	___	_____
Phase II: Applied Pressure Bandage—Second Nurse				
1. Quickly observed bleeding site and size.	___	___	___	_____
2. Observed area underneath patient for blood.	___	___	___	_____
3. Rapidly assessed vital signs and patient appearance.	___	___	___	_____
NURSING DIAGNOSIS				
1. Developed appropriate nursing diagnoses based on assessment data.	___	___	___	_____
PLANNING				
1. Identified expected outcomes.	___	___	___	_____
IMPLEMENTATION				
1. Applied gloves. Performed hand hygiene and provided privacy as patient's condition permitted.	___	___	___	_____
2. Pressed on site of bleeding (first person). Unwrapped roller bandage (second person).	___	___	___	_____
3. Cut lengths of tape (second person).	___	___	___	_____
4. Applied bandage quickly and correctly; maintained pressure, and secured with tape.	___	___	___	_____
5. Frequently checked circulation and patient's mental status.	___	___	___	_____
6. Removed gloves and performed hand hygiene.	___	___	___	_____
EVALUATION				
1. Immediately assessed patient's response to treatment.	___	___	___	_____
2. Identified unexpected outcomes.	___	___	___	_____

	S	U	NP	Comments

RECORDING AND REPORTING

1. Immediately evaluated and reported patient's status to physician. ___ ___ ___ _____

2. Recorded and implemented physician's orders, outcome, and patient status. ___ ___ ___ _____

Student _____ Date _____

Instructor _____ Date _____

PERFORMANCE CHECKLIST SKILL 39-3 **APPLYING A TRANSPARENT DRESSING**

	S	U	NP	Comments

ASSESSMENT

1. Assessed location and size of wound.

2. Reviewed health care provider's orders.

3. Assessed patient's level of comfort (1 to 10 scale, PQRST).

4. Assessed patient's knowledge of purpose of dressing.

5. Assessed patient's risk for wound healing problems.

NURSING DIAGNOSIS

1. Developed appropriate nursing diagnoses based on assessment data.

PLANNING

1. Identified expected outcomes.

2. Explained procedure to patient.

3. Positioned patient appropriately.

IMPLEMENTATION

1. Provided privacy, and exposed wound site only.

2. Correctly verified patient's identity.

3. Prepared supplies. Placed waterproof bag properly.

4. Performed hand hygiene and put on PPE.

5. Carefully removed old dressing, assessed drainage on dressing.

6. Properly disposed of soiled dressing, and removed and disposed of gloves. Performed hand hygiene.

7. Prepared dressing supplies.

8. Poured solution over 4 × 4s.

9. Applied clean or sterile gloves based on agency policy.

10. Cleansed wound area from least contaminated to most contaminated surface.

	S	U	NP	Comments

11. Patted dry and thoroughly inspected wound and periwound area.   —— —— —— _____

12. Applied transparent dressing per manufacturer's directions. Labeled dressing.   —— —— —— _____

13. Disposed of soiled supplies. Removed and disposed of PPE. Performed hand hygiene.   —— —— —— _____

14. Positioned patient comfortably.   —— —— —— _____

EVALUATION

1. Inspected appearance of wound and periwound area.   —— —— —— _____

2. Evaluated patient for pain.   —— —— —— _____

3. Identified unexpected outcomes.   —— —— —— _____

RECORDING AND REPORTING

1. Reported unexpected outcomes.   —— —— —— _____

2. Documented wound assessment and type of dressing selected.   —— —— —— _____

Student _____ Date _____

Instructor _____ Date _____

PERFORMANCE CHECKLIST SKILL 39-4 **APPLYING HYDROCOLLOID, HYDROGEL, FOAM, OR ABSORPTION DRESSINGS**

	S	U	NP	Comments
ASSESSMENT				
1. Assessed location and size of wound.	___	___	___	_____
2. Determined type of dressing to be used.	___	___	___	_____
3. Reviewed health care provider's orders.	___	___	___	_____
4. Assessed patient's comfort level (0 to 10 scale). Administered analgesic as needed.	___	___	___	_____
5. Assessed patient's knowledge of purpose of dressing.	___	___	___	_____
NURSING DIAGNOSIS				
1. Developed appropriate nursing diagnoses based on assessment data.	___	___	___	_____
PLANNING				
1. Identified expected outcomes.	___	___	___	_____
2. Explained procedure to patient.	___	___	___	_____
3. Positioned patient properly.	___	___	___	_____
IMPLEMENTATION				
1. Provided privacy. Verified patient's identity.	___	___	___	_____
2. Positioned patient comfortably. Exposed wound and draped patient.	___	___	___	_____
3. Placed cuffed disposable waterproof bag within reach.	___	___	___	_____
4. Performed hand hygiene and applied PPE.	___	___	___	_____
5. Gently removed old dressing.	___	___	___	_____
6. Disposed of soiled dressing and gloves in waterproof bag. Performed hand hygiene.	___	___	___	_____
7. Prepared sterile dressing supplies.	___	___	___	_____
8. Poured saline or prescribed solution over 4 × 4 sterile gauze dressings, or opened spray wound cleanser and applied to gauze.	___	___	___	_____
9. Applied clean or sterile gloves per agency policy.	___	___	___	_____
10. Gently cleansed area with moist 4 × 4s; swabbed exudate away from wound.	___	___	___	_____
11. Thoroughly dried area.	___	___	___	_____

	S	U	NP	Comments

12. Carefully inspected wound and periwound area.

13. Applied dressing according to manufacturer's directions. Labeled dressing.

   a. Hydrocolloid dressings

     (1) Applied hydrocolloid wafer over wound. Held in place for 30 to 60 seconds.

     (2) Applied a secondary dressing or secured hydrocolloid wafer with hypoallergenic tape around the edges.

   b. Foam dressings

     (1) Followed manufacturer's instructions for removal and application techniques.

     (2) Contoured dressing to extend 2.5 cm (1 inch) over periwound skin. Placed with proper surface to wound.

     (3) Applied secondary dressing per manufacturer's instructions.

   c. Absorption or alginate dressings

     (1) Loosely filled wound cavity one-half to two-thirds full, allowing for expansion.

     (2) Applied a secondary dressing.

14. Discarded soiled materials. Removed gloves properly. Removed PPE. Performed hand hygiene.

15. Assisted patient to comfortable position.

EVALUATION

1. Inspected condition of wound and characteristics of wound drainage.

2. Evaluated patient's comfort level.

3. Asked patient to describe wound care.

4. Identified unexpected outcomes.

RECORDING AND REPORTING

1. Reported and recorded unusual observations.

2. Recorded characteristics of wound and drainage.

3. Recorded and reported patient's tolerance to treatment.

432

Student _____ Date _____

Instructor _____ Date _____

PERFORMANCE CHECKLIST SKILL 39-5 **NEGATIVE PRESSURE WOUND THERAPY**

	S	U	NP	Comments

ASSESSMENT

1. Assessed location, appearance, and size of wound. ___ ___ ___ _____

2. Reviewed health care provider's orders. ___ ___ ___ _____

3. Assessed patient's level of comfort (0 to 10 scale). ___ ___ ___ _____

4. Assessed patient's and family's knowledge of purpose of dressing. ___ ___ ___ _____

5. Reviewed medication and allergy history. Assessed for sensitivity to irrigation solution. ___ ___ ___ _____

NURSING DIAGNOSIS

1. Developed appropriate nursing diagnoses based on assessment data. ___ ___ ___ _____

PLANNING

1. Identified expected outcomes. ___ ___ ___ _____

2. Explained procedure to patient. ___ ___ ___ _____

3. Positioned patient to allow access to dressing site. ___ ___ ___ _____

4. System set to "de-Vac" mode over a 45-minute period. ___ ___ ___ _____

5. Administered analgesic 30 minutes before dressing change if needed. ___ ___ ___ _____

IMPLEMENTATION

1. Provided privacy. Verified patient's identity. ___ ___ ___ _____

2. Positioned patient comfortably. Exposed wound site and draped patient. ___ ___ ___ _____

3. Properly cuffed and placed waterproof disposable bag. ___ ___ ___ _____

4. Performed hand hygiene and put on PPE. ___ ___ ___ _____

5. Pushed therapy on/off button on NPWT.

   a. Raised tubing connectors above the level of NPWT unit, and disconnected tubes to drain fluids into canister. ___ ___ ___ _____

   b. Tightened clamp on canister tube before lowering. ___ ___ ___ _____

	S	U	NP	Comments

6. Gently stretched transparent film horizontally and pulled up from skin.

7. Removed old NPWT dressing and observed appearance and drainage. Disposed of soiled dressings in waterproof bag. Removed and disposed of gloves. Performed hand hygiene.

8. Applied sterile or clean gloves per agency policy. Irrigated wound with normal saline or prescribed solution. Blotted dry.

9. Measured wound as ordered.

10. Applied skin protectant to periwound skin as ordered.

11. Removed and discarded gloves. Performed hand hygiene.

12. Applied sterile or new clean gloves per agency policy.

13. Selected appropriate foam dressing. Used sterile scissors to cut foam to exact wound size.

14. Gently placed foam in wound, covering entire wound base, margins, and tunneled areas.

15. Applied NPWT transparent dressing, covering foam and 3 to 5 cm of surrounding tissue. Removed all wrinkles from dressing. Secured tubing to transparent film to make an occlusive seal. Did not apply tension to drape and tubing.

16. Secured tubing several centimeters away from dressing.

17. Connected tubing from dressing to tubing from the canister and NPWT unit.

   a. Removed canister from sterile package and pushed into NPWT unit until click heard.

   b. Connected dressing tubing to the canister tubing, making sure that both clamps were open.

   c. Placed NPWT unit on level surface or hanging from foot of bed.

   d. Pressed in green-lit power button, and set pressure as ordered.

18. V.A.C. Instill option

   a. Verified the medication solution against prescriber's orders.

   b. Followed steps 1 through 15 (above).

434

	S	U	NP	Comments

   c. Placed the V.A.C. Instill pad at the highest point of the wound and the vacuum at the lowest, most dependent point of the wound.

   d. Connected the tubing from the vacuum pad to the V.A.C. Instill unit. Connected the tubing with the Luer-Lok to the irrigation solution bag. Labeled tubing.

   e. Using the touch screen on the V.A.C. Instill system, properly selected the therapy function and programmed as ordered.

   f. Checked all connections and lines and turned on the switch.

   g. Assessed, measured, and documented the solution instilled and drained during treatment. Emptied canister as needed.

19. Discarded soiled dressing materials. Performed hand hygiene.

20. Inspected NPWT system to verify negative pressure achieved.

   a. Verified display screen reading "Therapy On."

   b. Ensured clamps open and tubing patent.

   c. Identified air leaks with stethoscope or by moving hands around wound edges.

   d. Used strips of transparent film to patch areas around wound where leaks present.

   e. Labeled dressing.

21. Assisted patient to comfortable position. Patient may ambulate with a NPWT.

22. Removed and discarded gloves. Performed hand hygiene.

EVALUATION

1. Inspected condition of wound, drainage, and odor.

2. Evaluated patient's level of comfort.

3. Verified airtight dressing seal and correct negative pressure setting. Assessed dressing.

4. Monitored fluid balance and wound drainage.

5. Observed patient's or family member's ability to perform dressing change.

6. Identified unexpected outcomes.

	S	U	NP	Comments

RECORDING AND REPORTING

1. Reported and recorded unexpected outcomes, such as signs of infection, bleeding, or poor wound healing.   ___ ___ ___ _____

2. Recorded characteristics of wound and drainage, and presence of NPWT system.   ___ ___ ___ _____

3. Reported to oncoming shift nurses pertinent wound treatment, patient tolerance, and patient status.   ___ ___ ___ _____

Student _____ Date _____

Instructor _____ Date _____

PERFORMANCE CHECKLIST SKILL 39-6 **APPLYING GAUZE AND ELASTIC BANDAGES**

	S	U	NP	Comments

ASSESSMENT

1. Reviewed patient's medical records for specific orders related to required bandages. ___ ___ ___ _____

2. Applied clean gloves, if needed. Inspected skin in area to be bandaged. ___ ___ ___ _____

3. Inspected condition of any wound. ___ ___ ___ _____

4. Assessed circulation, edema, sensation, and movement of body part to be bandaged. ___ ___ ___ _____

5. Assessed for size and type of bandage. ___ ___ ___ _____

6. Assessed patient's and family's knowledge and ability related to application of bandages. ___ ___ ___ _____

NURSING DIAGNOSIS

1. Developed appropriate nursing diagnosis based on assessment data. ___ ___ ___ _____

PLANNING

1. Identified expected outcomes. ___ ___ ___ _____

2. Explained procedure to patient. ___ ___ ___ _____

3. Prepared to teach procedure to patient or family to guarantee continuation of care at home. ___ ___ ___ _____

IMPLEMENTATION

1. Provided for privacy. ___ ___ ___ _____

2. Assisted patient to a comfortable position. ___ ___ ___ _____

3. Performed hand hygiene and applied clean gloves, if needed. ___ ___ ___ _____

4. Applied gauze or elastic bandage as ordered.

  a. For gauze bandage:

   (1) Held roll of bandage in dominant hand and used other hand to hold beginning layer of bandage at distal body part. Wrapped twice to anchor. ___ ___ ___ _____

   (2) Applied bandage from distal point to proximal boundary using a variety of turns to cover shapes of body parts. ___ ___ ___ _____

   (3) Stretched bandage slightly while unrolling to improve venous circulation by compression. ___ ___ ___ _____

	S	U	NP	Comments

(4) Overlapped turns by one third to one half. Secured with clip or tape, before adding additional rolls if needed. ___ ___ ___ _____

(5) Applied additional rolls as needed, until skin surface covered. Secured end with clip. ___ ___ ___ _____

b. Applied elastic bandage for simple intermittent compression:

(1) Positioned patient in bed with leg elevated. ___ ___ ___ _____

(2) Held roll of bandage in dominant hand and used other hand to hold beginning layer at distal body part. Rolled bandage around body part. ___ ___ ___ _____

(3) Applied elastic conformable bandage using a figure-eight turn pattern. Applied from distal to most proximal boundary. ___ ___ ___ _____

(4) Stretched bandage slightly while applying to provide compression. Applied one layer of bandage. ___ ___ ___ _____

(5) Secured end with clip or tape. ___ ___ ___ _____

5. Removed gloves, if worn, and performed hand hygiene. ___ ___ ___ _____

6. Removed and reapplied elastic bandage once every 8 hours, or as directed by physician. ___ ___ ___ _____

7. Identified unexpected outcomes. ___ ___ ___ _____

EVALUATION

1. Evaluated distal circulation upon completion of application and at least twice per 8-hour period. ___ ___ ___ _____

2. Evaluated bandage for comfort, looseness, and drainage. ___ ___ ___ _____

3. Observed patient or family member demonstrating bandage application. ___ ___ ___ _____

RECORDING AND REPORTING

1. Recorded assessment of wound or skin, integrity of dressing, and patient status. ___ ___ ___ _____

2. Reported to nurse in charge or physician any changes in neurological or circulatory status. ___ ___ ___ _____

Student _____ Date _____

Instructor _____ Date _____

PERFORMANCE CHECKLIST SKILL 39-7 **APPLYING AN ABDOMINAL AND BREAST BINDER**

	S	U	NP	Comments

ASSESSMENT

1. Observed patient's need for support of thorax or abdomen. ___ ___ ___ _____

2. Reviewed medical record for order for binder. ___ ___ ___ _____

3. Inspected skin integrity in area where binder would be placed. ___ ___ ___ _____

4. Inspected surgical dressing, if present, for intactness. Changed soiled dressing as needed. ___ ___ ___ _____

5. Assessed patient's comfort level using scale of 0 to 10. Administered prescribed analgesic 30 minutes before dressing change. ___ ___ ___ _____

6. Gathered data on required size of binder appropriate to patient. ___ ___ ___ _____

7. Assessed patient's understanding of use of binder. ___ ___ ___ _____

NURSING DIAGNOSIS

1. Developed appropriate nursing diagnosis based on assessment data. ___ ___ ___ _____

PLANNING

1. Identified expected outcomes. ___ ___ ___ _____

2. Explained procedure to patient. ___ ___ ___ _____

3. Prepared to teach skill to patient or family member. ___ ___ ___ _____

IMPLEMENTATION

1. Provided privacy. ___ ___ ___ _____

2. Performed hand hygiene and applied clean gloves, if needed. ___ ___ ___ _____

3. Applied abdominal binder:

   a. Positioned patient in supine position with knees slightly flexed. ___ ___ ___ _____

   b. Assisted patient to roll on side, firmly supported by incision and dressing. ___ ___ ___ _____

   c. Placed binder on bed, fan-folded far side to middle of binder. ___ ___ ___ _____

	S	U	NP	Comments

d. Placed fan-folded ends under patient. Assisted patient in rolling over folded binder.

e. Unfolded and stretched ends out smoothly on both sides. Assisted patient to roll back to supine position.

f. Adjusted binder appropriately. Padded iliac prominences as needed.

g. Closed binder and secured.

h. Assessed patient's comfort and adjusted as needed.

4. Applied breast binder:

   a. Assisted patient to sitting position and placed arms through binder's armholes.

   b. Assisted patient to supine position as needed.

   c. Padded area under breasts as needed.

   d. Secured binder.

   e. Adjusted shoulder straps and waist darts to improve fit as needed.

   f. Assessed patient's comfort level, readjusted as needed.

5. Removed gloves and performed hand hygiene.

EVALUATION

1. Asked patient to rate pain on scale of 0 to 10.

2. Removed binder and dressings to assess skin and wound every 8 hours.

3. Evaluated patient's ability to breathe every 4 hours.

4. Evaluated patient's need for assistance in performing ADLs.

5. Identified unexpected outcomes.

RECORDING AND REPORTING

1. Recorded type and application of binder, skin assessment, circulatory status, and patient comfort level.

2. Reported any complications to nurse in charge.

3. Immediately reported any reduced lung expansion to health care provider.

440

Student _____   Date _____

Instructor _____   Date _____

PERFORMANCE CHECKLIST SKILL 40-1 **APPLICATION OF MOIST HEAT (COMPRESS AND SITZ BATH)**

	S	U	NP	Comments
ASSESSMENT				
1. Checked physician's orders for moist heat application. Reviewed institutional policies.	___	___	___	_____
2. Assessed condition of skin and/or wound before treatment and patient's level of sensation.	___	___	___	_____
3. Checked medical record for contraindications to therapy.	___	___	___	_____
4. Established baseline blood pressure and pulse.	___	___	___	_____
5. Assessed patient's mobility status and ability to position self.	___	___	___	_____
6. Assessed patient's level of comfort (scale 0 to 10, PQRST).	___	___	___	_____
7. Assessed patient's understanding of treatment.	___	___	___	_____
NURSING DIAGNOSIS				
1. Developed appropriate nursing diagnoses based on assessment data.	___	___	___	_____
PLANNING				
1. Identified expected outcomes.	___	___	___	_____
2. Prepared necessary equipment and supplies.	___	___	___	_____
3. Explained to patient procedure and expected types of sensations.	___	___	___	_____
IMPLEMENTATION				
1. Provided privacy.	___	___	___	_____
2. Performed hand hygiene.	___	___	___	_____
3. *Moist Sterile Compress*				
a. Assisted patient to a comfortable position and placed waterproof pad under area to be treated.	___	___	___	_____
b. Exposed body part to be covered with compress and draped patient.	___	___	___	_____
c. Applied clean gloves and removed existing dressing. Disposed of gloves and dressings in appropriate container.	___	___	___	_____
d. Assessed condition of wound and surrounding skin.	___	___	___	_____

	S	U	NP	Comments

e. Performed hand hygiene. ___ ___ ___ _____

f. Prepared compress:

   (1) Poured solution into sterile container. Warmed solution, if portable heating source available. ___ ___ ___ _____

   (2) Used sterile technique to drop gauze compress into solution. ___ ___ ___ _____

g. Prepared aquathermia pad or commercial heat pack according to manufacturer's instructions. ___ ___ ___ _____

h. Applied sterile or clean gloves, as appropriate. ___ ___ ___ _____

i. Picked up one layer of immersed gauze, removed excess moisture; applied gauze lightly to affected area only, avoiding surrounding skin. ___ ___ ___ _____

j. After a few seconds, lifted edge of gauze and assessed for redness. ___ ___ ___ _____

k. Packed wound snugly and completely, if tolerated by patient. ___ ___ ___ _____

l. Covered moist compress with dry sterile dressing and bath towel. Removed gloves. ___ ___ ___ _____

m. Applied aquathermia or waterproof heating pad over towel (optional). Kept in place for duration of application. ___ ___ ___ _____

n. Changed compress every 5 to 10 minutes, or as ordered by sterile technique, if aquathermia pad not used. ___ ___ ___ _____

o. Applied gloves after prescribed time. Removed pad, towel, and compress; assessed wound and skin; and replaced dry sterile dressing as ordered. ___ ___ ___ _____

p. Assisted patient to a comfortable position. ___ ___ ___ _____

q. Disposed of soiled compress, dressings, and supplies; performed hand hygiene. ___ ___ ___ _____

4. *Sitz Bath or Soak to Intact Open Skin*

   a. Applied clean gloves. Removed any existing dressing. Disposed of gloves and dressings. ___ ___ ___ _____

   b. Assessed condition of wound and skin. ___ ___ ___ _____

   c. Filled basin or tub with warmed solution. Checked temperature. ___ ___ ___ _____

   d. Assisted patient to immerse body part in tub or basin. ___ ___ ___ _____

   e. Assessed heart rate and assessed for lightheadedness. ___ ___ ___ _____

442

	S	U	NP	Comments

f. Covered patient with bath blanket or towel.

g. Maintained constant temperature throughout 15- to 20-minute soak.

   (1) Kept large sheet or blanket over container or basin.

   (2) Removed body part from soak and checked for burning sensation after 10 minutes. Emptied cooled solution, added new heated solution, and reimmersed body part.

h. Removed patient from soak or bath after 15 to 20 minutes. Thoroughly dried body parts. Used clean gloves if drainage present. Assessed body part.

i. Drained solution from basin or tub. Cleaned and stored reusable supplies. Disposed of contaminated linen and gloves. Performed hand hygiene.

EVALUATION

1. Inspected condition of skin and wound as treated.

2. Asked patient if burning sensation was felt.

3. Assessed vital signs and circulatory status.

4. Had patient explain and demonstrate application of heat.

5. Identified unexpected outcomes.

RECORDING AND REPORTING

1. Recorded type, location, and duration of procedure and name of person treating the area.

2. Recorded condition of wound and skin before and after treatment, and patient's response.

3. Recorded preprocedure and postprocedure vital signs and circulatory status.

4. Recorded instruction given and patient's ability to return verbalize/demonstrate.

5. Reported unusual findings to nurse in charge or physician.

Student _____ Date _____

Instructor _____ Date _____

PERFORMANCE CHECKLIST SKILL 40-2 **APPLYING AQUATHERMIA AND HEATING PADS**

	S	U	NP	Comments

ASSESSMENT

1. Reviewed physician's order for heat therapy and institutional policy for temperature recommendations. ___ ___ ___ _____

2. Assessed condition of patient's skin at site of heat application. ___ ___ ___ _____

3. Assessed and documented level of discomfort (scale 0 to 10, PQRST) and range of motion if applicable. ___ ___ ___ _____

4. Assessed skin for sensitivity to temperature, touch, and pain. ___ ___ ___ _____

5. Checked condition of electrical cords for safety hazards. ___ ___ ___ _____

6. Assessed patient's and family's knowledge of procedure. ___ ___ ___ _____

NURSING DIAGNOSIS

1. Developed appropriate nursing diagnoses based on assessment data. ___ ___ ___ _____

PLANNING

1. Identified expected outcomes. ___ ___ ___ _____

2. Prepared necessary equipment and supplies. ___ ___ ___ _____

3. Explained procedure and safety precautions to patient. ___ ___ ___ _____

IMPLEMENTATION

1. Provided privacy. ___ ___ ___ _____

2. Correctly identified patient. ___ ___ ___ _____

3. Performed hand hygiene. Positioned patient comfortably and exposed area to be treated. ___ ___ ___ _____

4. Protected patient's skin with towel or enclosed pad in a pillowcase. ___ ___ ___ _____

5. Placed pad over area to be treated; secured pad as needed. ___ ___ ___ _____

6. Checked temperature setting of pad. ___ ___ ___ _____

7. Monitored condition of skin and patient's response every 5 minutes. ___ ___ ___ _____

	S	U	NP	Comments
8. Removed pad after prescribed interval, usually after 20 to 30 minutes.	___	___	___	_____
9. Assisted patient to comfortable position, disposed of soiled linen, and performed hand hygiene.	___	___	___	_____

EVALUATION

	S	U	NP	Comments
1. Inspected condition of skin exposed to heat.	___	___	___	_____
2. Determined level of patient's discomfort (0 to 10 scale, PQRST).	___	___	___	_____
3. Noted patient's ability to move affected area (AROM).	___	___	___	_____
4. Observed patient's ability to apply pad correctly.	___	___	___	_____
5. Identified unexpected outcomes.	___	___	___	_____

RECORDING AND REPORTING

	S	U	NP	Comments
1. Recorded procedure and patient's response.	___	___	___	_____
2. Described instruction given and patient's ability to perform procedure.	___	___	___	_____
3. Reported unusual changes in condition of patient's skin to the nurse in charge.	___	___	___	_____

Student _____ Date _____

Instructor _____ Date _____

PERFORMANCE CHECKLIST SKILL 40-3 **APPLYING COLD APPLICATIONS**

	S	U	NP	Comments

ASSESSMENT

1. Reviewed physician's order and institutional policy on temperature settings. ___ ___ ___ _____

2. Assessed and documented condition of injured or affected part. ___ ___ ___ _____

3. Considered time at which injury occurred. ___ ___ ___ _____

4. Asked patient to describe pain, and documented character of pain (0 to 10 scale, PQRST). ___ ___ ___ _____

5. Assessed neurovascular status of affected area. ___ ___ ___ _____

6. Assessed patient's understanding of procedure. ___ ___ ___ _____

NURSING DIAGNOSIS

1. Developed appropriate nursing diagnoses based on assessment data. ___ ___ ___ _____

PLANNING

1. Identified expected outcomes. ___ ___ ___ _____

2. Prepared necessary equipment and supplies. ___ ___ ___ _____

3. Explained procedure and safety precautions to patient. ___ ___ ___ _____

IMPLEMENTATION

1. Provided privacy. ___ ___ ___ _____

2. Performed hand hygiene. ___ ___ ___ _____

3. Correctly identified patient. ___ ___ ___ _____

4. Positioned patient comfortably, with affected body part aligned properly and only the area to be treated exposed. ___ ___ ___ _____

5. Placed towel or pad under area to be treated. ___ ___ ___ _____

6. Applied clean gloves. ___ ___ ___ _____

7. Applied cold compress:

   a. Checked temperature of solution and submerged compress. Wrung out excess moisture. ___ ___ ___ _____

   b. Applied compress to affected area. ___ ___ ___ _____

8. Applied electronically controlled cooling device:

	S	U	NP	Comments

a. Wrapped cooling pad in towel or pillow-case. ___ ___ ___ _____

b. Wrapped enclosed cooling pad around affected part, set temperature, and secured in place. ___ ___ ___ _____

9. Applied ice bag or collar:

   a. Filled bag/collar with cool water, capped, and inverted. Emptied water. Filled bag/collar two-thirds full with ice chips. Pressed out air and secured cap. ___ ___ ___ _____

   b. Wrapped bag/collar with towel or pillowcase; applied and secured over affected area. ___ ___ ___ _____

10. Applied ice pack:

    a. Squeezed commercial cold pack to activate. ___ ___ ___ _____

    b. Covered pack with towel or pillowcase. Applied to affected area. ___ ___ ___ _____

11. Removed and disposed of gloves. ___ ___ ___ _____

12. Inspected condition of skin and neurovascular status every 5 minutes during application. ___ ___ ___ _____

13. Applied clean gloves; removed cooling application after 15 to 20 minutes (or as ordered), and dried area. ___ ___ ___ _____

14. Assisted patient to comfortable position. ___ ___ ___ _____

15. Emptied and stored basin, disposed of used linens and gloves, and performed hand hygiene. ___ ___ ___ _____

EVALUATION

1. Inspected condition of skin. ___ ___ ___ _____

2. Gently palpated affected area. ___ ___ ___ _____

3. Measured patient's level of comfort. ___ ___ ___ _____

4. Asked patient to demonstrate cold application and explain risks of treatment. ___ ___ ___ _____

5. Identified unexpected outcomes. ___ ___ ___ _____

RECORDING AND REPORTING

1. Recorded procedure and patient's response. ___ ___ ___ _____

2. Described instruction given and patient's ability to perform procedure. ___ ___ ___ _____

3. Reported undesirable skin changes to nurse in charge or physician. ___ ___ ___ _____

Student_____ Date_____

Instructor_____ Date_____

PERFORMANCE CHECKLIST SKILL 40-4 **CARING FOR PATIENTS REQUIRING HYPOTHERMIA OR HYPERTHERMIA BLANKETS**

	S	U	NP	Comments
ASSESSMENT				
1. Verified physician's orders, and rechecked patient's current body temperature.	___	___	___	_____
2. Assessed vital signs, neurovascular and mental status.	___	___	___	_____
3. Verified that less intensive measures were not effective in returning body temperature to normal.	___	___	___	_____
4. Assessed patient's skin on bony prominences and other susceptible areas before therapy.	___	___	___	_____
NURSING DIAGNOSIS				
1. Developed appropriate nursing diagnoses based on assessment data.	___	___	___	_____
PLANNING				
1. Identified expected outcomes.	___	___	___	_____
2. Explained procedure to patient.	___	___	___	_____
3. Positioned patient comfortably.	___	___	___	_____
4. Prepared blanket per agency policy and manufacturer's instructions.	___	___	___	_____
IMPLEMENTATION				
1. Performed hand hygiene and applied clean gloves.	___	___	___	_____
2. Correctly verified patient's identity.	___	___	___	_____
3. Obtained baseline vital signs.	___	___	___	_____
4. Applied lanolin/cold cream to patient's skin.	___	___	___	_____
5. Turned on blanket and set on desired temperature. Observed that the "cool" or "warm" light was on.	___	___	___	_____
6. Verified that pad temperature limits were set correctly.	___	___	___	_____
7. Placed sheet or thin blanket between the patient and the thermal blanket.	___	___	___	_____
8. Placed blanket on patient. Wrapped patient's hands, feet, and scrotum in towels or gauze before applying hypothermia blanket.	___	___	___	_____

	S	U	NP	Comments

9. Lubricated rectal probe and inserted into patient's rectum.

10. Repositioned patient regularly and checked linens for moisture.

11. Double-checked fluid thermometer on blanket control panel.

12. Removed gloves and performed hand hygiene.

EVALUATION

1. Monitored patient's temperature and vital signs at appropriate time intervals.

2. Verified accuracy of automatic temperature control device visually every 30 minutes, and by taking rectal temperature every 4 hours.

3. Observed the skin for injuries or changes.

4. Observed patient for signs of shivering.

5. Determined patient's level of comfort.

6. Identified unexpected outcomes.

RECORDING AND REPORTING

1. Recorded baseline data, time that therapy was initiated, temperature control setting, and patient's response to therapy.

2. Charted repeated readings for patient's temperature and vital signs.

3. Reported any unexpected outcomes to nurse in charge or physician.

450

Student _____ Date _____

Instructor _____ Date _____

PERFORMANCE CHECKLIST SKILL 41-1 **MODIFYING SAFETY RISKS IN THE HOME ENVIRONMENT**

	S	U	NP	Comments
ASSESSMENT				
1. Reviewed previous findings and/or conducted sensory and neuromuscular assessments.	___	___	___	_____
2. Determined patient's history of falls or other injuries in the home (SPLATT).	___	___	___	_____
3. Had patient with near or actual fall maintain a diary.	___	___	___	_____
4. Conducted a Timed Up & Go (TUG) test.	___	___	___	_____
5. Reviewed medical and medication history and increasing risk factors for accidents in the home.	___	___	___	_____
6. Determined if patient had fear of falling.	___	___	___	_____
7. Conducted a complete home safety assessment with patient and family: Front and back entrances, walkways, stairways, kitchen, bathroom, bedroom, living room, basement, around the house, fire and electrical safety.	___	___	___	_____
8. Assessed patient's financial resources. Determined need for social services referral.	___	___	___	_____
9. Assessed patient's and family's ability and willingness to make changes.	___	___	___	_____
10. Determined importance of independence to patient.	___	___	___	_____
NURSING DIAGNOSIS				
1. Developed appropriate nursing diagnoses based on assessment data.	___	___	___	_____
PLANNING				
1. Identified expected outcomes.	___	___	___	_____
2. Prioritized with patient and family the greatest personal and environmental risks to safety.	___	___	___	_____
3. Recommended calling a reliable contractor if major home repairs required.	___	___	___	_____
IMPLEMENTATION				
1. Took steps to reduce physical hazards that predispose to falls, focusing on space, lighting, and safety devices.	___	___	___	_____
2. Had patient use padding or clothing to cushion bony prominences.	___	___	___	_____

	S	U	NP	Comments
3. Made modifications to promote safe practice of activities of daily living.	——	——	——	———————
4. Instructed patient and family on infection control practices focusing on kitchen and bathroom.	——	——	——	———————
5. Took steps to eliminate fire hazards and injuries from burns.	——	——	——	———————
6. Took steps to prevent carbon monoxide exposure.	——	——	——	———————

EVALUATION

	S	U	NP	Comments
1. Had patient and family member(s) identify potential safety risks.	——	——	——	———————
2. Asked patient to discuss on subsequent visits plans for modifications and observed changes made.	——	——	——	———————
3. During follow-up visit or call, asked if patient experienced any injuries or falls.	——	——	——	———————
4. Reassessed for deterioration of mental status.	——	——	——	———————
5. Identified unexpected outcomes.	——	——	——	———————

RECORDING AND REPORTING

	S	U	NP	Comments
1. Retained copy of home safety assessment in patient's home health record.	——	——	——	———————
2. Recorded any instruction given, patient's response, and changes made in the home environment.	——	——	——	———————
3. Recorded any referrals made.	——	——	——	———————

Student _____   Date _____

Instructor _____   Date _____

PERFORMANCE CHECKLIST SKILL 41-2 **ADAPTING THE HOME SETTING FOR PATIENTS WITH COGNITIVE DEFICITS**

	S	U	NP	Comments
ASSESSMENT				
1. Conducted assessment during short session while maintaining sensitivity to patient's needs or disabilities.	___	___	___	_____
2. Met with patient and family in quiet, uninterrupted environment.	___	___	___	_____
3. Asked patient to describe level of health and its effects on ability to perform self-care tasks.	___	___	___	_____
4. Asked how patient is doing with home management.	___	___	___	_____
5. Assessed medications taken by patient, availability and storage of medications. Reviewed patient's medication list for current/updated orders.	___	___	___	_____
6. Determined if patient has family member or friend who assists with self-care or home management.	___	___	___	_____
7. Determined patient's resources and quality of support.	___	___	___	_____
8. Observed patient's appearance and behavior during discussion.	___	___	___	_____
9. Observed for signs and symptoms of abuse or neglect.	___	___	___	_____
10. Observed physical aspect of home environment.	___	___	___	_____
11. Completed a mini-mental examination if cognitive or mental status change is suspected (Folstein's examination for dementia, Short Geriatric Depression Scale-SGDS).	___	___	___	_____
12. Observed behaviors to determine if patient "wandering."	___	___	___	_____
13. Assessed current environmental strategies for dealing with wandering.	___	___	___	_____
14. Determined caregiver's needs for assistance.	___	___	___	_____
NURSING DIAGNOSIS				
1. Developed appropriate nursing diagnoses based on assessment data.	___	___	___	_____

	S	U	NP	Comments

PLANNING

1. Identified expected outcomes. ___ ___ ___ _____

2. Referred family to occupational therapy, home-maker services, and/or respite care if patient has difficulty with self-care skills. ___ ___ ___ _____

3. Recommended assistive devices as appropriate. ___ ___ ___ _____

4. Considered patient's level of cognitive impairment before implementing strategies. ___ ___ ___ _____

5. Determined best time of day for specific approaches. ___ ___ ___ _____

IMPLEMENTATION

1. Created and discussed methods to assist patient in remembering task performance and organizing activities. ___ ___ ___ _____

2. Found ways to consolidate and simplify tasks. ___ ___ ___ _____

3. Assisted patient and caregiver to determine a routine schedule for self-care activities and home management tasks. ___ ___ ___ _____

4. Assisted patient and caregiver to focus on patient's abilities rather than his or her disabilities. ___ ___ ___ _____

5. Had caregiver assist with setting up tasks that the patient can complete. ___ ___ ___ _____

6. Reviewed medication taken by patient and discussed with patient, caregiver, and physician/primary care provider options for scheduling multiple medications. ___ ___ ___ _____

7. Instructed caregiver about use of simple and direct communication. ___ ___ ___ _____

8. Kept clocks, calendars, and personal mementos throughout the house. ___ ___ ___ _____

9. Had caregiver routinely orient patient. ___ ___ ___ _____

10. Encouraged regular naps or rest periods throughout the day. ___ ___ ___ _____

11. Had caregiver encourage and support frequent short visits by family and significant others and encouraged participation in social activities as tolerated. ___ ___ ___ _____

12. Provided a safe place for person to wander. ___ ___ ___ _____

13. Provided signs or cues to guide patient to a desired location, such as the bathroom. ___ ___ ___ _____

14. Recommended that family of the wandering patient should install different kinds of locks or motion/light sensors at doorways. ___ ___ ___ _____

454

	S	U	NP	Comments

15. Assisted in creating a calm and safe environment with consideration for patient's abilities.

16. Monitored patient for personal comfort and needs.

17. Recommended installation of alarm at exit of residence.

EVALUATION

1. During follow-up visit, asked patient to review daily personal and home management activities.

2. Reviewed with patient and caregiver schedule for medication administration.

3. Had caregiver keep track of medication doses taken over a week and any adverse reactions.

4. Asked caregiver to show you and to describe approaches used to enhance patient's success in self-care and home management activities.

5. Had family caregivers report approaches taken to minimize episodes of wandering.

6. Identified unexpected outcomes.

RECORDING AND REPORTING

1. Recorded assessment of patient's cognitive and mental status, interventions, and patient's and caregiver's responses.

2. Reported to physician any changes in patient's behavior that reflect a possible decline in cognitive or mental status.

Student _____ Date _____

Instructor _____ Date _____

PERFORMANCE CHECKLIST SKILL 41-3 **MEDICATION AND MEDICAL DEVICE SAFETY**

	S	U	NP	Comments

ASSESSMENT

1. Assessed patient's sensory, musculoskeletal, and neurological function. ___ ___ ___ _____

2. Assessed ability of caregiver to assist the patient. ___ ___ ___ _____

3. Assessed medication schedule. ___ ___ ___ _____

4. Asked patient to identify where medications are kept in the home. Assessed safety and temperature of storage area. Looked at each container. ___ ___ ___ _____

5. Had patient describe daily schedule for drug administration and pertinent information related to medication. ___ ___ ___ _____

6. Asked patient to show you the area where self-injection supplies are stored and how supplies are disposed of, if applicable. ___ ___ ___ _____

7. Asked patient to identify where glucose monitor and supplies are stored and how lancets are disposed of, if applicable. ___ ___ ___ _____

8. Asked patient to identify where dressings are stored and how/where soiled dressings are disposed of, if applicable. ___ ___ ___ _____

NURSING DIAGNOSIS

1. Developed appropriate nursing diagnoses based on assessment data. ___ ___ ___ _____

PLANNING

1. Identified expected outcomes. ___ ___ ___ _____

IMPLEMENTATION

1. Instructed patient and caregiver about principles to follow to ensure that medications are safe to use. ___ ___ ___ _____

2. Recommended approaches to facilitate preparation of medications and hand hygiene practices:

   a. Well-lit and clean area for preparation. ___ ___ ___ _____

   b. Large labels and screw-on tops. For blind patients, use Braille labels on all medications. ___ ___ ___ _____

   c. Color-coded system. ___ ___ ___ _____

	S	U	NP	Comments

d. Syringes with larger numbers and spring-loaded injection aid. ___ ___ ___ _____

e. Wash hands before and after preparation. ___ ___ ___ _____

3. Recommended approaches to ensure that medications and supplies are safely and properly stored.

   a. Discussed safety issues if patient has children or grandchildren in the home. ___ ___ ___ _____

   b. Instructed patients and caregiver to store liquids or parenteral medications in cool area (away from food, in plastic storage bin). ___ ___ ___ _____

   c. Instructed patient and caregiver to use new needle with each medication administration. ___ ___ ___ _____

4. Reviewed with patient and caregiver proper techniques for disposal of sharps and other medical supplies.

   a. Provided instruction on disposal of unused drugs or outdated drugs in sink or toilet. ___ ___ ___ _____

   b. Provided instruction on disposal of all sharps in an approved sharps container or a small-neck plastic bottle with cover. ___ ___ ___ _____

   c. Cautioned against overfilling sharps container. ___ ___ ___ _____

   d. Instructed patient and caregiver to store in areas away or protected from children. ___ ___ ___ _____

   e. Instructed patient and caregiver to double-bag soiled dressings and supplies. ___ ___ ___ _____

   f. Instructed patient and caregiver to consult with local health department regarding proper disposal. ___ ___ ___ _____

EVALUATION

1. Had patient or caregiver describe steps to take to ensure that medications are safe to use. ___ ___ ___ _____

2. Observed patient preparing and administering a medication dose. ___ ___ ___ _____

3. Observed home setting for location of medications and supplies. ___ ___ ___ _____

4. Had patient describe disposal of sharps and other medical supplies. ___ ___ ___ _____

5. Performed pill counts at regular intervals. ___ ___ ___ _____

6. Identified unexpected outcomes. ___ ___ ___ _____

RECORDING AND REPORTING

1. Recorded recommendations provided to patient and caregiver and their responses. ___ ___ ___ _____

458

Student _____ Date _____

Instructor _____ Date _____

PERFORMANCE CHECKLIST SKILL 42-1 **TEACHING BODY TEMPERATURE MEASUREMENT**

	S	U	NP	Comments
ASSESSMENT				
1. Assessed patient's ability to hold and read thermometer.	___	___	___	_____
2. Assessed patient's knowledge about temperature ranges, risk for fever, and type of thermometer to use. Assessed for signs and symptoms of fever or hypothermia.	___	___	___	_____
3. Determined patient's knowledge of criteria for selecting appropriate type of thermometer.	___	___	___	_____
4. Assessed patient's previous knowledge and technique for measuring temperature. Had patient return demonstrate.	___	___	___	_____
NURSING DIAGNOSIS				
1. Developed appropriate nursing diagnoses based on assessment data.	___	___	___	_____
PLANNING				
1. Identified expected outcomes.	___	___	___	_____
2. Selected setting in home for patient to measure temperature.	___	___	___	_____
3. Instructed patient/caregiver about normal temperature ranges and proper positioning for checking temperature.	___	___	___	_____
IMPLEMENTATION				
1. Demonstrated steps for preparation, insertion, and reading of thermometer.	___	___	___	_____
2. Performed hand hygiene. Instructed patient to use only rectal thermometer for rectal temperature measurement. Lubricated tip and inserted into rectum carefully for recommended time.	___	___	___	_____
3. Guided patient each step of the way without rushing.	___	___	___	_____
4. Discussed when to take temperature and factors that influence results.	___	___	___	_____
5. Discussed common symptoms of fever.	___	___	___	_____
6. Discussed signs and symptoms of hypothermia.	___	___	___	_____
7. Discussed importance of notifying nurse/physician when fever develops and discussed methods for controlling fever.	___	___	___	_____
8. Instructed in proper storage of thermometer.	___	___	___	_____

	S	U	NP	Comments

	S	U	NP	Comments
9. Provided written guidelines for reference.	___	___	___	_____
10. Provided log book or paper to record times and temperature measurements.	___	___	___	_____

EVALUATION

1. Had patient measure body temperature and demonstrate ability to read thermometer and record measurements independently.	___	___	___	_____
2. Observed patient cleaning and storing equipment.	___	___	___	_____
3. Had patient discuss and identify normal temperature range and factors influencing temperature.	___	___	___	_____
4. Had patient describe signs and symptoms and management of fever and hypothermia.	___	___	___	_____
5. Observed patient record in log book. Checked log book periodically.	___	___	___	_____
6. Identified unexpected outcomes.	___	___	___	_____

RECORDING AND REPORTING

1. Recorded information taught and patient's response.	___	___	___	_____
2. Recorded temperature in patient log and home care record.	___	___	___	_____

Student _____ Date _____

Instructor _____ Date _____

PERFORMANCE CHECKLIST SKILL 42-2 **TEACHING BLOOD PRESSURE AND PULSE MEASUREMENT**

	S	U	NP	Comments

ASSESSMENT

1. Assessed patient's visual and motor ability to manipulate equipment and determine reading. ___ ___ ___ _____

2. Assessed patient's knowledge of normal blood pressure (BP) and pulse ranges and symptoms and common causes of high or low readings. ___ ___ ___ _____

3. Assessed patient's knowledge of the significance of the BP/pulse measurement and its variations. ___ ___ ___ _____

4. Assessed patient's knowledge and asked for demonstration of technique if patient had previous experience. ___ ___ ___ _____

5. Determined best place in the house for BP/pulse measurement. ___ ___ ___ _____

NURSING DIAGNOSIS

1. Developed appropriate nursing diagnoses based on assessment data. ___ ___ ___ _____

PLANNING

1. Identified expected outcomes. ___ ___ ___ _____

2. Encouraged patient to perform BP/pulse measurements on a regular schedule, and log results. ___ ___ ___ _____

3. Encouraged patient to avoid activities or factors that increase BP/pulse before measurement. ___ ___ ___ _____

4. Had patient perform measurement in a comfortable position and environment. ___ ___ ___ _____

5. Explained procedure to patient and had patient rest 5 minutes before measurement. ___ ___ ___ _____

6. Had patient describe symptoms that would indicate the need to measure BP and pulse. ___ ___ ___ _____

IMPLEMENTATION

1. Blood pressure measurement:

   a. Discussed with patient the most appropriate sites for BP measurements. ___ ___ ___ _____

   b. Discussed reasons to avoid particular site. ___ ___ ___ _____

   c. Demonstrated steps for BP measurement for manual and electronic blood pressure measuring devices. ___ ___ ___ _____

	S	U	NP	Comments

2. Pulse measurements:

   a. Discussed with patient or caregiver how to assess a radial and carotid pulse.

   b. Demonstrated technique of palpating pulses and locating landmarks with caution not to press hard over pulse site.

   c. Instructed to use a watch/clock with a second hand and check pulse for 60 seconds.

3. Discussed with patient or caregiver normal desired BP and pulse ranges, the purpose for monitoring, when to check, and when to report to physician.

4. Had patient perform skill on nurse or caregiver and on self.

5. Instructed to continue monitoring, although BP and pulse may be within normal range.

6. Provided with appropriate written and/or pictorial instructions for reference and a log book.

7. Instructed and demonstrated to patient how to care for equipment.

EVALUATION

1. Observed patient demonstrating technique for BP/pulse measurement on at least three different occasions.

2. Asked patient if BP/pulse readings were within normal range and when should findings be reported to physician.

3. Asked patient to describe the rationale for BP/pulse monitoring and related medications.

4. Had patient demonstrate care of equipment.

5. Identified unexpected outcomes.

RECORDING AND REPORTING

1. Recorded teaching and patient responses in home care record.

2. Recorded BP/pulse in home care record and patient's documentation system.

3. Reported abnormal readings and related symptoms to health care provider and/or physician.

Student _____ Date _____

Instructor _____ Date _____

PERFORMANCE CHECKLIST SKILL 42-3 **TEACHING INTERMITTENT SELF-CATHETERIZATION**

	S	U	NP	Comments
ASSESSMENT				
1. Reviewed patient's medical history for genitourinary alterations, existing medical and surgical history, and daily fluid intake and voiding pattern.	___	___	___	_____
2. Assessed patient's level of consciousness, sensory and cognitive.	___	___	___	_____
3. Assessed patient's or caregiver's knowledge and understanding about procedure.	___	___	___	_____
NURSING DIAGNOSIS				
1. Developed appropriate nursing diagnosis based on assessment data.	___	___	___	_____
PLANNING				
1. Identified expected outcomes.	___	___	___	_____
2. Selected appropriate home setting to perform CIC.	___	___	___	_____
3. Helped patient or caregiver select a catheter of appropriate size and equipment needed.	___	___	___	_____
IMPLEMENTATION				
1. Discussed infection control and proper hand hygiene.	___	___	___	_____
2. Assisted to a comfortable position in a well-lit room.	___	___	___	_____
3. Discussed technique to clean urethral meatus:				
a. Female patient:				
(1) Spread labia and performed perineal care.	___	___	___	_____
(2) Found a comfortable position. Used mirror to help find meatus for catheterization.	___	___	___	_____
b. Male patient:				
(1) Retracted foreskin if not circumcised.	___	___	___	_____
(2) Held penis perpendicular to body and cleansed urethral opening.	___	___	___	_____
4. Instructed patient on catheter insertion:				
a. For female: Insert catheter 5 to 10 cm (2 to 4 inches) into meatus until urine begins to flow.	___	___	___	_____

	S	U	NP	Comments

b. For male:

   (1) Lubricate tip of catheter 13 to 18 cm (5 to 7 inches). _____ _____ _____ _____

   (2) Insert lubricated tip into the meatus 15 to 20 cm (6 to 8 inches) until urine began to flow. _____ _____ _____ _____

5. Instructed to hold catheter in place while urine flows into container/toilet. _____ _____ _____ _____

6. Removed slowly and gently when urine flow stopped and performed hand hygiene. _____ _____ _____ _____

7. Assisted patient in recording characteristics of urine. _____ _____ _____ _____

8. Instructed patient to clean catheter with warm, soapy water, rinse thoroughly, and store in wrapped towel or brown paper bag. _____ _____ _____ _____

9. Discussed appropriate replacement and disposal of used supplies. _____ _____ _____ _____

EVALUATION

1. Observed patient independently demonstrating CIC. _____ _____ _____ _____

2. Had patient identify catheterization schedule, technique, and whom to call when problems arise. _____ _____ _____ _____

3. Reviewed patient's log book periodically. _____ _____ _____ _____

RECORDING AND REPORTING

1. Recorded in home care record information taught and patient's response. _____ _____ _____ _____

2. Recorded urinary output. _____ _____ _____ _____

Student _____ Date _____

Instructor _____ Date _____

PERFORMANCE CHECKLIST SKILL 42-4 **USING HOME OXYGEN EQUIPMENT**

	S	U	NP	Comments
ASSESSMENT				
1. Determined patient's or caregiver's ability to use oxygen equipment correctly while still in the hospital. Reassessed for appropriate use in the home.	___	___	___	_____
2. Assessed patient's home environment for adequate electrical power for oxygen concentrator.	___	___	___	_____
3. Assessed patient's or caregiver's knowledge of oxygen therapy and ability to recognize signs and symptoms of hypoxia.	___	___	___	_____
4. Determined readily available resource for assistance with home oxygen systems.	___	___	___	_____
5. Determined backup system in the event of power failure. A spare oxygen tank will be available in the home. EMS will be notified, if needed.	___	___	___	_____
NURSING DIAGNOSIS				
1. Developed appropriate nursing diagnoses based on assessment data.	___	___	___	_____
PLANNING				
1. Identified expected outcomes.	___	___	___	_____
2. Selected setting in home where patient is more likely to use oxygen.	___	___	___	_____
IMPLEMENTATION				
1. Performed hand hygiene.	___	___	___	_____
2. Placed oxygen delivery system in safe place in the home. Discussed safety measures and proper storage.	___	___	___	_____
3. Demonstrated steps for preparation and completion of oxygen therapy.				
a. Compressed oxygen system:				
(1) Turned cylinder valve counterclockwise two to three turns with wrench.	___	___	___	_____
(2) Checked cylinders by reading amount on pressure gauge.	___	___	___	_____
(3) Stored wrench with oxygen tank or in other safe place.	___	___	___	_____
b. Oxygen concentrator system:				

	S	U	NP	Comments
(1) Plugged concentrator into appropriate outlet.	___	___	___	_____
(2) Turned on power switch. Alarm sounds momentarily until it reaches proper pressure.	___	___	___	_____

c. Liquid oxygen system:

	S	U	NP	Comments
(1) Checked liquid system by depressing button and reading dial on stationary reservoir or ambulatory tank.	___	___	___	_____
(2) Collaborated with equipment provider on instruction for refilling ambulatory tank.	___	___	___	_____
4. Connected oxygen delivery device (nasal cannula/mask) to oxygen delivery system.	___	___	___	_____
5. Adjusted liter flow and placed on patient.	___	___	___	_____
6. Performed hand hygiene.	___	___	___	_____
7. Instructed patient or caregiver not to change oxygen flow rate.	___	___	___	_____
8. Guided patient or caregiver through each step.	___	___	___	_____
9. Provided and discussed written materials given.	___	___	___	_____
10. Instructed patient or caregiver to recognize signs and symptoms of hypoxia and URI, and instructed when to notify physician. Asked for verbal feedback.	___	___	___	_____
11. Discussed emergency plan for respiratory distress, power failure, or natural disaster. Instructed to activate 9-1-1.	___	___	___	_____
12. Instructed patient to place "No Smoking—Oxygen in Use" sign at each entrance to the home.	___	___	___	_____
13. Recorded teaching plan and documented patient's learning.	___	___	___	_____

EVALUATION

	S	U	NP	Comments
1. Monitored oxygen delivery rate.	___	___	___	_____
2. Evaluated patient's or caregiver's ability and any problem with oxygen at home.	___	___	___	_____
3. Had patient or caregiver verbalize safety guidelines and emergency plans.	___	___	___	_____
4. Identified unexpected outcomes.	___	___	___	_____

466

	S	U	NP	Comments

RECORDING AND REPORTING

1. Recorded in the care plan teaching plan and information provided. ____ ____ ____ _____

2. Recorded learning progress. ____ ____ ____ _____

3. Communicated with other staff regarding learning activity and progress. ____ ____ ____ _____

4. Recorded type of oxygen delivery system, supplies, and flow rate. ____ ____ ____ _____

Student _____   Date _____

Instructor _____   Date _____

PERFORMANCE CHECKLIST SKILL 42-5 **TEACHING HOME TRACHEOSTOMY CARE AND SUCTIONING**

	S	U	NP	Comments
ASSESSMENT				
1. Assessed patient's ability to perform tracheostomy care and suctioning. Instructed caregiver for emergency situations.	___	___	___	_____
2. Assessed patient's or caregiver's recognition of physical signs and symptoms that indicate need for suctioning and tracheostomy care.	___	___	___	_____
3. Observed patient or caregiver performing suctioning and tracheostomy care.	___	___	___	_____
NURSING DIAGNOSIS				
1. Developed appropriate nursing diagnoses based on assessment data.	___	___	___	_____
PLANNING				
1. Identified expected outcomes.	___	___	___	_____
2. Selected most appropriate setting in home for tracheostomy care.	___	___	___	_____
3. Discussed and demonstrated proper position for procedure.	___	___	___	_____
IMPLEMENTATION				
1. Suctioning:				
a. Verified health care provider's order.	___	___	___	_____
b. Performed hand hygiene. Applied sterile gloves.	___	___	___	_____
c. Demonstrated step-by-step aseptic preparation and technique of suctioning.	___	___	___	_____
d. Demonstrated nasal and oral suction: To be done after tracheal suctioning followed by assisting with oral hygiene, as needed.	___	___	___	_____
e. Had patient take two or three deep breaths to indicate if airway was now clear.	___	___	___	_____
f. Disconnected suction catheter: if catheter to be cleansed for reuse, set aside, otherwise coiled and disposed of catheter.	___	___	___	_____
g. Removed and disposed of gloves. Performed hand hygiene.	___	___	___	_____

	S	U	NP	Comments

2. Trach care:

   a. Discussed and demonstrated trach care and replacement of ties.

   b. Cleaned reusable equipment in warm soapy water. Rinsed and dry thoroughly. Stored supplies in loosely closed plastic bag.

   c. Removed gloves and performed hand hygiene.

   d. Disinfected reusable supplies once a week by using *one* of the following methods:

      (1) *Method 1*: Boil supplies for 15 minutes. Cool and dry thoroughly before storing.

      (2) *Method 2*: Soak supplies in equal parts of white vinegar and water for 30 minutes. Remove, rinse, and dry thoroughly before storing.

      (3) *Method 3*: Soak supplies in prepared solutions of quarternary ammonium chloride compounds. Remove, rinse, and dry thoroughly before storing.

3. Caregiver performed each step with guidance from nurse.

4. Discussed signs and symptoms of the following:

   a. Stoma infection

   b. Respiratory tract infection

   c. Transesophageal fistula

5. Emphasized importance of recognizing symptoms and notifying health care provider.

EVALUATION

1. Had patient or caregiver state signs and symptoms of complications.

2. Observed patient or caregiver demonstrating suctioning and trach care independently.

3. Identified unexpected outcomes.

RECORDING AND REPORTING

1. Recorded instructions and skills demonstrated and accuracy of care rendered by patient or caregiver.

2. Developed a system of recording performance of care by patient or caregiver.

Student _____   Date _____

Instructor _____   Date _____

PERFORMANCE CHECKLIST PROCEDURAL GUIDELINE 42-1 **CHANGING A TRACHEOSTOMY TUBE AT HOME**

	S	U	NP	Comments
STEPS				
1. Held tube feeding for an hour or maintained NPO for an hour before procedure.	___	___	___	_____
2. Explained procedure to patient before starting.	___	___	___	_____
3. Performed hand hygiene and applied clean gloves.	___	___	___	_____
4. Prepared sterile supplies. Removed inner cannula and inserted obturator into outer cannula. Attached clean ties and checked integrity of cuff.	___	___	___	_____
5. Suctioned trach; had bag-valve mask and face mask available.	___	___	___	_____
6. Loosened trach ties and deflated trach cuff (if present).	___	___	___	_____
7. Removed old trach by pulling out with gentle, steady pressure in the same direction as an inner cannula would be removed.	___	___	___	_____
8. Applied sterile gloves and pushed new trach into tracheostomy site, using gentle force, while pushing back and then down. Removed obturator. Allowed air to flow, then inserted inner cannula.	___	___	___	_____
9. Attached new trach ties, inflated cuff, and placed dressing around stoma if necessary.	___	___	___	_____

Student _____ Date _____

Instructor _____ Date _____

PERFORMANCE CHECKLIST SKILL 42-6   **TEACHING MEDICATION SELF-ADMINISTRATION**

	S	U	NP	Comments
ASSESSMENT				
1. Assessed patient's cognitive, sensory, and motor function, level of consciousness, literacy, willingness to learn/participate in support group.	___	___	___	_____
2. Assessed patient's resources for obtaining medications.	___	___	___	_____
3. Assessed patient's and caregiver's knowledge of drug therapy and drug interactions.	___	___	___	_____
4. Assessed patient's cultural and religious beliefs and past experiences with drug therapy.	___	___	___	_____
5. Reviewed patient's prescribed, OTC, herbal, and nutritional supplements. Discussed compliance.	___	___	___	_____
6. Reviewed history of food and drug sensitivities and allergies.	___	___	___	_____
7. Assessed patient's understanding of drug-drug, drug-food, and drug-herb interactions.	___	___	___	_____
NURSING DIAGNOSIS				
1. Developed appropriate nursing diagnoses based on assessment data.	___	___	___	_____
PLANNING				
1. Identified expected outcomes.	___	___	___	_____
2. Prepared environment for teaching session.	___	___	___	_____
3. Provided useful teaching materials that complemented patient's learning ability.	___	___	___	_____
4. Had patient wear glasses or hearing aid during teaching session, if appropriate.	___	___	___	_____
5. Consulted with physician to simplify prescribed medications.	___	___	___	_____
6. Included caregiver in teaching program.	___	___	___	_____
IMPLEMENTATION				
1. Presented information in a clear, concise manner.	___	___	___	_____
2. Offered frequent opportunities for patient or caregiver to ask questions.	___	___	___	_____

	S	U	NP	Comments

3. Discussed with patient or caregiver relevant information pertaining to safe drug administration, related side effects, and management of effects, as well as when to call health care provider and implications of noncompliance. ____ ____ ____ _____

4. Discussed appropriate routes for medications. ____ ____ ____ _____

5. Discussed and reinforced information over several short sessions. Provided patient with written materials and charts for dosage schedule. ____ ____ ____ _____

6. Provided information on prescribed, OTC, and herbal supplements. Provided graphic/written learning aids for reference. ____ ____ ____ _____

7. Assisted patient or caregiver with preparation of medications. ____ ____ ____ _____

8. Arranged with pharmacy to have large-print labels for medication bottles and containers that are easy to open. ____ ____ ____ _____

9. Arranged for pharmacy to receive prescriptions and refills in a timely manner. Arranged for pharmacy to deliver, if needed. ____ ____ ____ _____

EVALUATION

1. Had patient or caregiver explain purpose, route, action, and timing of each prescribed medication, plus potential interactions. ____ ____ ____ _____

2. Identified patient's problem-solving abilities. ____ ____ ____ _____

3. Had patient or caregiver independently prepare dosages of all medications. ____ ____ ____ _____

4. Asked patient or caregiver to explain medication safety. ____ ____ ____ _____

5. Offered additional opportunity for patient to ask questions. ____ ____ ____ _____

6. Identified unexpected outcomes. ____ ____ ____ _____

RECORDING AND REPORTING

1. Documented instruction provided to patient or caregiver and learning outcomes. ____ ____ ____ _____

2. Developed a system of recording medication administered by patient or caregiver. ____ ____ ____ _____

Student _____ Date _____

Instructor _____ Date _____

PERFORMANCE CHECKLIST SKILL 42-7 **MANAGING FEEDING TUBES IN THE HOME**

	S	U	NP	Comments
ASSESSMENT				
1. Assessed patient's medical history, including factors contributing to fatigue and discomfort and ability to manage home feedings independently.	___	___	___	_____
2. Assessed patient's or caregiver's ability to perform procedure and availability of resources.	___	___	___	_____
3. Assessed environmental conditions of home.	___	___	___	_____
4. Assessed patient's or caregiver's understanding of the purpose of enteral nutrition.	___	___	___	_____
5. Assessed patient's or caregiver's understanding of the storage, management, and acquisition of supplies.	___	___	___	_____
6. Assessed patient's or caregiver's ability to administer feedings.	___	___	___	_____
NURSING DIAGNOSIS				
1. Developed appropriate nursing diagnoses based on assessment data.	___	___	___	_____
PLANNING				
1. Identified expected outcomes.	___	___	___	_____
IMPLEMENTATION				
1. Performed hand hygiene.	___	___	___	_____
2. Discussed patient's or caregiver's understanding of enteral feeding and nutritional health.	___	___	___	_____
3. Assisted patient or caregiver in determining feeding schedule.	___	___	___	_____
4. Demonstrated technique to verify NGT placement.	___	___	___	_____
5. Observed patient or caregiver return demonstrate NGT placement.	___	___	___	_____
6. Observed patient or caregiver aspirating gastric contents. Discussed potential problems and solutions, and when to notify health care provider.	___	___	___	_____
7. Discussed asepsis in preparing and administering feedings. Observed patient or caregiver preparing and administering feeding and cleaning and storing supplies.	___	___	___	_____

	S	U	NP	Comments
8. Observed patient or caregiver administering medication and flushing tube.	___	___	___	_____
9. Discussed and observed use of infusion pump, if indicated.	___	___	___	_____
10. Discussed measures to stabilize the NGT/PEG tube and to maintain skin integrity.	___	___	___	_____
11. Provided contact information for equipment or supplies in case of equipment failure.	___	___	___	_____
12. Discussed signs and symptoms of aspiration and emergency plan in the event of aspiration.	___	___	___	_____
13. Discussed whom to contact and when for signs of diarrhea, constipation, or weight loss.	___	___	___	_____
14. Performed hand hygiene.	___	___	___	_____

EVALUATION

	S	U	NP	Comments
1. Asked patient or caregiver to state purpose of home enteral nutrition therapy.	___	___	___	_____
2. Observed patient or caregiver performing medical asepsis technique, checking tube placement, aspirating and checking residual, administering medications, and using equipment.	___	___	___	_____
3. Asked patient or caregiver to state measures to prevent and manage complications, and when to call health care provider,	___	___	___	_____
4. Asked patient or caregiver how to care for open formula cans.	___	___	___	_____
5. Asked patient about community contacts for supplies, equipment, and emergency care.	___	___	___	_____
6. Identified unexpected outcomes.	___	___	___	_____

RECORDING AND REPORTING

	S	U	NP	Comments
1. Documented in home care record teaching provided and patient's or caregiver's response.	___	___	___	_____
2. Documented specifics of enteral feeding plan.	___	___	___	_____
3. Reviewed home documentation by patient or caregiver of enteral feeding and patient status.	___	___	___	_____

Student _____ Date _____

Instructor _____ Date _____

PERFORMANCE CHECKLIST SKILL 42-8 **MANAGING PARENTERAL NUTRITION IN THE HOME**

	S	U	NP	Comments
ASSESSMENT				
1. Assessed patient's nutritional status and risks for malnutrition.	___	___	___	_____
2. Obtained vital signs, height, and weight.	___	___	___	_____
3. Reviewed blood test pertaining to nutritional status.	___	___	___	_____
4. Assessed patency of patient's peripheral VAD or central VAD.	___	___	___	_____
5. Measured and marked arm if patient had a PICC.	___	___	___	_____
6. Verified prescriber's order and compared label versus order.	___	___	___	_____
7. Assessed patient's or caregiver's ability and readiness to learn.	___	___	___	_____
8. Determined understanding of purpose of parenteral feeding.	___	___	___	_____
NURSING DIAGNOSIS				
1. Developed appropriate nursing diagnoses based on assessment data.	___	___	___	_____
PLANNING				
1. Identified expected outcomes.	___	___	___	_____
2. Selected most appropriate setting at home for parenteral nutrition.	___	___	___	_____
IMPLEMENTATION				
1. Provided resources and contact information for 24-hour support 7 days a week in the event of problems.	___	___	___	_____
2. Explained all components of PN storage and administration.	___	___	___	_____
3. Guided patient or caregiver through every step of preparation and administration.	___	___	___	_____
4. Suggested to have solution at room temperature for at least 30 to 60 minutes before administration.	___	___	___	_____
5. Performed hand hygiene.	___	___	___	_____
6. Explained need to inspect fluid in bag for color and precipitates.	___	___	___	_____

	S	U	NP	Comments

7. Demonstrated connection of IV bag to filter and tubing and priming and loading of tubing into pump. ___ ___ ___ _____

8. Applied clean gloves. Wiped CVC port with alcohol and demonstrated flushing CVC and connecting tubing port. ___ ___ ___ _____

9. Explained how to program and use infusion pump. ___ ___ ___ _____

10. When infusion was completed, performed hand hygiene and applied gloves. ___ ___ ___ _____

11. Disconnected IV tubing, flushed CVC. Cleaned and stored infusion pump. Discarded used supplies in appropriate containers and discussed Standard Precautions. ___ ___ ___ _____

12. Demonstrated proper care of CVC site, dressing changes, and signs and symptoms of infection. ___ ___ ___ _____

13. Instructed patient or caregiver on how to recognize signs and symptoms of complications and when to call for help. ___ ___ ___ _____

14. Discussed importance and use of self–blood glucose monitor, normal values, and what to do for abnormal values. ___ ___ ___ _____

15. Discussed signs and symptoms of hypoglycemia and hyperglycemia, how to intervene, and when to call the health care provider. ___ ___ ___ _____

16. Provided with a log book and discussed how to record PN, I&O, weights, and blood glucose levels. ___ ___ ___ _____

17. Provided patient or caregiver with available resources to order equipment and supplies and emergency services. ___ ___ ___ _____

18. Discussed home safety plan and secondary plan for environmental disasters or emergencies. ___ ___ ___ _____

EVALUATION

1. Had patient or caregiver independently perform techniques for administration, infusion, and CVC site care. Cleaned and stored equipment and supplies. ___ ___ ___ _____

2. Asked patient or caregiver to identify expectations of PN. ___ ___ ___ _____

3. Had patient or caregiver describe signs and symptoms of complications, how to intervene, and when to call a health care provider. ___ ___ ___ _____

4. Observed patient or caregiver record information in log book. Reviewed patient's log book periodically. ___ ___ ___ _____

	S	U	NP	Comments

RECORDING AND REPORTING

1. Recorded in home care record information taught and patient's/caregiver's response. ____ ____ ____ _____

2. Recorded information pertinent to PN administration. ____ ____ ____ _____

3. Recorded and reported to health care provider any changes in condition or unexpected outcomes. ____ ____ ____ _____

Student _____ Date _____

Instructor _____ Date _____

PERFORMANCE CHECKLIST SKILL 43-1 **URINE SPECIMEN COLLECTION: MIDSTREAM, STERILE
URINARY CATHETER**

	S	U	NP	Comments
ASSESSMENT				
1. Assessed patient's or caregiver's understanding of test and method of collection.	___	___	___	_____
2. Assessed for signs and symptoms of urinary tract infection.	___	___	___	_____
3. Reviewed medical record for history of urinary infection and risk factors.	___	___	___	_____
4. Reviewed agency policy for specimen collection procedures. For clean voided specimen, assessed patient's ability to cooperate and assist.	___	___	___	_____
5. Assessed type of indwelling urinary catheter, if present.	___	___	___	_____
NURSING DIAGNOSIS				
1. Developed appropriate nursing diagnoses based on assessment data.	___	___	___	_____
PLANNING				
1. Identified expected outcomes.	___	___	___	_____
2. Offered patient fluids before specimen collection.	___	___	___	_____
3. Explained procedure to patient or family.	___	___	___	_____
IMPLEMENTATION				
1. Identified patient correctly. Verified type of specimen needed.	___	___	___	_____
2. Performed hand hygiene. Labeled specimen container.	___	___	___	_____
3. Provided privacy. Assisted ambulatory patient to bathroom.	___	___	___	_____
4. Collected clean voided specimen:				
a. Assisted patient as needed with perineal care.	___	___	___	_____
b. Assisted bedridden patient onto bedpan.	___	___	___	_____
c. Opened sterile package and prepared collection kit.	___	___	___	_____
d. Applied sterile gloves.	___	___	___	_____
e. Prepared sterile collection kit with specimen container.	___	___	___	_____
f. Cleansed perineum with antiseptic solution.	___	___	___	_____

	S	U	NP	Comments

g. Began collection after stream initiated and collected 30 to 60 ml of urine. If assistance was needed:

  (1) Male patient

    (a) Nurse/patient held penis and cleansed with antiseptic solution.   —— —— —— —————————————

    (b) After initiating stream, passed collection device into stream and collected 30 to 60 ml.   —— —— —— —————————————

  (2) Female patient

    (a) Nurse/patient separated labia and cleansed urethral area with antiseptic solution.   —— —— —— —————————————

    (b) After initiating stream in bedpan or toilet, passed collection device into stream and collected 30 to 60 mL.   —— —— —— —————————————

h. Had patient complete voiding in bedpan or toilet.   —— —— —— —————————————

i. Secured specimen container top tightly and cleansed outside of container.   —— —— —— —————————————

j. Disposed of soiled supplies. Removed gloves. Performed hand hygiene.   —— —— —— —————————————

5. Collected sterile urinary catheter specimen.

a. Drainage tube clamped for 30 minutes.   —— —— —— —————————————

b. Returned to room. Explained to patient that procedure will begin.   —— —— —— —————————————

c. Performed hand hygiene. Applied gloves.   —— —— —— —————————————

d. Positioned patient so catheter was accessible.   —— —— —— —————————————

e. Cleansed entry port with antiseptic and allowed to dry.   —— —— —— —————————————

f. Used sterile syringe to draw up necessary quantity of urine for scheduled test. Unclamped Foley catheter tubing and allowed urine to flow into drainage bag.   —— —— —— —————————————

g. Transferred urine into sterile specimen container.   —— —— —— —————————————

6. Disposed of soiled supplies. Removed and discarded gloves and performed hand hygiene.   —— —— —— —————————————

7. Attached laboratory requisition to specimen.   —— —— —— —————————————

8. Sent specimen to laboratory within 15 to 20 minutes or refrigerated for no longer than 2 hours before sending.   —— —— —— —————————————

	S	U	NP	Comments

EVALUATION

1. Observed specimen for characteristics of urine and presence of contaminants. ___ ___ ___ _____

2. Reviewed and compared results of U/A and C & S. ___ ___ ___ _____

3. Observed urinary drainage system. ___ ___ ___ _____

4. Asked patient to describe procedure for urine collection. ___ ___ ___ _____

5. Identified unexpected outcomes. ___ ___ ___ _____

RECORDING AND REPORTING

1. Recorded collection data of specimen. ___ ___ ___ _____

2. Recorded characteristics of urine and patient status. ___ ___ ___ _____

3. Reported to health care provider any significant changes or positive reports. ___ ___ ___ _____

Student _____ Date _____

Instructor _____ Date _____

PERFORMANCE CHECKLIST PROCEDURAL GUIDELINE 43-1 **COLLECTING A TIMED URINE SPECIMEN**

	S	U	NP	Comments
PROCEDURAL STEPS				
1. Explained procedure to patient.	___	___	___	_____
2. Placed specimen collection containers in the bathroom, in a pan of ice if indicated. Posted signs reminding staff and patient of timed urine collection.	___	___	___	_____
3. Applied clean gloves, collected and discarded first voided specimen. Indicate time on laboratory requisition. Collected urine from designated time.	___	___	___	_____
4. Measured volume of each voiding and calculated I&O.	___	___	___	_____
5. Placed all voided urine in collection bottle. Reminded patient not to discard urine or drop toilet paper into bottle.	___	___	___	_____
6. Encouraged patient to empty bladder during the last 15 minutes of urine collection period.	___	___	___	_____
7. At completion time, sent labeled specimen to laboratory.	___	___	___	_____
8. Removed signs and notified patient that specimen collection period was over.	___	___	___	_____

Student _____ Date _____

Instructor _____ Date _____

PERFORMANCE CHECKLIST PROCEDURAL GUIDELINE 43-2 **MEASURING CHEMICAL PROPERTIES OF URINE: GLUCOSE, KETONES, PROTEIN, BLOOD, AND pH**

	S	U	NP	Comments
PROCEDURAL STEPS				
1. Determined if double-voided specimen was needed for testing. If so:				
a. Asked patient to collect random specimen and discard.	___	___	___	_____
b. Had patient drink a glass of water.	___	___	___	_____
c. Collected another specimen 30 to 45 minutes later.	___	___	___	_____
2. Performed hand hygiene and applied gloves.	___	___	___	_____
3. Used Multistix reagent test strip to assess for up to 10 chemical properties.				
a. Immersed end of chemically impregnated test strip into urine.	___	___	___	_____
b. Removed strip from container immediately, and tapped it gently against side of container.	___	___	___	_____
c. Timed for number of seconds specified on container, and compared color of strip versus color chart.	___	___	___	_____
4. Removed and discarded gloves: Performed hand hygiene.	___	___	___	_____
5. Recorded results immediately on appropriate testing flowsheet. Reported reading to nurse or health care provider.	___	___	___	_____

Student _____ Date _____

Instructor _____ Date _____

PERFORMANCE CHECKLIST SKILL 43-2 **MEASURING OCCULT BLOOD IN STOOL**

	S	U	NP	Comments

ASSESSMENT

1. Assessed patient's or family's understanding of need for stool test. ___ ___ ___ _____

2. Assessed patient's ability to cooperate and collect specimen. ___ ___ ___ _____

3. Assessed medical history for bleeding, gastrointestinal disorder, and hemorrhoids. ___ ___ ___ _____

4. Reviewed patient medications to identify those with potential to increase bleeding. ___ ___ ___ _____

5. Referred to health care provider's orders for medication or dietary modifications before test. ___ ___ ___ _____

NURSING DIAGNOSIS

1. Developed appropriate nursing diagnoses based on assessment data. ___ ___ ___ _____

PLANNING

1. Identified expected outcomes. ___ ___ ___ _____

2. Explained procedure and purpose of test and method by which patient could assist. Feces must be free of urine and toilet tissue. ___ ___ ___ _____

3. Arranged for necessary dietary and medication restrictions. ___ ___ ___ _____

IMPLEMENTATION

1. Performed hand hygiene and applied clean gloves. ___ ___ ___ _____

2. Obtained uncontaminated stool specimen. ___ ___ ___ _____

3. With tip of wooden applicator, obtained small amount of feces. ___ ___ ___ _____

4. Measured for occult blood.

   a. Hemoccult slide test:

     (1) Applied thin smear of stool on paper in first box. ___ ___ ___ _____

     (2) Obtained second fecal specimen from different portion of stool, and applied thinly to second box. ___ ___ ___ _____

     (3) Closed slide cover and turned over. Applied 2 drops of Hemoccult developing solution to each box of guaiac paper. ___ ___ ___ _____

	S	U	NP	Comments

(4) Read results after 30 to 60 seconds. Disposed of slides properly. Noted results. ___ ___ ___ _____

5. Performed test using Hematest tablets.

   a. Placed stool on guaiac paper and Hematest tablet on top of specimen. ___ ___ ___ _____

   b. Applied 2 to 3 drops of tap water to tablet, allowing water to flow onto guaiac paper. ___ ___ ___ _____

   c. Observed color of guaiac paper within 2 minutes. ___ ___ ___ _____

   d. Disposed of tablet and paper in proper receptacle. ___ ___ ___ _____

6. Discarded wooden applicator wrapped in paper towel. Removed gloves properly and disposed of everything in proper container. ___ ___ ___ _____

7. Performed hand hygiene. ___ ___ ___ _____

EVALUATION

1. Asked patient to explain collection procedure. ___ ___ ___ _____

2. Noted character of stool. ___ ___ ___ _____

3. Noted color changes in guaiac paper. ___ ___ ___ _____

4. Identified unexpected outcomes. ___ ___ ___ _____

RECORDING AND REPORTING

1. Recorded test results. ___ ___ ___ _____

2. Recorded unusual stool characteristics. ___ ___ ___ _____

3. Reported positive test results to health care provider. ___ ___ ___ _____

Student _____ Date _____

Instructor _____ Date _____

PERFORMANCE CHECKLIST SKILL 43-3 **MEASURING OCCULT BLOOD IN GASTRIC SECRETIONS (GASTROCCULT)**

	S	U	NP	Comments

ASSESSMENT

1. Assessed patient's, family members' understanding of need for test. ___ ___ ___ _____

2. Assessed patient's medical history for GI bleeding or other disorders. ___ ___ ___ _____

3. Assessed medications that may increase risk for bleeding. ___ ___ ___ _____

NURSING DIAGNOSIS

1. Developed appropriate nursing diagnoses based on assessment data. ___ ___ ___ _____

PLANNING

1. Identified expected outcomes. ___ ___ ___ _____

2. Explained procedure to patient. ___ ___ ___ _____

IMPLEMENTATION

1. Performed hand hygiene. Applied clean gloves. ___ ___ ___ _____

2. Verified NGT placement, if present. ___ ___ ___ _____

3. Obtained specimen by attaching bulb syringe to NGT, if present, and aspirating 5 to 10 mL of gastric secretions. If no NGT, of vomitus. ___ ___ ___ _____

4. Used tip of wooden tip applicator to obtain sample of secretions from emesis basin. ___ ___ ___ _____

5. Performed Gastroccult slide test.

   a. Applied 1 drop of gastric sample to Gastroccult test paper. ___ ___ ___ _____

   b. Applied 2 drops of developer solution over sample and 1 drop to performance monitors. ___ ___ ___ _____

   c. Verified performance monitor turned blue after 30 seconds. ___ ___ ___ _____

   d. Read test results correctly within 60 seconds. ___ ___ ___ _____

   e. Disposed of soiled supplies correctly. ___ ___ ___ _____

6. Performed hand hygiene. ___ ___ ___ _____

	S	U	NP	Comments

EVALUATION

1. Asked patient to explain reason for procedure. —— —— —— _____

2. Assessed quantity and character of gastric secretions. —— —— —— _____

3. Noted color changes in Gastroccult. —— —— —— _____

4. Identified unexpected outcomes. —— —— —— _____

RECORDING AND REPORTING

1. Recorded test, source of specimen, and results. —— —— —— _____

2. Recorded characteristics of gastric contents. —— —— —— _____

3. Reported positive results to health care provider. —— —— —— _____

Student _____   Date _____

Instructor _____   Date _____

PERFORMANCE CHECKLIST SKILL 43-4   **COLLECTING NOSE AND THROAT SPECIMENS FOR CULTURE**

	S	U	NP	Comments
ASSESSMENT				
1. Assessed patient's understanding of procedure and ability to cooperate. Assessed mental status.	___	___	___	_____
2. Assessed condition and drainage from nasal mucosa and sinuses.	___	___	___	_____
3. Assessed patient for symptoms of URI, seasonal allergies, and systemic infections.	___	___	___	_____
4. Assessed condition of posterior pharynx.	___	___	___	_____
5. Assessed patient for systemic signs of infection.	___	___	___	_____
6. Reviewed health care provider's orders for type of culture needed.	___	___	___	_____
NURSING DIAGNOSIS				
1. Developed appropriate nursing diagnoses based on assessment data.	___	___	___	_____
PLANNING				
1. Identified expected outcomes.	___	___	___	_____
2. Planned to do culture before meals or at least 1 hour after meals.	___	___	___	_____
3. Explained procedure to patient and family members.	___	___	___	_____
4. Explained common sensations felt during collection.	___	___	___	_____
IMPLEMENTATION				
1. Correctly verified patient's identity. Verified type of procedure scheduled.	___	___	___	_____
2. Assisted patient to required position.	___	___	___	_____
3. Prepared swab and tube.	___	___	___	_____
4. Collected throat culture:				
a. Performed hand hygiene and applied clean gloves.	___	___	___	_____
b. Had patient tilt head back.	___	___	___	_____
c. Asked patient to open mouth and say "ah."	___	___	___	_____
d. Swabbed tonsillar area from side to side without touching other areas.	___	___	___	_____
e. Immediately placed swab in culture tube securely and activated culture medium.	___	___	___	_____

	S	U	NP	Comments

f. Removed and disposed of gloves and used supplies correctly. Performed hand hygiene. ___ ___ ___ _____

5. Collected nasal culture:

a. Performed hand hygiene and applied clean gloves. ___ ___ ___ _____

b. Encouraged patient to blow nose. Checked condition of nostrils and nasal mucosa. ___ ___ ___ _____

c. Had patient tilt head back. ___ ___ ___ _____

d. Inserted speculum and swab through center of speculum. ___ ___ ___ _____

e. Rotated swab; avoided touching sides of speculum or outside of nose when removing. ___ ___ ___ _____

f. Inserted swab into culture tube and activated culture medium. ___ ___ ___ _____

g. Removed speculum and offered patient a tissue. ___ ___ ___ _____

h. Removed gloves. Performed hand hygiene. ___ ___ ___ _____

6. Collected nasopharyngeal culture:

a. Followed steps for nasal culture. ___ ___ ___ _____

b. Used special swab with flexible wire. Nasopharynx reached via nose. ___ ___ ___ _____

7. Placed swab into collection tube and activated culture medium. ___ ___ ___ _____

8. Discarded supplies and gloves. Performed hand hygiene. ___ ___ ___ _____

9. Attached label to culture tube and affixed requisition. Identified antibiotic use, if applicable. ___ ___ ___ _____

10. Sent specimen immediately to laboratory, or refrigerated specimen. ___ ___ ___ _____

EVALUATION

1. Checked laboratory record for test results. ___ ___ ___ _____

2. Inspected patient's nose for evidence of bleeding. ___ ___ ___ _____

3. Identified unexpected outcomes. ___ ___ ___ _____

RECORDING AND REPORTING

1. Recorded specimen collection data. ___ ___ ___ _____

2. Described appearance of nasal and oral mucosa. ___ ___ ___ _____

3. Reported positive test results to health care provider. ___ ___ ___ _____

494

Student _____   Date _____

Instructor _____   Date _____

PERFORMANCE CHECKLIST SKILL 43-5 **OBTAINING VAGINAL OR URETHRAL DISCHARGE SPECIMENS**

	S	U	NP	Comments
ASSESSMENT				
1. Assessed understanding of need for specimen and ability to cooperate.	___	___	___	_____
2. Assessed condition of patient's external genitalia.	___	___	___	_____
3. Assessed patient for symptoms of urinary, vaginal, or STD infection.	___	___	___	_____
4. Collected sexual history of patient, when appropriate.	___	___	___	_____
5. Referred to health care provider's orders for type of culture.	___	___	___	_____
NURSING DIAGNOSIS				
1. Developed appropriate nursing diagnoses based on assessment data.	___	___	___	_____
PLANNING				
1. Identified expected outcomes.	___	___	___	_____
2. Explained procedure to patient.	___	___	___	_____
3. Maintained nonjudgmental attitude.	___	___	___	_____
IMPLEMENTATION				
1. Correctly verified patient's identity. Verified type of scheduled test.	___	___	___	_____
2. Performed hand hygiene. Closed bed curtains or room door and placed "Do Not Enter" sign on door.	___	___	___	_____
3. Assisted patient to required position and draped.	___	___	___	_____
4. Applied clean gloves.	___	___	___	_____
5. Directed light onto perineum.	___	___	___	_____
6. Opened culture tube and held swab in dominant hand.	___	___	___	_____
7. Instructed patient to breathe slowly during procedure.	___	___	___	_____
8. Obtained specimen(s):				
a. Female				
(1) Exposed vaginal or urethral orifice.	___	___	___	_____
(2) Inserted swabs 1 to 2.5 cm (½-1 inch).	___	___	___	_____

	S	U	NP	Comments
(3) Avoided touching labia. Applied swab to area of discharge.	——	——	——	————————
b. Male				
(1) Grasped penis. Retracted foreskin, if present.	——	——	——	————————
(2) Gently swabbed urinary meatus. If no discharge visible, gently inserted swab into urethra.	——	——	——	————————
(3) Returned foreskin to natural position.	——	——	——	————————
9. Returned swab(s) to culture tube and activated medium.	——	——	——	————————
10. Properly removed and discarded gloves.	——	——	——	————————
11. Labeled each culture tube. Sent to laboratory with requisition.	——	——	——	————————
12. Assisted patient to a comfortable position. Assisted with personal hygiene as needed. Disposed of used supplies in proper container.	——	——	——	————————
13. Performed hand hygiene.	——	——	——	————————

EVALUATION

	S	U	NP	Comments
1. Reviewed laboratory results.	——	——	——	————————
2. Noted characteristics of discharge.	——	——	——	————————
3. Observed specimen for presence of feces.	——	——	——	————————
4. Identified unexpected outcomes.	——	——	——	————————

RECORDING AND REPORTING

	S	U	NP	Comments
1. Recorded specimen-related data.	——	——	——	————————
2. Described characteristics of discharge and appearance of vaginal orifice and urethra.	——	——	——	————————
3. Reported laboratory test results.	——	——	——	————————

Student _____   Date _____

Instructor _____   Date _____

PERFORMANCE CHECKLIST PROCEDURAL GUIDELINE 43-3 **COLLECTING A SPUTUM SPECIMEN BY EXPECTORATION**

	S	U	NP	Comments

STEPS

1. Explained purpose of procedure to patient. Indicated importance of deep cough to bring up sputum for testing.   ___ ___ ___ _____

2. Provided opportunity to rinse mouth with water before taking sample.   ___ ___ ___ _____

3. Applied clean gloves, provided sputum cup, and instructed patient not to touch inside of cup.   ___ ___ ___ _____

4. Instructed patient to take three to four deep breathes before coughing. Asked patient to cough forcefully and expectorate sputum into container.   ___ ___ ___ _____

5. Repeated until 5 to 10 mL of sputum was collected.   ___ ___ ___ _____

6. Secured top on container, wiped exterior with disinfectant, if needed.   ___ ___ ___ _____

7. Offered patient tissue to wipe mouth followed by mouth care. Disposed of tissue appropriately.   ___ ___ ___ _____

8. Removed and disposed of gloves.   ___ ___ ___ _____

9. Attached correct identification label and laboratory requisition to side of specimen container.   ___ ___ ___ _____

10. Enclosed specimen container in plastic biohazard bag.   ___ ___ ___ _____

11. Sent specimen immediately to laboratory.   ___ ___ ___ _____

Student _____ Date _____

Instructor _____ Date _____

PERFORMANCE CHECKLIST SKILL 43-6   **COLLECTING SPUTUM SPECIMENS BY SUCTION**

	S	U	NP	Comments
ASSESSMENT				
1. Reviewed health care provider's orders for type of sputum analysis and specifications.	___	___	___	_____
2. Assessed patient's understanding of procedure.	___	___	___	_____
3. Checked when patient last ate.	___	___	___	_____
4. Determined type of assistance needed in producing specimen.	___	___	___	_____
5. Assessed patient's respiratory status.	___	___	___	_____
NURSING DIAGNOSIS				
1. Developed appropriate nursing diagnoses based on assessment data.	___	___	___	_____
PLANNING				
1. Identified expected outcomes.	___	___	___	_____
2. Explained procedure to patient.	___	___	___	_____
IMPLEMENTATION				
1. Correctly verified patient's identity. Verified type of test ordered.	___	___	___	_____
2. Performed hand hygiene. Provided privacy.	___	___	___	_____
3. Positioned patient correctly. Assisted patient to splint painful area, if necessary.	___	___	___	_____
4. Applied clean glove to nondominant hand and prepared equipment.	___	___	___	_____
5. Correctly applied sterile glove to dominant hand.	___	___	___	_____
6. Inserted suction catheter, without applying suction through nasopharynx, ET tube, or trach.	___	___	___	_____
7. Suctioned 5 to 10 seconds while patient coughed. Collected 2 to 10 mL of sputum.	___	___	___	_____
8. Removed catheter without applying suction.	___	___	___	_____
9. Detached catheter from sputum trap. Detached and disposed of suction catheter.	___	___	___	_____
10. Secured top of container or sputum trap.	___	___	___	_____
11. Cleansed outside of container with disinfectant if needed.	___	___	___	_____

	S	U	NP	Comments
12. Offered patient facial tissues. Performed oral care.	___	___	___	_____
13. Removed and disposed of gloves.	___	___	___	_____
14. Performed hand hygiene.	___	___	___	_____
15. Labeled specimen. Placed in protective specimen collection plastic bag.	___	___	___	_____
16. Attached requisition and sent to laboratory.	___	___	___	_____

EVALUATION

	S	U	NP	Comments
1. Assessed patient's respiratory status during procedure.	___	___	___	_____
2. Noted presence of anxiety or discomfort.	___	___	___	_____
3. Observed character of sputum.	___	___	___	_____
4. Reviewed laboratory results.	___	___	___	_____
5. Asked patient to describe/demonstrate procedure.	___	___	___	_____
6. Identified unexpected outcomes.	___	___	___	_____

RECORDING AND REPORTING

	S	U	NP	Comments
1. Recorded data related to specimen collection.	___	___	___	_____
2. Described characteristics of sputum.	___	___	___	_____
3. Described patient's tolerance of procedure.	___	___	___	_____
4. Reported unusual sputum characteristics.	___	___	___	_____
5. Reported abnormal test results.	___	___	___	_____

Student _____   Date _____

Instructor _____   Date _____

PERFORMANCE CHECKLIST SKILL 43-7   **OBTAINING WOUND DRAINAGE SPECIMENS**

	S	U	NP	Comments
ASSESSMENT				
1. Assessed patient's understanding of need for wound culture and ability to cooperate.	___	___	___	_____
2. Assessed patient for systemic signs of infection. Reviewed laboratory results.	___	___	___	_____
3. Assessed pain level (scale 0 to 10, PQRST) and need for analgesics.	___	___	___	_____
4. Determined schedule for dressing change.	___	___	___	_____
5. Reviewed health care provider's orders for culture.	___	___	___	_____
6. Applied clean gloves and assessed condition of wound.	___	___	___	_____
NURSING DIAGNOSIS				
1. Developed appropriate nursing diagnoses based on assessment data.	___	___	___	_____
PLANNING				
1. Identified expected outcomes.	___	___	___	_____
2. Determined patient's need for analgesic before dressing change or specimen collection.	___	___	___	_____
3. Explained procedure to patient.	___	___	___	_____
4. Explained that patient may feel tickling sensation when wound is swabbed.	___	___	___	_____
IMPLEMENTATION				
1. Correctly verified patient's identity. Verified type of test ordered.	___	___	___	_____
2. Performed hand hygiene. Provided privacy.	___	___	___	_____
3. Applied clean gloves. Removed current dressing carefully, assessed characteristics of drainage.	___	___	___	_____
4. Cleansed periwound area with antiseptic.	___	___	___	_____
5. Disposed of antiseptic swab and gloves. Performed hand hygiene.	___	___	___	_____
6. Prepared sterile dressing supplies and culture tubes.	___	___	___	_____
7. Applied sterile gloves.	___	___	___	_____

	S	U	NP	Comments

8. Cleansed wound with normal saline and collected cultures:

  a. Aerobic culture

    (1) Inserted tip of swab into wound and coated gently with fresh secretions.   ___ ___ ___ _____

  b. Anaerobic cultures

    (1) Inserted tip of swab deeply into wound and rotated gently.   ___ ___ ___ _____

    (2) Or....Syringe aspiration: Inserted tip of syringe (without needle) into wound and aspirated exudates. Injected drainage into culture tube.   ___ ___ ___ _____

9. Returned swab to culture tube and activated medium.   ___ ___ ___ _____

10. Asked staff member to label tubes separately, affix requisitions, and send to laboratory immediately.   ___ ___ ___ _____

11. Repeated wound cleansing, if needed. Applied medicated solutions/dressings, if ordered.   ___ ___ ___ _____

12. Disposed of gloves and soiled supplies.   ___ ___ ___ _____

13. Secured dressing.   ___ ___ ___ _____

14. Assisted patient to comfortable position.   ___ ___ ___ _____

15. Performed hand hygiene.   ___ ___ ___ _____

EVALUATION

1. Reviewed laboratory report for culture results.   ___ ___ ___ _____

2. Assessed wound characteristics.   ___ ___ ___ _____

3. Asked patient about purpose of culture.   ___ ___ ___ _____

4. Identified unexpected outcomes.   ___ ___ ___ _____

RECORDING AND REPORTING

1. Recorded specimen-related data.   ___ ___ ___ _____

2. Recorded wound assessment and wound care, patient's need for analgesia and tolerance to procedure.   ___ ___ ___ _____

3. Reported evidence of infection to nurse in charge or health care provider.   ___ ___ ___ _____

Student _____   Date _____

Instructor _____   Date _____

PERFORMANCE CHECKLIST SKILL 43-8 **COLLECTING BLOOD SPECIMENS AND BLOOD CULTURES BY VENIPUNCTURE (SYRINGE METHOD, VACUTAINER METHOD)**

	S	U	NP	Comments
ASSESSMENT				
1. Determined patient's understanding of procedure.	___	___	___	_____
2. Determined if specific conditions are required before specimen collection.	___	___	___	_____
3. Reviewed patient's history for contraindications to venipuncture.	___	___	___	_____
4. Identified site contraindications for venipuncture.	___	___	___	_____
5. Reviewed health care provider orders for type of test(s).	___	___	___	_____
NURSING DIAGNOSIS				
1. Developed appropriate nursing diagnoses based on assessment data.	___	___	___	_____
PLANNING				
1. Identified expected outcomes.	___	___	___	_____
2. Explained procedure to patient.	___	___	___	_____
IMPLEMENTATION				
1. Correctly verified patient's identity. Verified prescriber's order.	___	___	___	_____
2. Performed hand hygiene. Prepared equipment at bedside.	___	___	___	_____
3. Prepared supplies needed at bedside.	___	___	___	_____
4. Assisted patient to a comfortable position.	___	___	___	_____
5. Applied tourniquet. Asked patient to slowly open and close fists several times and leave fists gently clenched.	___	___	___	_____
6. Inspected extremity for best site.	___	___	___	_____
7. Gently palpated selected vein with fingers.	___	___	___	_____
8. Selected two sites for blood cultures (opposite extremity).	___	___	___	_____
9. Performed hand hygiene. Applied clean gloves.	___	___	___	_____

		S	U	NP	Comments

10. Obtained blood sample:

a. Syringe method

(1) Prepared syringe with needle securely attached. Relocated vein. ___ ___ ___ _____

(2) Cleansed site. Used antiseptic swab only when drawing for blood alcohol levels and blood cultures. ___ ___ ___ _____

(3) Removed needle cover. ___ ___ ___ _____

(4) Pulled skin taut with thumb or forefinger 2.5 cm (1 inch) below site. ___ ___ ___ _____

(5) Held syringe and needle at 15- to 30-degree angle. ___ ___ ___ _____

(6) Slowly inserted needle into vein. ___ ___ ___ _____

(7) Held syringe securely and pulled back on plunger. Watched for blood return. ___ ___ ___ _____

(8) Obtained desired amount of blood. ___ ___ ___ _____

(9) Released tourniquet after specimen obtained. ___ ___ ___ _____

(10) Applied pressure with 2- × 2-inch gauze, then withdrew needle from vein. ___ ___ ___ _____

(11) Properly discarded uncapped needle. ___ ___ ___ _____

(12) Followed recommended CLSI and OSHA practice standards. ___ ___ ___ _____

(13) Filled blood tubes and inverted if additives present. ___ ___ ___ _____

b. Vacutainer method ___ ___ ___ _____

(1) Relocated vein. ___ ___ ___ _____

(2) Attached double-ended needle to vacuum tube. ___ ___ ___ _____

(3) Placed blood specimen tube in Vacutainer without puncturing rubber stopper. ___ ___ ___ _____

(4) Followed procedure for syringe method for venipuncture. ___ ___ ___ _____

(5) Held Vacutainer securely and advanced specimen tube onto needle in Vacutainer. ___ ___ ___ _____

(6) Noted blood flow. ___ ___ ___ _____

(7) Removed specimen tube after filled; inserted additional tubes, if necessary. ___ ___ ___ _____

(8) Released tourniquet after last sample obtained. ___ ___ ___ _____

504

	S	U	NP	Comments
(9) Applied 2- × 2- gauze pad over site, withdrew needle, and applied pressure.	___	___	___	_____
c. Blood cultures				
(1) Relocated vein and swabbed site. Allowed to dry completely.	___	___	___	_____
(2) Cleansed tops of culture bottles.	___	___	___	_____
(3) Collected 10 to 15 mL of blood from site.	___	___	___	_____
(4) Safely discarded used needle. Replaced with sterile needle to transfer sample to culture bottle.	___	___	___	_____
(5) Inoculated anaerobic first, if both aerobic and anaerobic cultures needed. Mixed gently after inoculation.	___	___	___	_____
d. CVC blood collection				
(1) Selected appropriate port. Turned off all IV pumps.	___	___	___	_____
(2) Wiped cap with alcohol or antiseptic swab. Aspirated 5 ml of blood with syringe and discarded syringe, or used Vacutainer and discarded specimen tube.	___	___	___	_____
(3) When sampling completed, discarded supplies in appropriate receptacle.	___	___	___	_____
(4) Wiped port and flushed with 10 ml NS using push-pause method.	___	___	___	_____
(5) Gently rotated any tubes containing additives.	___	___	___	_____
(6) Removed gloves and performed hand hygiene.	___	___	___	_____
11. Applied gauze with tape to puncture site.	___	___	___	_____
12. Checked tubes, wiped with alcohol if necessary.	___	___	___	_____
13. Assisted patient to comfortable position.	___	___	___	_____
14. Labeled every tube.	___	___	___	_____
15. Properly disposed of used supplies and soiled equipment.	___	___	___	_____
16. Bagged specimens and cleaned up any spills.	___	___	___	_____
17. Removed and disposed of gloves.	___	___	___	_____
18. Sent specimens to laboratory or refrigerated until sent (for no longer than 30 minutes.)	___	___	___	_____

	S	U	NP	Comments

EVALUATION

1. Reassessed venipuncture site.

2. Determined if patient remained anxious or fearful.

3. Reviewed laboratory results.

4. Asked patient to explain purpose of test.

5. Identified unexpected outcomes.

RECORDING AND REPORTING

1. Recorded data related to specimen collected.

2. Described venipuncture site and patient's response.

3. Reported "stat" test results to health care provider.

4. Reported any abnormal findings to health care provider.

Student _____ Date _____

Instructor _____ Date _____

PERFORMANCE CHECKLIST SKILL 43-9 **BLOOD GLUCOSE MONITORING**

	S	U	NP	Comments
ASSESSMENT				
1. Assessed patient's understanding of procedure.	___	___	___	_____
2. Determined if specific conditions had to be met before procedure.	___	___	___	_____
3. Determined risks or contraindications for performing procedure.	___	___	___	_____
4. Assessed area of skin to be used as puncture site.	___	___	___	_____
5. Reviewed health care provider's ordered schedule.	___	___	___	_____
6. Assessed diabetic patient's ability to handle skin puncture device.	___	___	___	_____
NURSING DIAGNOSIS				
1. Developed appropriate nursing diagnoses based on assessment data.	___	___	___	_____
PLANNING				
1. Identified expected outcomes.	___	___	___	_____
2. Explained procedure to patient.	___	___	___	_____
IMPLEMENTATION				
1. Performed hand hygiene.	___	___	___	_____
2. Instructed patient to perform hand hygiene.	___	___	___	_____
3. Positioned patient comfortably.	___	___	___	_____
4. Removed reagent strip. Checked expiration date.	___	___	___	_____
5. Activated glucometer.	___	___	___	_____
6. Inserted strip into glucometer. Followed manufacturer's recommendations. Made adjustments if necessary.	___	___	___	_____
7. Removed reagent strip from meter and placed on clean, dry surface.	___	___	___	_____
8. Applied clean gloves.	___	___	___	_____
9. Selected puncture site, avoiding central area of finger.	___	___	___	_____
10. Gently massaged finger to be punctured in dependent position.	___	___	___	_____

	S	U	NP	Comments
11. Cleansed site with antiseptic swab and allowed to dry.	——	——	——	_____
12. Removed cover of lancet or blood-letting device.	——	——	——	_____
13. Used lancet or lancet-holding device to quickly puncture finger or heel.	——	——	——	_____
14. Wiped away first droplet of blood with cotton ball, or as manufacturer's directions describe.	——	——	——	_____
15. Squeezed puncture site lightly until droplet formed.	——	——	——	_____
16. Applied drop of blood to reagent strip test pad. Obtained results.	——	——	——	_____
17. Turned meter off, and disposed of test strip, lancet, and gloves.	——	——	——	_____
18. Discussed results with patient.	——	——	——	_____

EVALUATION

	S	U	NP	Comments
1. Reinspected puncture site for bleeding or tissue injury.	——	——	——	_____
2. Compared glucose meter reading versus normal levels.	——	——	——	_____
3. Asked patient to describe/demonstrate procedure.	——	——	——	_____
4. Determined if patient had any questions or concerns.	——	——	——	_____
5. Identified unexpected outcomes.	——	——	——	_____

RECORDING AND REPORTING

	S	U	NP	Comments
1. Recorded procedure, glucose level, and action taken for abnormal range.	——	——	——	_____
2. Described patient's response and appearance of puncture site.	——	——	——	_____
3. Described any explanations or teaching provided for patient.	——	——	——	_____
4. Reported abnormal blood glucose levels to health care provider.	——	——	——	_____

Student _____ Date _____

Instructor _____ Date _____

PERFORMANCE CHECKLIST SKILL 43-10 OBTAINING AN ARTERIAL SPECIMEN FOR BLOOD GAS MEASUREMENT

	S	U	NP	Comments
ASSESSMENT				
1. Determined need to obtain ABG sample. Verified health care provider's order.	___	___	___	_____
2. Identified factors that could alter sample.	___	___	___	_____
3. Performed physical assessment of thorax and lungs.	___	___	___	_____
4. Identified any medications that may influence ABG measurement.	___	___	___	_____
5. Reviewed criteria for choosing site for sample collection.	___	___	___	_____
6. Assessed collateral blood flow. Performed Allen test. Assessed arterial sites.	___	___	___	_____
7. Determined patient's baseline arterial blood gases.	___	___	___	_____
8. Determined patient's knowledge of procedure.	___	___	___	_____
NURSING DIAGNOSIS				
1. Developed appropriate nursing diagnoses based on assessment data.	___	___	___	_____
PLANNING				
1. Identified expected outcomes.	___	___	___	_____
2. Prepared heparinized syringe.	___	___	___	_____
3. Explained procedure to patient.	___	___	___	_____
IMPLEMENTATION				
1. Verified patient's identity. Verified health care provider's order.	___	___	___	_____
2. Performed hand hygiene and applied clean gloves.	___	___	___	_____
3. Palpated selected arterial site.	___	___	___	_____
4. Stabilized chosen arterial site appropriately.	___	___	___	_____
5. Applied gloves. Cleansed area with alcohol swab or antiseptic swab.	___	___	___	_____
6. Held 2- × 2-inch gauze, with fingers palpating artery.	___	___	___	_____
7. Kept fingertip on artery.	___	___	___	_____

	S	U	NP	Comments
8. Correctly performed arterial stick, inserting needle at 45-degree angle.	___	___	___	_____
9. Stopped advancing needle when blood noted.	___	___	___	_____
10. Allowed arterial pulsations to pump 2 to 3 mL of blood into syringe.	___	___	___	_____
11. Removed needle, holding gauze over site.	___	___	___	_____
12. Applied pressure over site for 3 to 5 minutes or as indicated.	___	___	___	_____
13. Inspected site for signs of bleeding.	___	___	___	_____
14. Palpated artery distal to puncture site.	___	___	___	_____
15. Removed gloves and performed hand hygiene.	___	___	___	_____
16. Expelled air bubbles from syringe.	___	___	___	_____
17. Prepared syringe for laboratory according to agency policy using common principles such as the following:				
a. Labeled syringe properly.	___	___	___	_____
b. Placed sample on ice.	___	___	___	_____
c. Prepared laboratory requisition.	___	___	___	_____
d. Indicated on requisition patient's FIO_2, use of oxygen, and temperature.	___	___	___	_____
18. Immediately sent sample to laboratory.	___	___	___	_____

EVALUATION

	S	U	NP	Comments
1. Inspected area distal to puncture site for complications.	___	___	___	_____
2. Reviewed results as soon as possible.	___	___	___	_____
3. Identified unexpected outcomes.	___	___	___	_____

RECORDING AND REPORTING

	S	U	NP	Comments
1. Recorded Allen's test, puncture site assessment, and disposition of specimen to laboratory.	___	___	___	_____
2. Reported ABG results to health care provider.	___	___	___	_____
3. Recorded ventilator settings if applicable.	___	___	___	_____
4. Recorded test results and condition of puncture site.	___	___	___	_____

Student _____ Date _____

Instructor _____ Date _____

PERFORMANCE CHECKLIST SKILL 44-1 **INTRAVENOUS MODERATE SEDATION DURING A DIAGNOSTIC PROCEDURE**

	S	U	NP	Comments
ASSESSMENT				
1. Verified patient's identity using two forms of identifiers. Verified type of procedure scheduled and procedure site. Determined patient's understanding of procedure.	___	___	___	_____
2. Verified that a preprocedure history and physical examination were completed.	___	___	___	_____
3. Verified that informed consent was obtained.	___	___	___	_____
4. Assessed patient's history of adverse reaction to IV sedation.	___	___	___	_____
5. Verified the patient's ASA Physical Status Classification.	___	___	___	_____
6. Assessed patient's past history for substance abuse.	___	___	___	_____
7. Verified that patient did not eat or drink for at least 4 hours, or per agency requirements.	___	___	___	_____
8. Assessed the patient's history of medication/ latex allergies.	___	___	___	_____
9. Assessed patient's understanding of procedure.	___	___	___	_____
10. Assessed baseline vital signs, oxygen saturation, pain level, and level of consciousness.	___	___	___	_____
11. Determined patient's height and weight.	___	___	___	_____
12. Assessed and documented patient's baseline status using the Aldrete score system.	___	___	___	_____
NURSING DIAGNOSIS				
1. Developed appropriate nursing diagnoses based on assessment data.	___	___	___	_____
PLANNING				
1. Identified expected outcomes.	___	___	___	_____
2. Explained effects of IV sedation.	___	___	___	_____
3. Explained that close monitoring will occur throughout procedure.	___	___	___	_____
4. Explained the major steps of the procedure.	___	___	___	_____
5. Positioned patient as needed for the procedure.	___	___	___	_____
6. Explained "Time Out."	___	___	___	_____

	S	U	NP	Comments

IMPLEMENTATION

1. Established IV access.

2. Applied monitoring leads, blood pressure cuff, and pulse oximetry to patient.

3. Monitored for verbal and nonverbal evidence of pain.

4. Monitored level of consciousness.

5. Assessed level of sedation using the Modified Ramsay Sedation Scale.

EVALUATION

1. Monitored according to the type of procedure performed using the Modified Ramsay Sedation Scale.

2. Monitored airway, vital signs, SpO_2, pain level, and level of consciousness every 5 minutes for at least 30 minutes, then every 15 minutes for an hour, then every 30 minutes until patient met discharge criteria.

3. Determined level of patient's understanding by return verbalization of instructions given pre-procedure and postprocedure.

4. Had patient's caregiver explain postprocedure discharge instructions.

5. Identified unexpected outcomes.

RECORDING AND REPORTING

1. Recorded preprocedure and postprocedure patient assessment, as well as postprocedure monitoring until discharge.

2. Recorded medication administered (pain management) after the procedure, including any IV fluids and blood products.

3. Recorded and reported significant patient reactions during and after procedure, interventions, and patient status.

4. Recorded any teaching or instructions given, and patient's feedback and understanding.

5. Reported unusual findings to nurse in charge or physician.

512

Student _____ Date _____

Instructor _____ Date _____

	S	U	NP	Comments

ASSESSMENT

1. Verified patient's identity and the type of procedure scheduled.

2. Verified that informed consent was obtained.

3. Determined if patient is taking anticoagulants.

4. Determined if patient is allergic to iodine dye, latex, and shellfish; if so, notified appropriate physician.

5. Assessed for any risk factors or contraindications to procedure.

6. Assessed vital signs, including peripheral pulses. Marked arterial pulses for arterial procedures. Auscultated heart and lungs and obtained weight for cardiac catheterization.

7. Assessed hydration status. Reviewed laboratory results, including bleeding and coagulation studies.

8. Assessed patient's understanding of the procedure.

9. Removed all patient's jewelry and other metal objects.

10. Verified bowel prep completed, if appropriate.

11. Determined type of arteriogram scheduled.

12. Verified NPO status and noted last time food/fluid was ingested.

    Exception: Patients at high risk for contrast media–induced renal impairment may have been instructed to drink increased fluids before procedure.

13. Reviewed physician's orders for preprocedure medications.

14. Reviewed orders for IV sedation during procedure.

NURSING DIAGNOSIS

1. Developed appropriate nursing diagnoses based on assessment data.

	S	U	NP	Comments

PLANNING

1. Identified expected outcomes. ___ ___ ___ _____

2. Explained to patient/family purpose of procedure. ___ ___ ___ _____

3. Verified availability of emergency cardiac surgery facility before cardiac catheterization. ___ ___ ___ _____

IMPLEMENTATION

1. Performed hand hygiene and applied PPE. ___ ___ ___ _____

2. Had patient empty bladder. ___ ___ ___ _____

3. Prepared monitoring equipment; checked vital signs, height, and weight; and palpated, marked, and noted peripheral pulses (for arterial procedures). ___ ___ ___ _____

4. Provided IV access using a large-bore cannula. ___ ___ ___ _____

5. Assisted in positioning patient comfortably on x-ray table and immobilizing appropriate extremity. ___ ___ ___ _____

6. Participated in "Time Out" verification. ___ ___ ___ _____

7. Prepared patient for the sensation that may be felt during dye injection, and instructed patient to reported symptoms. ___ ___ ___ _____

8. Demonstrated knowledge of physician's responsibilities and proper technique in the procedural suite. ___ ___ ___ _____

9. Anesthetized skin over arterial puncture site. ___ ___ ___ _____

10. Observed patient for signs of anaphylaxis. ___ ___ ___ _____

11. Assisted with measuring cardiac volumes and pressures during cardiac catheterization. ___ ___ ___ _____

12. Patient's level of sedation and level of consciousness monitored by personnel administering IV sedation. ___ ___ ___ _____

13. Applied manual pressure to catheterization site for 5 to 15 minutes post procedure. ___ ___ ___ _____

14. Demonstrated knowledge of alternative methods of vascular closure and interventions. ___ ___ ___ _____

15. Carefully assessed patient for presence of cardiac sheaths. ___ ___ ___ _____

16. Removed gloves and performed hand hygiene. ___ ___ ___ _____

17. Post procedure:

    a. Maintained affected extremity immobilized for time period ordered. ___ ___ ___ _____

514

	S	U	NP	Comments

b. Emphasized need to lie flat for 6 to 12 hours post procedure. ___ ___ ___ _____

c. Encouraged patient to increase fluid intake. ___ ___ ___ _____

d. Provided emotional support during immobilized recovery phase. ___ ___ ___ _____

EVALUATION

1. Assessed patient's body position and comfort level. ___ ___ ___ _____

2. Performed respiratory, cardiac, and neurovascular checks on recommended schedule. ___ ___ ___ _____

3. Monitored for complications and possible delayed reactions to dye. ___ ___ ___ _____

4. Determined levels of sedation and oxygenation. ___ ___ ___ _____

5. Assessed postprocedure laboratory values. ___ ___ ___ _____

6. Observed for signs of discomfort. ___ ___ ___ _____

7. Identified unexpected outcomes. ___ ___ ___ _____

RECORDING AND REPORTING

1. Recorded preprocedure and postprocedure assessments and vital signs. ___ ___ ___ _____

2. Recorded type of procedure, type of dressing applied, any drainage, and presence of pain. ___ ___ ___ _____

3. Recorded and reported to physician immediately critical changes in vital signs, peripheral pulses, and laboratory values. ___ ___ ___ _____

Student _____   Date _____

Instructor _____   Date _____

PERFORMANCE CHECKLIST SKILL 44-3 **ASSISTING WITH ASPIRATIONS: BONE MARROW ASPIRATION/
BIOPSY, LUMBAR PUNCTURE, PARACENTESIS, AND THORACENTESIS**

	S	U	NP	Comments
ASSESSMENT				
1. Verified patient's identity. Reviewed physician's orders for type of procedure scheduled, purpose, and site of procedure.	___	___	___	_____
2. Verified signature on informed consent.	___	___	___	_____
3. Reviewed medical record for contraindications to procedure.	___	___	___	_____
4. Assessed patient's ability to remain still in the position required for procedure.	___	___	___	_____
5. Assessed vital signs and pain level, and performed baseline-focused assessment of the body system associated with the procedure.	___	___	___	_____
6. Instructed patient to empty bladder.	___	___	___	_____
7. Assessed patient's coagulation status. Determined last time anticoagulants were taken.	___	___	___	_____
8. Determined if patient is allergic to antiseptic, latex, or anesthesia.	___	___	___	_____
9. Assessed patient's understanding of procedure and any concerns.	___	___	___	_____
10. Obtained baseline pain level.	___	___	___	_____
NURSING DIAGNOSIS				
1. Developed appropriate nursing diagnoses based on assessment data.	___	___	___	_____
PLANNING				
1. Identified expected outcomes.	___	___	___	_____
2. Explained steps to patient.	___	___	___	_____
3. Verified recent chest x-ray, if thoracentesis ordered.	___	___	___	_____
IMPLEMENTATION				
1. Performed hand hygiene.	___	___	___	_____
2. Premedicated for pain, if ordered.	___	___	___	_____
3. Set up sterile tray or opened supplies for physician.	___	___	___	_____
4. Took "time out" with patient to verify patient identity, procedure, and procedure site.	___	___	___	_____

	S	U	NP	Comments

5. Assisted patient in maintaining correct position; reassured patient during procedure.

6. Explained that discomfort may occur when analgesia administered.

7. Assessed patient's condition during procedure.

8. Noted characteristics of specified aspirate.

9. Labeled all specimens correctly and transported to laboratory.

10. Assisted with application of pressure at site, as needed.

EVALUATION

1. Monitored vital signs.

2. Inspected dressing over puncture site.

3. Assessed patient's pain level.

4. Identified unexpected outcomes.

RECORDING AND REPORTING

1. Recorded procedure, location of puncture site, characteristics of aspirate, tests ordered, type of dressing, and patient assessment.

2. Reported unexpected outcomes to physician.

Student _____ Date _____

Instructor _____ Date _____

PERFORMANCE CHECKLIST SKILL 44- 4 **ASSISTING WITH BRONCHOSCOPY**

	S	U	NP	Comments

ASSESSMENT

1. Correctly verified patient identity. ___ ___ ___ _____

2. Verified informed consent. ___ ___ ___ _____

3. Assessed patient's history for inability to tolerate interruption of high-flow oxygen. ___ ___ ___ _____

4. Assessed vital signs and patient's knowledge about procedure. ___ ___ ___ _____

5. Assessed respiratory status. ___ ___ ___ _____

6. Determined purpose of procedure. ___ ___ ___ _____

7. Determined if patient is allergic to local anesthetic. ___ ___ ___ _____

8. Assessed need for preprocedure medication. ___ ___ ___ _____

9. Determined time patient last ingested food. ___ ___ ___ _____

10. Assessed patient's understanding of procedure. ___ ___ ___ _____

NURSING DIAGNOSIS

1. Developed appropriate nursing diagnoses based on assessment data. ___ ___ ___ _____

PLANNING

1. Identified expected outcomes. ___ ___ ___ _____

2. Explained procedure to patient. ___ ___ ___ _____

3. Assisted patient with maintaining position. ___ ___ ___ _____

4. Removed and stored dentures. ___ ___ ___ _____

IMPLEMENTATION

1. Performed hand hygiene. ___ ___ ___ _____

2. Assessed IV access, established new IV if required. ___ ___ ___ _____

3. Assisted patient in maintaining position. ___ ___ ___ _____

4. Took "time out" with patient to verify patient identity, procedure, and procedure site. ___ ___ ___ _____

5. Placed suction catheter near patient's mouth. ___ ___ ___ _____

6. Instructed patient not to swallow as local anesthetic is sprayed. ___ ___ ___ _____

7. Attached bronchoscope to machine to provide light. ___ ___ ___ _____

	S	U	NP	Comments
8. Explained each step to patient as it occurs.	___	___	___	_____
9. Reassessed respiratory status continually throughout procedure.	___	___	___	_____
10. Noted characteristics of suctioned material.	___	___	___	_____
11. Wiped patient's mouth and nose to remove lubricant after bronchoscope was removed.	___	___	___	_____
12. Maintained NPO until gag reflex returns.	___	___	___	_____
13. Removed and disposed of PPE. Performed hand hygiene.	___	___	___	_____

EVALUATION

1. Monitored vital signs and SpO_2.	___	___	___	_____
2. Observed sputum production.	___	___	___	_____
3. Observed airway and respiratory status.	___	___	___	_____
4. Instructed patient not to try to swallow sputum until gag reflex returns.	___	___	___	_____
5. Asked patient to describe postprocedure normal and abnormal symptoms.	___	___	___	_____
6. Identified unexpected outcomes.	___	___	___	_____

RECORDING AND REPORTING

1. Recorded procedure and pertinent information related to the procedure, patient assessment and tolerance to procedure, and return of gag reflex.	___	___	___	_____
2. Reported unexpected outcomes to physician immediately.	___	___	___	_____

Student _____ Date _____

Instructor _____ Date _____

PERFORMANCE CHECKLIST SKILL 44-5 **ASSISTING WITH GASTROINTESTINAL ENDOSCOPY**

	S	U	NP	Comments

ASSESSMENT

1. Verified patient's identity. Verified type of procedure scheduled and the procedure site. ___ ___ ___ _____

2. Verified informed consent. ___ ___ ___ _____

3. Determined presence of gastrointestinal bleeding and contraindications to procedure. ___ ___ ___ _____

4. Determined purpose of procedure. ___ ___ ___ _____

5. Verified that patient was NPO for at least 8 hours before upper GI endoscopy. ___ ___ ___ _____

6. Verified that patient was on a clear liquid diet for 2 days for lower GI examination. ___ ___ ___ _____

7. Assessed patient's understanding of procedure. Addressed concerns. ___ ___ ___ _____

NURSING DIAGNOSIS

1. Developed appropriate nursing diagnoses based on assessment data. ___ ___ ___ _____

PLANNING

1. Identified expected outcomes. ___ ___ ___ _____

2. Explained procedure to patient. ___ ___ ___ _____

3. Administered preprocedure medication. ___ ___ ___ _____

IMPLEMENTATION

1. Performed hand hygiene and applied PPE. ___ ___ ___ _____

2. Removed patient's dentures and partial bridges. ___ ___ ___ _____

3. Participated in "Time Out" process. ___ ___ ___ _____

4. Assessed present IV or established IV access with large-bore cannula. ___ ___ ___ _____

5. Assisted patient during procedure:

   a. Assisted in maintaining comfort during procedure. ___ ___ ___ _____

   b. Explained what is happening as it happens. ___ ___ ___ _____

   c. Placed tissue specimens in proper laboratory containers. ___ ___ ___ _____

   d. Assisted patient in maintaining comfortable position. ___ ___ ___ _____

	S	U	NP	Comments

6. Demonstrated knowledge of physician's responsibilities.
— — — _____

7. Administered atropine, if ordered.
— — — _____

8. Positioned tip of suction catheter for easy access to patient's mouth. Suctioned as needed.
— — — _____

9. Provided slides and containers for specimens. Placed and labeled tissue specimens in proper containers.
— — — _____

10. Assisted patient to comfortable position after completion of procedure.
— — — _____

12. Instructed patient to remain NPO until gag reflex returns.
— — — _____

EVALUATION

1. Monitored vital signs, SpO_2, level of consciousness, and level of pain.
— — — _____

2. Assessed for return of gag reflex and need for suctioning.
— — — _____

3. Evaluated character of emesis or aspirate.
— — — _____

4. Assisted with oral hygiene after gag reflex returns.
— — — _____

5. Asked patient to state postprocedure dietary and activity limitations.
— — — _____

6. Identified unexpected outcomes.
— — — _____

RECORDING AND REPORTING

1. Recorded pertinent information related to procedure, specimen collection, patient assessment, and patient's tolerance.
— — — _____

2. Reported unexpected outcomes to physician.
— — — _____

3. Reported pertinent findings to nurse in charge.
— — — _____

Student _____ Date _____

Instructor _____ Date _____

PERFORMANCE CHECKLIST SKILL 44-6 **OBTAINING A CARDIOGRAM**

	S	U	NP	Comments
ASSESSMENT				
1. Verified patient's identity. Verified physician's order for test.	___	___	___	_____
2. Determined rationale for ECG.	___	___	___	_____
3. Assessed patient's level of understanding and ability to follow directions.	___	___	___	_____
NURSING DIAGNOSIS				
1. Developed appropriate nursing diagnoses based on assessment data.	___	___	___	_____
PLANNING				
1. Identified expected outcomes.	___	___	___	_____
2. Provided privacy.	___	___	___	_____
3. Prepared patient for procedure.	___	___	___	_____
IMPLEMENTATION				
1. Performed hand hygiene.	___	___	___	_____
2. Cleansed and prepared patient's skin as needed. Assessed skin sensitivities.	___	___	___	_____
3. Applied self-sticking electrodes and attached leads to chest and extremities.	___	___	___	_____
4. Turned the ECG machine on, entered demographic information, and obtained tracing.	___	___	___	_____
5. Inspected printout for clarity. Repeated if necessary.	___	___	___	_____
6. Disconnected leads, cleansed skin, repositioned patient, and performed hand hygiene.	___	___	___	_____
7. Delivered ECG tracing to appropriate laboratory, health care provider, or physician.	___	___	___	_____
EVALUATION				
1. Assessed patient's response to procedure.	___	___	___	_____
2. Assessed for chest discomfort.	___	___	___	_____
3. Identified unexpected outcomes.	___	___	___	_____
RECORDING AND REPORTING				
1. Recorded procedure, baseline vital signs, and patient's status.	___	___	___	_____
2. Recorded and reported where or to whom the ECG was delivered.	___	___	___	_____
3. Reported any unexpected outcomes.	___	___	___	_____